DATE			

Spatial Hearing

Tag	Ind 1	Ind 2	Field Data
000			00741nam 2200229 a 4500
001			81117
003			DLC
008			960304s1997 maua b 001 0 eng
010			‡a 96012637
020			‡a 0262024136 ‡c $38.00
041	1		‡a eng ‡h ger
049			‡aKVCG ‡l m-991566 10/98
050	0	0	‡a QP469 ‡b .B5413 1997
100	1		‡a Blauert, Jens.
240	1	0	‡a R"aumliches H"oren. ‡l English
245	1	0	‡a Spatial hearing : ‡b the psychophysics of human sound localization / ‡c Jens Blauert.
250			‡a Rev. ed.
260			‡a Cambridge, Mass. : ‡b MIT Press, ‡c c1997.
300			‡a xiii, 494 p. : ‡b ill. ; ‡c 24 cm.
504			‡a Includes bibliographical references (p. [423]-480) and indexes.
590			‡a PHY 100 PHY 111 PHY 221
650		0	‡a Directional hearing.
035			‡q 0262024136

Spatial Hearing
The Psychophysics of Human Sound Localization

Revised edition

Jens Blauert

The MIT Press
Cambridge, Massachusetts
London, England

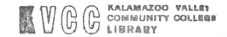

New material and English translation © 1997, 1983 Massachusetts Institute of Technology

Original edition published under the title *Räumliches Hören* by S. Hirzel Verlag, Stuttgart. © 1974 by S. Hirzel Verlag.

Chapters 1–4 translated by John S. Allen

This book was set in Times Roman by Asco Trade Typesetting Ltd., Hong Kong and was printed and bound in the United States of America.

Library of Congress Cataloging-in-Publication Data

Blauert, Jens.
  [Räumliches Hören. English]
  Spatial hearing : the psychophysics of human sound localization /
  Jens Blauert; chapters 1–4 translated by John S. Allen. — [Rev. ed.]
    p. cm.
  Includes bibliographical references and index.
  ISBN 0-262-02413-6 (hardcover : alk. paper)
  1. Directional hearing. I. Title.
QP469.B5413   1996
152.1′58—dc20   96-12637
                                                        CIP

Contents

Preface to the Revised Edition

The original German edition of this book appeared in 1974. At that time, digital signal processing in industry and university laboratories was performed almost exclusively on mainframe computers. To execute a simple fast-Fourier transform, a researcher may well have had to wait a couple of days: he punched a stack of cards, took them to the computer center, and waited for the output — maybe only to discover that he had punched a few holes wrong and had to do the job all over again. Nevertheless, many of the basic concepts of spatial hearing were already known at that time, and some key applications were possible, mainly by using mechanical (acoustic) hardware and analog electric circuitry.

About a decade later minicomputers had made their way into the laboratories, and researchers and developers were now able to do digital signal processing on the spot. As a result, it became possible to carry the old concepts of spatial hearing further and test them rigorously via computer simulations — though not in real time. The minicomputer as a laboratory tool made the field of spatial hearing an attractive research ground for many, and the number of publications on the subject increased considerably. Feeling the necessity to amend the original body of the book for the 1983 American edition, I had to give up the idea of completely covering the field — as I had attempted to do in the original edition — in favor of elaborating on general progress and prominent trends. I had a presentiment, however, that progress in signal processing — especially through miniaturization and increase in computer speed — would soon pave the way for a great variety of novel applications of the principles of spatial hearing in science and industry.

Today, another decade later, this notion has become true and a new industry has evolved under the general label of "binaural technology." Binaural technology has established itself as an important enabling technology in fields such as information and communication systems, measurement technology, hearing aids, speech technology, multimedia systems, and virtual reality. The field of spatial hearing has virtually exploded over the last 10 years, and it would be futile to try to cover it all in a single book.

Nevertheless, it seems appropriate to use the occasion of the preparation of this revised edition to at least comment on a recent dramatic evolution in the field of spatial hearing. To this end, a new chapter, namely chapter 5, has been added. After the introduction (section 5.1), section 5.2 deals with "auditory virtual reality," an important field of application which is mainly based on the physics of spatial hearing. Section 5.3 is devoted to signal processing in the peripheral auditory system and deals with modeling speech enhancement by binaural hearing (the so-called cocktail-party effect). This topic is also of great technological interest. Finally, section 5.4 discusses new research concerning the precedence effect — formerly known as the law of the first wavefront (see section 3.1). Recent research in the precedence effect provides clear experimental evidence that cognition plays a significant role in spatial hearing.

I am especially indebted to my doctoral students over the years, particularly to Drs. M. Bodden, J.-P. Col, H. Els, W. Gaik, H. Lehnert, U. Letens, W. Lindemann, Ch. Pösselt, W. Pompetzki, D. Schlichthärle, J. Schroeter, H. Slatky, S. Wolf, and N. Xiang, whose work provided a major basis for the new chapter. Mrs. R. Leopold prepared most of the new figures.

The new chapter provides examples of progress with respect to the three basic aspects of spatial hearing, namely, the physical, the psychophysical, and the psychological. It is hoped that the book, in its new form, will find its way to the desk of everybody interested in the fascinating field of spatial hearing.

Bochum
November 1995

Preface to the American Edition

The goal of the original German edition of this book, published in 1974, was to offer readers an introductory survey and analysis of the fundamentals of spatial hearing. It has been gratifying to hear from my students and other readers that the book is indeed serving its intended purpose, both as an introductory text and as a reference work. The book has been well received outside German-speaking countries, too. A Russian edition was published in 1980, and a Japanese edition is now being prepared.

I am especially pleased that an English-language edition is now available as well. The interest of many colleagues was extremely helpful in making this edition possible. The energetic work of my friends Professors Campbell Searle and Steven Colburn, and also Wayne Gatehouse, deserves special thanks. I also especially thank Mr. John Allen, who showed fine sensitivity to shades of meaning in translating the text, as well as a thorough knowledge of the subject, even correcting a few errors in the original edition. Further thanks are due to The MIT Press for most careful copy editing.

Except for a few minor changes, the main part of this book corresponds to the German original. The fourth chapter, however, is new. This chapter examines selected experimental results and trends since 1972. I have placed special emphasis on work being done in Germany, some of which has not hitherto been easily accessible to English-speaking readers.

Bochum
March 1982

Preface to the German Edition

It is the task of telecommunications engineering to gather up whatever is to be communicated, to process it, and to transmit it across space and time. A typical example of this task is to bring about in a person an auditory perception that originated at another place and time, perhaps as it was experienced by another person. At the end of the telecommunications chain signals must be generated whose result is that the listener hears what is intended.

If an attempt is to be made to create the auditory illusion that the listener is present at the point of origin of the transmission and directly experiencing the original auditory events, then the directions and distances of what is heard must correspond as closely as possible to those at the point of origin. This requirement has led an increasing number of telecommunications engineers to become interested in the spatial attributes of auditory perceptions and in the signals that accompany these attributes, which is to say in what we shall call "spatial hearing."

Interest in spatial hearing is interdisciplinary. Important contributions to research on the subject have come from fields as diverse as psychology, psychophysics, physiology, and medicine on the one hand, and engineering, physics, and musical analysis on the other.

The first of these groups consists of fields that, from the outset, concern themselves with the human being as a consciously perceiving being. The differences between psychology, psychophysics, and physiology in this regard are, after all, only methodological. Psychology and psychophysics attempt to draw conclusions from externally observable behavior about the internal processes of the human being before, during, and after auditory experiences; physiology deals with these internal processes through direct observation. Medicine uses both methods but is especially concerned with abnormal processes and with distinguishing them from normal ones. There is special interest in spatial hearing in the fields of otology and audiology.

The second group consists of fields in which the person perceiving the auditory event is seen as the last link of a transmission chain, that is, as the recipient of the information. Among the branches of engineering, telecommunications takes the greatest note of, and makes the greatest use of, the phenomenon of spatial hearing, though applications occur also in the technologies of measurement and of noise control. When applied to design problems in architectural acoustics, physics runs up against the problem that the quality of the "acoustics" of a room must ultimately be determined according to human judgments. Musical analysis, finally, is interested in the relationship between the spatial ambience created during the performance of a work and the artistic impression obtained in subsequent reproduction. It should be apparent to anyone who listens to music that contemporary composers— of popular as well as "serious" music—make increasing use of spatial effects as an artistic element.

Because of this diversity of sources of interest, knowledge about spatial hearing is widely dispersed and not readily accessible to a specialist in any particular field. The few works that contain detailed summaries (indicated by asterisks in the bibliography) are of limited scope, and their perspectives are those of one particular field.

The present study attempts to bring together the currently known fundamentals of spatial hearing and to explain them clearly enough so that readers will gain at least a preliminary overview of the subject. The numerous source notes and bibliographical references in the text are intended to provide easy access to the more detailed literature on specific problems. The number of relevant works is, however, enormous, and some of these are not readily accessible. A complete bibliography is therefore impossible.

This monograph is based primarily on literature in the fields of psychology, psychophysics, otology and audiology, telecommunications, and physics. Although physiological details are not explained, the material presented here will nonetheless be of interest to the physiologist, who is faced with the especially difficult task of bringing the results of behavioral studies into line with knowledge about physiological processes. Also, details of electroacoustic transmission systems are not discussed, since there are already a good number of surveys of works in this field. Reference is made to these in the text where appropriate.

Research in spatial hearing is based for the most part on auditory experiments using human subjects. At least for engineers and physicists, it is unusual for data to be available only by way of the descriptions by subjects being tested. Often descriptions by several subjects, based on identical experimental conditions, will differ considerably from one another. In order to arrive at quantitative results despite these problems, psychology and psychophysics have developed special "psychometric" methods of measurement. A brief explanation of these techniques, and of the models upon which they are based, is given in the first chapter.

The first chapter also includes a few remarks on test signals and on sound fields. These will be familiar to physicists and engineers, but the remarks may make it easier for other readers to understand the physical and acoustical context of spatial hearing.

The human being has two ears. The acoustic signals presented to the two ears are by far the most important physical parameters of spatial hearing. It would be appropriate to discuss spatial hearing in terms of these signals alone, thus making possible an organization of the text based on the categories of signal theory. However, experimental results are currently available only for certain classes of ear input signals: mostly for ones that occur in a free sound field or in enclosed spaces. For this reason the present study preserves the traditional classification according to the number of sources of sound. This choice has the advantage of conforming to common practice.

I have had an opportunity to do both theoretical and experimental work in the field of spatial hearing for a number of years at the Institute of Electrical Telecommunications Engineering of the Rheinisch Westfälische Technische Hochschule Aachen. I wish to express sincere appreciation to my honored teacher, the Director of the Institute for many years, Prof. Dr.-Ing. V. Aschoff, who has given strong support to my work and who encouraged me to compile it in the present form.

I would also like to thank Prof. Dr.-Ing. L. Cremer of the Technische Universität Berlin, who read a preliminary version of the manuscript and suggested a number of important corrections.

I would further thank two colleagues, Dr.-Ing. P. Laws and Dipl.-Ing. R. Hartmann, whose encouragement and criticisms contributed to this work. Dipl.-Ing. H.-J. Platte evaluated large numbers of experimental results.

Aachen
August 1972

1 Introduction

The present monograph deals mostly with the results of auditory experiments: those which, under defined conditions, examine auditory perceptions. Here and throughout this work, we restrict ourselves to *conscious* perceptions.

The different branches of science approach perceptual phenomena from different perspectives. Fundamental distinctions are between:

1. The approach from the perspective of the theory of cognition: "What are perceptions?"
2. The approach from the perspective of the natural and technical sciences: "How do (particular) perceptions come about?"

The first question concerns the essence of perception. The answer to it indicates that, at the moment of perception, the perceived and the perceiver encounter each other in such a way that the perceiver becomes conscious of what is perceived. If the common terms "subject" and "object" replace the terms "perceiver" and "perceived," one arrives at the statement that perception is the conjunction-in-opposition of subject and object or, briefly, the "subject-object relationship" (Lungwitz 1923, 1933a, Bense 1961). There is no perception without both a subject and an object.

The second question concerns the physical, physiological, and psychological details of perception. Since perception is inseparably linked to the physiological processes of organisms, the question may be asked in a more detailed way: "What conditions must be fulfilled inside and outside an organism for a particular object to appear in the sensory world of that organism?" This is the general question that underlies the present study. The organisms to be studied are the human subjects of the auditory experiments; the external conditions are the stimuli (for the most part sound signals) presented to these subjects; and what the subjects hear are the objects of interest.

1.1 Auditory Events and Auditory Space

Human beings are primarily visually oriented. Compared with the visual world of the human being, the worlds of the other senses (auditory, tactile, etc.) are much less highly developed. Correspondingly, concepts and descriptions are based primarily on visual objects (Becker 1971). For example, we say "the bell sounds" and not "the sound bells"; similar observations may be made about scientific and technical descriptions.

The German Standard DIN 1320 (1959) defines "sound" from this perspective as "mechanical vibrations and waves of an elastic medium, particularly in the frequency range of human hearing (16 Hz to 20 kHz)." This is a description of physically measurable changes of position, primarily perceived visually. What is heard, what is perceived auditorily, is only implicitly included in the final phrase "particularly in the frequency range of human hearing."

Satisfactory description of auditory experiments requires a more thorough analysis of the state of affairs that underlies this definition. The underlying assumption is that a normal human being generally hears something when in a medium in which vibratory or wave phenomena are occurring whose frequency is between 16 Hz and 20 kHz. This does not, however, mean that the vibrations and waves of the medium are what is heard. For example, if the ears of a human experimental subject were temporarily plugged or were to suffer from a loss in sensitivity, then this person would hear nothing, although the vibrations and waves of the medium would still be perceptible (for example, by means of physical measuring instruments).

For the sake of terminological clarity, and as has been proposed previously (Blauert 1966), the word "sound," as defined in the DIN standard, will be used in this monograph to describe the physical aspect of the phenomena of hearing—particularly in the compound "sound event." Terms such as "sound source," "sound signal," and "sound wave" will always be used to describe physical phenomena that are characteristic of sound events. What is perceived auditorily will be denoted by the adjective "auditory," as in the term "auditory object" or, preferably, "auditory event."

It is commonly believed that auditory events are caused, determined, or elicited by sound events. Auditory events, however, also occur without corresponding mechanical vibrations or waves. Examples are the ringing in the ears that occurs under certain disease conditions (tinnitus) and the auditory events perceived when the acoustic nerve is artificially stimulated. More generally, the fact that a sound event does not necessarily produce an auditory event, and that not every auditory event is connected with a sound event, must exclude the interpretation that one leads to the other in a causal sense. The human visual system is more highly differentiated than the human auditory system, and so the visual world is more highly differentiated than the auditory world. The common belief that sound events cause auditory events is, consequently, understandable, but nonetheless incorrect.

A careful description would go no farther than to say that particular precisely definable sound events and particular precisely definable auditory events occur with one another or one after the other under certain precisely definable conditions (Blauert 1969a,b). It may also be said that sound events and auditory events are related to each other, associated with each other, or classified in relation to each other.

Sound events and auditory events are distinct in terms of time, space, and other attributes (Lungwitz 1933b); that is, they occur only at particular times, at particular places, and with particular attributes. The concept of "spatial hearing" acquires its meaning in this context. Since this concept implies that auditory events are inherently spatially distinct, it is in fact tautological; there is no "nonspatial hearing." Defined more narrowly, the concept of spatial hearing embraces the relationships between the locations of auditory events and other parameters—particularly those of sound events, but also others such as those related to the physiology of the brain.

The "locatedness" of auditory events may be more or less precise.* Thus, for example, the position and spatial extent of the auditory event called a "sustained tone" in a reverberant room cannot be determined with any precision. The locatedness of the tone is diffuse. A click in an anechoic chamber, on the other hand, is precisely located and sharply limited in extent. The locatedness of an auditory event is described in terms of its position and extent, as evaluated in comparison with the

---

*We introduce the new term "locatedness" for the spatial distinction in order to avoid certain misunderstandings that might arise from use of "localization" at this point (see Blauert 1969a). The word "localization" will be newly defined in another context in section 2.1.

positions and extents of other objects of perception, which might be other auditory events or the objects of other senses—in particular, visual objects.

Auditory events may occur at positions where nothing is visible: in connection with sounds inside one's own body or another opaque object, behind walls, beyond the horizon, in the dark, and so forth. Auditory events, in contrast to what is perceived visually, occur not only in front of the observer, but in all directions from the person who is perceiving them. Similar comparisons may be made with what is perceived via the other senses, such as the tactile, olfactory, and gustatory senses. The totality of all possible positions of auditory events constitutes auditory space. The word "space" used in this expression is to be understood in the mathematical sense, as a set of points between which distances can be defined.

Especially in the older literature, the opinion is frequently expressed that locatedness is not an inherent characteristic of auditory events, but that it develops only during the course of the differentiation of the organism and, specifically, to the degree that the human being learns by experience to ascribe the "correct" location to auditory events. The "correct" location is taken to be the position of the sound source. This approach implies that there exist auditory events which, so to speak, wait in a "nonspace" to be ascribed, and only by an experienced individual, to a particular location. The error of such a point of view has long been a matter of record (see, e.g., Hornbostel 1926). The actual situation is the following: During the development of the individual, the auditory world differentiates itself. Auditory events, at first relatively diffuse in their locatedness, become more precisely defined spatially; the correspondence to the visual world and to the other senses also becomes more precise.

It is certainly true that the position of the auditory event and the position of the vibrating body that radiates the sound waves (the sound source) frequently coincide. Nonetheless, the conclusion that the position of the sound source is also the intrinsically correct position of the auditory event is, at the very least, problematic. The sound source and the auditory event are both sensory objects, after all. If their positions differ, it is an idle question to ask which is false.

The telecommunications engineer, of course, is especially interested in just those cases in which the positions of the sound source and the auditory event do not coincide. The telecommunications engineer seeks to reproduce the auditory events that occur at the point where a recording or transmission originates, using the smallest possible number of sound sources (e.g., loudspeakers). Sound events must be generated at the receiving end of the electroacoustic telecommunications chain in such a way that auditory events occur in the same directions and at the same distances as at the point of origin. Auditory events must, therefore, also occur at other positions besides those of the loudspeakers.

1.2 Systems Analysis of the Auditory Experiment

Generally, in an auditory experiment, a sound event with a known spatial and temporal structure is presented in a precisely defined way to an experimental subject. The subject then describes, with regard to the particular attributes that are of interest, the auditory events that occur under these conditions. Description may be in the form of verbal statements, but may also consist of actions such as hand gestures, operation of electrical contact switches, or note-taking. It is, however, essential that the description allow a quantitative evaluation of the auditory attributes of interest.

Two fundamentally different types of auditory experiments may be distinguished: those in which the experimenter is also the subject and those in which one or more other persons are the subjects. Experiments performed on oneself are useful only for preliminary investigations. But in an experiment in which another person is the subject, the auditory events perceived by the subject are accessible to the experimenter only indirectly, by way of the subject's own description. From this description, the conclusion may be drawn (by analogy with the experimenter's own experience) that, with a certain degree of probability, the subject has perceived a given auditory event. The experimenter can never perceive the subject's auditory event directly!

Except in physiology and medicine, the physiological processes within the subject are also, as a rule, not observable for the purposes of the experiments. The experimental arrangement may, however, be represented symbolically by a "black box" in the sense of systems theory, which in the simplest case treated here has three ports: one input port and two output ports (figure 1.1). Note, however, that the black box

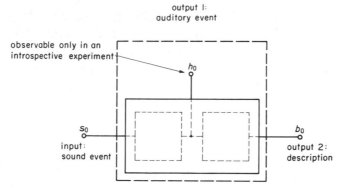

Figure 1.1
A simple schematic representation of the subject of an auditory experiment.

serves here only as a way of portraying functional relationships and is not to be taken as a physiological model of the subject.

Now let us suppose that a sound event with a certain attribute of interest, s_0, is present at the input port. An auditory event with the (spatial) attribute h_0 appears at the output port. This auditory event appears in its location in auditory space, at a position that is only in unusual cases inside the subject's body (see section 2.3.2). The auditory event is directly accessible only when the experimenter himself is also the subject. The two system elements and their connections inside the black box that are drawn with dashed lines at this stage of the discussion are intended only to indicate that the outputs h_0 and b_0 are not defined as identical. If more than one auditory experiment is to be considered, whether with one or more subjects, the following sets of inputs and outputs may be distinguished:

1. The set of the attributes of sound events S_0, whose elements are s_0.
2. The set of attributes of auditory events H_0, whose elements are h_0.
3. The set of descriptions of the attributes of the auditory events B_0, whose elements are b_0.

These "fundamental" sets are related: the sets H_0 and B_0 are both functions of the set S_0. The goal of auditory experiments is to arrive at quantitative statements about these sets, or about subsets of them. Before this goal can be achieved, certain intermediate steps are necessary.

Clearly, if there are to be quantitative statements, measurements must be taken.

Measurement, defined generally, is the assignment of numbers to objects according to consistent rules (Campbell 1938, Stevens 1951). "Consistent rules" means, in this context, that the assignment must be undertaken in such a way that isomorphic relationships exist between the attributes under consideration that form the fundamental sets and between the numbers. In each specific case, a set of numbers is first chosen which can be correlated with the elements of a fundamental set, or a subset of it, in such a way that each element under consideration can be assigned to a number. Such a set of numbers is called a "scale." The elements of the scale are used to describe the elements of the fundamental set in a quantitative manner.

In the theory of measurement, distinctions are made between scales of different complexity, namely, nominal, ordinal, interval, and ratio scales. These scales differ according to which of the following properties of numbers are applied: identity (each number is identical only with itself), rank order (the numerals are arranged in a specified order), and additivity (rules for addition are defined).

Nominal scales are based only on the property of identity. A number is used only as a label for an element or a group of elements of a fundamental set that are identical with respect to the attribute under consideration. The number has no other meaning. For example, auditory events can be ordered into groups numbered 1 and 2, depending on whether they are impulsive or sustained.

Ordinal scales use identity and also rank order. A group of n auditory events, for example, can be denoted by the numbers 1 through n corresponding to increasing distance from the experimental subject. A higher number corresponds to a greater distance, but the differences in distance between auditory events need not be equal; that is, the steps of the scale are not necessarily equidistant.

Interval scales use the properties of identity, rank order, and additivity of intervals. What is not required is that the attribute of the particular element corresponding to the number zero be equal to zero; that is, no "absolute" zero of the scale is required. A well-known example is the Celsius scale of temperature.

In *ratio scales,* finally, all three of the listed properties of numbers are true for the elements of the fundamental sets assigned to the numbers

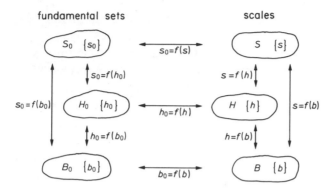

Figure 1.2
Relationships between fundamental sets and scales in an auditory experiment.

in the scales; for example, the distance of two auditory events from one another is denoted by zero when it disappears. The distance denoted by the number two is twice as great as that denoted by the number one, and so forth. The great majority of physical measurements are based on ratio scales.

The type of scale used in a measurement procedure determines which mathematical operations may be used in interpreting the measured results. Guilford (1954), Siegel (1956), and Sixtl (1967), among others, examine this topic in more detail.

In connection with the schematic representation of the experimental subject in figure 1.1, three scales may be established with which to measure the three fundamental sets:

1. A scale of sound events S with the numbers s.
2. A scale of auditory events H with the numbers h.
3. A scale of descriptions B with the numbers b.

In figure 1.2, the three fundamental sets and the scales pertaining to them are represented by enclosed areas. Also shown are the relationships between elements of the different sets:

1. Scaling functions—essentially the rules of measurement, indicating how the assignment of the elements of the fundamental sets to the numbers that form the scales is to be carried out.
2. Psychophysical functions—represented vertically in the diagram, these indicate the relationships between the elements of the fundamental sets

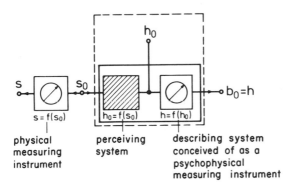

Figure 1.3
Measurement of the psychophysical function $h = f(s)$.

and, in a narrower sense, the corresponding relationships between the scales.

In practice, every measurement is of limited accuracy; the number that, according to a rule of measurement, corresponds to an element of a fundamental set may be determined only within certain limits. When measurements are repeated, it also becomes clear that reproducibility is limited; the results of repeated measurements differ more or less from one another. Problems relating to the accuracy of measurement and to reproducibility occur in several ways in auditory experiments; figure 1.3 indicates where they occur. Let us take as an example the determination of the psychophysical function $h = f(s)$, representing the relationships between measured values of specific attributes of sound events and auditory events.

The measurement of a specific attribute s_0 of a sound event at the input is undertaken by means of a physical measuring instrument and corresponds to the measurement procedure effected through this instrument: $s = f(s_0)$. The attribute h_0 of the auditory event that appears at output port 1 is not accessible to direct measurement. Its measurement is undertaken indirectly, in this way: The subject is considered schematically as being divided into two parts, which are interposed into the system. The first of these is the "perceiving part" and the second the "describing part." The subject in the experiment is instructed to give a numerical description of the attribute of interest of the auditory event according to consistent rules, or is at least instructed to give a description from which a numerical result can be derived. The methods that make this possible are described in section 1.3.1. In our schematic representation, the output b_0 represents a numerical description of h_0, that is, a measured value. We can then say that $b_0 = h$. The subject serves at the same time as an object being measured in the experiment (the perceiving part) and as a psychophysical measuring instrument (the describing part).

If this experimental situation is examined with regard to accuracy and reproducibility of measurement, it can be seen that inaccuracies occur twice: once in the physical measuring instrument, and independently in the psychophysical measuring instrument. Limited reproducibility of measurement also occurs twice, as variations in the measured values of the attributes of the sound events and of those of the auditory events. These variations are not independent of one another, since the sound events and auditory events are related as the inputs and outputs of the system. If s_0 varies, so does h_0. The perceiving part of the system also usually changes from one experimental run to the next, whether several measurements are performed using a single subject, or measurements are performed on each of several subjects; h_0 would vary, then, even if s_0 could be held constant.

In practice, it is possible to simplify the treatment of these relatively difficult relationships, because in most cases the following assumptions may be made:

1. The reproducibility of sound events and the accuracy of measuring them is so great that s_0 may be taken as being constant during an auditory experiment.
2. The psychophysical measurement procedures are chosen and the subject is instructed in such a way that the psychophysical measuring instrument may be regarded as nearly invariant from one experimental run to another or between subjects.

If these assumptions are made, variations in the attributes of auditory events, and of their measured values, are to be explained only as resulting from variations in the perceiving part of the system.

Changes in the perceiving part with regard to measurement, however, are neither predictable in the case of each individual experimental run nor controllable by choice of experimental procedure; therefore, the measured results must be regarded as being influenced by a random variable. The collection of these results, then, must use the methods of descriptive statistics, and their interpretation must use statistical methods of parameter estimation and tests of significance (see, e.g., Guilford 1950, Siegel 1956, Graf et al. 1966, Kreyszig 1967).

These statistical procedures rest on the assumption that the available measured values are samples taken randomly and independently of one another from a specified ensemble. The subjects in auditory experiments should fulfill these conditions; for example, they might be chosen at random from a given population. However, these conditions are as a rule not fulfilled in an ideal sense, since the experimenter is usually limited to volunteer subjects. From these volunteers, the suitable ones—e.g., those with normal hearing—will be chosen. In any particular experiment, failure to fulfill the conditions for a statistical sample may reduce the validity of a generalization of the results of the measurements.

Another point that deserves brief mention is the question of whether any general validity, or "objectivity," can be attributed to measured results obtained by means of statements made by individual experimental subjects. With physical measuring techniques it is assumed as a rule that measured results are independent of the experimenter and thus have general validity. This assumption rests on the presumed ability of most persons to arrive at the same results when bringing an indicating needle of a meter into line with a mark on its dial, or when reading a number off the dial. A closer look at this situation, however, reveals that each person is, in fact, describing his own indicating needle and his own number—his own objects of perception. Consequently, there is no difference between physical and psychophysical measurements such that the one may be called, in principle, "objective" and the other "subjective." Differences exist only in the degree of agreement among descriptions given by different persons.

Indices of this degree of agreement, known as "indices of objectivity," have consequently become a common feature of the technique of psychophysical measurement. According to these indices, objectivity is complete when the measured result is always the same, either over several measurements using one subject or over one measurement using each of several subjects. Another way of expressing this is to say that objectivity is complete when the hypothesis holds true that the system under test is ergodic. Measurements of objectivity are seldom provided along with the conclusions about spatial hearing in the published literature; the general validity of many hypothesis must therefore be held in doubt.

In the schematic representation of the experimental subject (figures 1.1–1.3), it was assumed that the inputs are attributes of sound events. At this point, however, we generalize the sets of inputs to include all attributes of physical phenomena and processes that might correlate in any way with the location of an auditory event. The relevant phenomena and processes are sought out by asking which of the experimental subject's senses take part in the creation of the physiological situation in the brain that is related to the formation of an auditory event. Attributes may be correlated if they are suitable for particular senses, that is, if they are received by particular sensory organs and result in transmission of nerve impulses to the central nervous system. These are called "adequate stimuli."

Table 1.1 lists the physical phenomena and processes for which a correlation to the position of auditory events has been proven or hypothesized. The first column lists the physical processes and phenomena. The second lists the sensory organs involved in receiving and processing these. The third gives the usual name for the psychophysical theory of spatial hearing that describes the relationship between the particular physical attribute and the location of the auditory event. The fourth shows several ways of categorizing these theories. Thus, for example, theories of sound transmitted through air are categorized as the basic theories; every theory of spatial hearing is based on sound transmitted through air to the eardrums. Only in cases in which the location of the auditory event is not unequivocally correlated with the sound signals at the eardrums are further physical characteristics drawn into consideration, through supplementary theories. According to whether one or more senses are involved, theories of spatial hearing are categorized as homosensory or heterosensory. Finally, theories are categorized according to whether they apply to experimental subjects whose head is held still (fixed-position theories) or whether they require head movements (motional theories).

1.3 Remarks Concerning Experimental Procedures

In the following discussion of experimental procedures, it should be noted that references to position in connection with spatial hearing

Table 1.1
Psychophysical theories of spatial hearing.

Physical phenomena and processes considered	Participating sensory organs	Usual designation	Categorization
Sound conducted through the air to one or both eardrums	Hearing (one ear suffices)	Monaural theories for air-conducted sound	B, Ho, F
Interaural differences for air-conducted sound at both eardrums	Hearing (both ears necessary)	Binaural theories for air-conducted sound	B, Ho, F
Sound conducted through the air to the eardrums and sound conducted through bone in the skull (generated by air-conducted sound)	Hearing	Bone-conduction theories	S, Ho, F
Sound conducted through the air to the eardrums and light on the retinas	Hearing, vision	Visual theories	S, He, F
Sound conducted through the air to the eardrums and to the cochlea and vestibular organ	Hearing, sense of balance	Vestibular theories	S, He, F
Sound conducted through the air to the eardrums and sound received by tactile receptors (such as the hair at the nape of the neck)	Hearing, sense of touch	Tactile theories	S, He, F
Head movements during which air-conducted sounds are modified at the eardrums	Hearing, sense of balance; receptors of tension, position, and orientation; vision	Motional theories	S, He, M

Categories: Basic (B) vs. Supplemental (S); Homosensory (Ho) vs. Heterosensory (He); Fixed-position (F) vs. Motional (M).

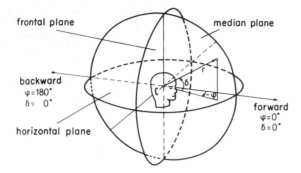

frontal plane   median plane

backward
φ=180°
δ= 0°

forward
φ=0°
δ=0°

horizontal plane

Figure 1.4
A head-related system of coordinates used in auditory experiments; r is distance, φ is the azimuth, and δ is the elevation.

(position of the auditory event, position of the sound source, point of measurement, etc.) are usually made in terms of a head-related system of spherical coordinates. In other words, the system of coordinates shifts in conjunction with movements of the subject's head. The system of coordinates is also practically constant relative to the position of the ears, since we humans are almost incapable of moving our ears with relation to our heads.

In this book, unless otherwise noted, the system shown in figure 1.4 will be assumed. Angles will be denoted as shown. The origin of the system of coordinates lies halfway between the upper margins of the entrances to the two ear canals. These, with the lower margins of the eye sockets, define the horizontal plane, in conformity with international standards for measurement of the skull. The frontal plane intersects the upper margins of the entrances to the ear canals and lies at right angles to the horizontal plane. The median plane (median sagittal plane) lies at right angles to the horizontal and frontal planes. The three planes intersect at the origin. If the head may be assumed symmetrical, it is then symmetrical about the median plane.

1.3.1 Psychometric methods

Psychophysical and psychological measuring techniques, to which the name "psychometric methods" has been given, may be categorized in different ways. For example, they may be categorized according to the level of judgment the experimental subject is required to make. Corresponding to the four levels of complexity of the measurement scales, measuring methods are distinguished as requiring nominal, ordinal, interval, or ratio judgments. Or they may be categorized according to how the inputs (e.g., sound signals) are presented to the subject.

With regard to the latter ways of categorizing, there are two principal possibilities. It is a prerequisite of the first that the input attribute under consideration be continuously variable. This attribute is then adjusted during the experiment until the experimental subject perceives a given judgment as being fulfilled. It is of secondary importance in this respect whether the adjustment is carried out by the experimenter, the subject, or automatically. Methods using this procedure are called "methods of adjustment." They are especially efficient when different subjects are used successively for a series of auditory experiments.

The second possibility is to present to the subject an input whose attribute of interest remains constant throughout each interval of presentation. From a consistently organized list of judgments, the subject chooses the one that seems most appropriate for each presentation. The experiment is repeated several times, with variations in the input attribute each time. The judgments are then evaluated statistically using suitable procedures. The variations in the input attribute follow a pattern unknown to the subject; usually they are stochastic. Methods of this type are called "constant methods" or "interrogative methods." They are especially efficient when auditory experiments are conducted using several subjects simultaneously.

Here we shall confine ourselves to discussion of a few methods commonly used in conducting auditory experiments. Additional methods and further details are given by Fechner (1860), Stevens (1951, 1958), Guilford (1954), Sixtl (1967), and Robinson and Jackson (1972). Because the results of measurements with experimental subjects depend to some extent upon the measuring technique, the method used should always be indicated along with the results.

The most important methods in auditory experiments are based on nominal and ordinal judgments. These methods are especially well adapted to determine thresholds of perceptibility, difference thresholds, and points of perceptual equality. Figure 1.5 clarifies these concepts.

Let us take as an example an auditory experiment seeking to determine the relationship between the intensity of a sound and the loudness of the corresponding auditory event. The scales appropriate to such an

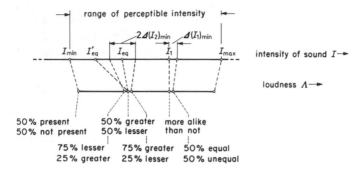

Figure 1.5
Definitions of thresholds of perceptibility, difference thresholds, and points of perceptual equality.

experiment are one-dimensional: a scale of intensity for the sound events and a scale of loudness for the auditory events. Thresholds of perceptibility are, in this example, the two points I_{min} and I_{max} on the scale of intensity, which set the limits for the range of readily perceivable intensities. We shall not discuss I_{max} here; it may be understood as a threshold of discomfort or pain. For the measurement of the lower threshold of perceptibility I_{min}, the subject is required to make the nominal judgment whether an auditory event is "present" or "not present." The threshold of perceptibility is defined as the point on the intensity scale where both judgments occur with equal probability (0.5).

Difference thresholds are segments of the intensity scale corresponding to a just noticeable difference in loudness; for example, $\Delta(I_1)_{min}$ and $\Delta(I_2)_{min}$. The subject is required to make either nominal or ordinal judgments. For example, if the judgments "equal" or "unequal" loudness are required, then the difference threshold corresponds to the segment of the intensity scale from a point I_1 to another point at which the probability of the answer "unequal" becomes 0.5. If the ordinal judgments "greater" or "lesser" are required, then the two points at which the probability of one or the other judgment is 0.75 define the limits of a segment that corresponds to twice the difference threshold. (These two procedures can produce different measured values for the difference threshold; there is no agreement in the literature as to which procedure is preferable.)

Points of perceptual equality are, in the example, the points I_{eq} and I'_{eq} that correspond to auditory events of equal loudness. Let us take

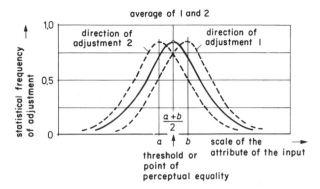

Figure 1.6
Evaluation of results obtained by using the method of adjustment.

as an example two sound sources whose outputs are pure sinusoids, one of 1,000 Hz and the other of 200 Hz. Let us say that the auditory events corresponding to the two sources are equally loud when the intensity of the 1,000 Hz tone is 10 dB and that of the 200 Hz tone is 15 dB. Ordinal judgments are required of the subject. If only the answers "greater" and "lesser" are permitted, then the point of perceptual equality is where each of these answers occurs with equal probability.

Two of the better-known methods of adjustment suited to determining thresholds of perceptibility, difference thresholds, and points of perceptual equality are the method of average error and the method of minimal changes. When the method of average error is used, the subject adjusts the variable attribute of the input until a given judgment is fulfilled. In the method of minimal changes, the input variation, in small increments, is effected by the experimenter, until the subject indicates that a given judgment is fulfilled. The experimenter repeats this measurement procedure several times, until the relative frequency of each of the judgments, as given by the subject, can be plotted against a variable that characterizes the input attribute of interest. This usually leads to a function resembling a normal (Gaussian) distribution. According to whether the input attribute was varied toward higher or lower values, two different curves may result, from which an average curve may be calculated (figure 1.6). For example, in measuring a threshold of perceptibility, the input attribute of interest may be varied

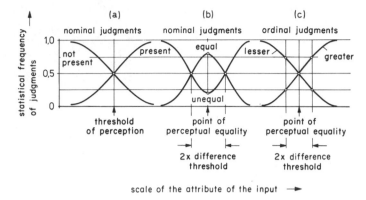

Figure 1.7
Evaluation of results obtained by using the constant method.

first from lower to higher values until the subject gives the response that an auditory event is present; then the input attribute may be varied from higher to lower values until the subject indicates that the perception of an auditory event has disappeared. The final, calculated value for the threshold is the peak of the averaged curve. To measure difference thresholds and points of perceptual equality, a similiar procedure is used, with the subject giving the answers "equal" or "unequal," "greater" or "lesser." A useful variation of the methods of adjustment is von Békésy's (1947) method of oscillating adjustment (see also section 2.2.3).

When the constant method is used to determine thresholds and points of perceptual equality, a series of inputs is presented successively to the subject, each of which includes the attribute of interest to a different degree. The order of the series is unknown to the subject. For example, if a threshold of perceptibility is to be measured, the subject is required to answer whether the auditory event is present or not. It is evident that the series of different inputs must be chosen by means of preliminary experimentation so that the range of the attribute of interest in which the threshold is expected will be as evenly covered as possible. After several repetitions of the series of inputs, it becomes possible to derive a curve of the relative frequencies of the two answers as a function of the input attribute, as shown in more detail in the curves of figure 1.7a. The 50-percent point of both curves is the calculated value for the threshold. In order to measure difference thresholds and points of perceptual equality, on the other hand, at least two inputs that contain the attribute of interest to a different degree must be presented either simultaneously or successively. One input (the standard) remains the same for all test runs, and the other input is varied from one run to the next. According to whether the judgments "equal" or "unequal," "lesser" or "greater" are required, the curve of the relative frequencies of judgments of figure 1.7b or 1.7c may be calculated. The figures also show how the calculated values for difference thresholds and points of perceptual equality are derived. A sometimes-used variation on the constant method is the method of triads, in which three inputs—two equal and one different—are presented to subjects who are then required to identify the auditory event corresponding to the input that is different.

The foregoing methods do not without additional assumptions allow assignment of one particular point on a scale of attributes of auditory events (a perceptual scale) to a scale of input attributes (e.g., a physical scale) and vice versa. In other words, these methods do not by themselves permit a point-by-point assignment between the two scales. This task may, however, be undertaken directly by means of techniques based on interval and ratio judgments. These techniques differ from those already described in the following important way: the subjects, when making judgments, ascribe numerical values "directly" to attributes of auditory events, or else, when using a constant procedure, numerical values among which they can choose are prescribed by the experimenter. These methods are therefore called "direct methods of measurement."

In the methods based on interval judgments, subjects are instructed to pay attention to differences between auditory events. An auditory event to whose attribute of interest a subject assigns the number 2 should, with regard to this attribute, differ equally from other events to which the subject ascribes the numbers 1 and 3. Two procedures lead to particularly good reproducibility of results. In the method of equal perceptual intervals, a number of inputs are presented to the subject, either successively or simultaneously. The subject must place each corresponding auditory event into one of a group of numbered categories, which are usually organized so as to appear equidistant along a scale. In the halving method, the subject's task is to adjust an input attribute so that, with respect to the auditory attribute of interest, the corresponding auditory event lies exactly in the middle on a scale between two other, fixed auditory events.

The basic assumption underlying methods based on ratio judgments is that the subject is capable of distinguishing ratios between attributes of interest. Here, for example, is one outline of a measurement procedure: An input is presented to the subject, and it is explained that the attribute of interest of the corresponding auditory event has the numerical value 1. Then another input is presented, and the subject is asked for the new value of the attribute of interest. It is also possible to ask by what factor, ratio, or percentage the new attribute is different from the one presented first. The judging is made easier if the instructions are for the subject to represent the relationship between the two characteristics so that their sum is 100—as 50/50 for 1/1 and 80/20 for 4/1. This is called the method of constant sums. The corresponding method of adjustment requires the subject, by varying an input attribute, to adjust an auditory event so that the attribute of interest is changed according to a given ratio, or until the attribute exhibits a given ratio with respect to a standard, which may be presented simultaneously or successively.

This has been a general review of psychometric methods, but we must now consider how these techniques may be applied to spatial attributes, that is, to the locations of auditory events. These are the positions of the auditory events and, with spatially extended auditory events, all positions within and on the surfaces of the spaces occupied by these events. It has already been noted that positions and their descriptions cannot be absolute, but must always be in terms of angle and distance relative to another position. What is measured is, in the final analysis, quantities such as distance and angle. A complete description of these requires a three-dimensional coordinate system, such as the one in figure 1.4.

In such a coordinate system, the scales of distance and angle are ratio scales. Consequently, all four classes of judgments—nominal, ordinal, interval, and ratio—are possible, and all of the previously described measuring methods are usable.

When measuring thresholds of angles and distances, it is pointless to deal with thresholds of perceptibility separately from difference thresholds, since these two types of thresholds can be converted into each other by means of a transformation of coordinates. What is meant, in each case, is the smallest change in the input attribute of interest that leads to a change in the position (direction and/or distance) of the auditory event. In section 2.1 we shall designate this threshold by the term "localization blur." One way to measure it, for example, is to use two sound sources that emit the same sound signal in alternation and are capable of being displaced from each other spatially. It is important for the subject to pass judgment only about spatial changes in the auditory event and to pay no attention to changes in loudness, tone color, or other variable attributes.

So-called pointer methods are the most widely used in determining points of perceptual equality for spatial attributes of perceptual events. The task of the subject may be to identify a pointer that indicates exactly the direction of an auditory event and/or whose length corresponds to the distance of an auditory event. Visual and tactile pointers, as well as auditory ones, may be used. An example of a method using an auditory pointer is for the subject to displace a movable sound source until the auditory event that corresponds to it is in the same position as another auditory event to which it is to be compared. As one example of a visual pointer, consider a movable source of light; the position of the visual event corresponding to it may be compared with that of the auditory event. The pointer is also primarily a visual one if the subject points toward the auditory event with a finger or a stick. Von Békésy (1930a) gives as an example of a tactile pointer the use of a small nozzle to direct a stream of air onto the forehead of the subject. Using pointer methods, it is, for example, possible to measure differences between the positions of different sound sources, or between sound sources and light sources whose corresponding perceptual objects are equivalent with respect to a certain spatial attribute. The pointer method is, however, insufficient to assign the position of a sound source to that of an auditory event. The direction of an auditory event cannot be determined from what the subject indicates by pointing unless the relationship between the physically measurable direction of the pointer and the direction of the perceptual event corresponding to the pointer is known. This important consideration is often not taken clearly into account.

For both direction and distance, direct measurement of the location of auditory events as related to attributes of sound events is in all cases possible using interval and ratio judgments. One common method is to have the subject displace a sound source so that the auditory event appears in an agreed direction or at an agreed distance. Another method is to give the subject the task of making an interval or ratio judgment for the direction or distance of a given auditory event. A third procedure belonging to this same class of methods is for the subject to organize auditory events into defined, adjacent categories according to their direction and distance. All of these methods make it possible to determine the position of the auditory event in a system of spatial coordinates, though some of them are more accurate than others.

1.3.2 Signals and sound fields

In an auditory experiment, let a sound event be presented to a subject. The sound event consists of one or more sound signals, which may be the same or different, radiated into space by one sound source or by multiple sources at different positions in space. The signals propagate as sound waves in the medium surrounding the sources, usually air, finally reaching the eardrums of the subject. The signals at the eardrums can be described as functions of sound pressure against time. The sound pressure at the eardrum, $p(t)$, depends, for a given subject, upon such parameters as determine the spatial and temporal structure of sound fields; namely, upon the type, number, and position of the sound sources and upon the sound signals radiated by these sources.

In theory, sound fields of any desired complexity may be used in auditory experiments. Because complicated fields present great difficulties in analysis, however, most experiments employ sound fields of the simplest possible temporal and spatial structure, though these are chosen so as to allow the furthest possible extrapolation of measured results to more complex sound fields. Some factors that play a role in the choice of signals and sound sources in this context will be examined below. Many textbooks give detailed explanations of signal theory, for example: Lee (1960), Küpfmüller (1968), Fischer (1969), and Unbehauen (1969); with regard to the theory of sound sources, see Skudrzyk (1954), Meyer and Neumann (1967), Reichardt (1968), and Cremer (1971), among others.

Almost any function $x(t)$ whose independent variable is time, whether x represents sound pressure, velocity, voltage, or any other variable, can be decomposed into series of elementary signals, which are commonly used as test signals in auditory experiments. For example, a

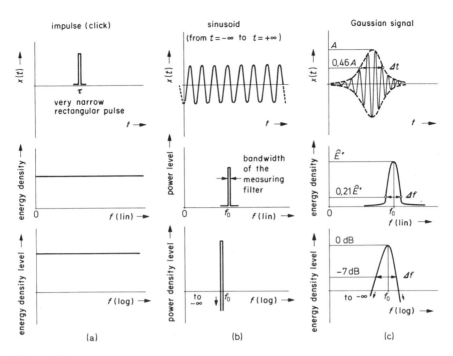

Figure 1.8
Temporal functions and energy or power density spectra of three elementary signals.
Note that the lowest row of drawings are log-log representations.

given time function can be analyzed into a series of very short impulses.
This analysis is based on the superposition integral

$$x(t) = \int_{-\infty}^{+\infty} x(\tau)\, \delta(t - \tau)\, d\tau, \tag{1.1}$$

where $\delta(t - \tau)$ represents the so-called unit impulse, or Dirac impulse,
at the time t. The unit impulse is a fictional concept that can be approximated by decreasing to zero the duration of an actual impulse
while the area under it, 1, remains constant. A short impulse has the
property as a test signal that its energy is concentrated at a definite
point in time but is distributed evenly over all frequencies. The time
function and energy density spectrum (energy per bandwidth) of a short
impulse are represented in figure 1.8a. In practice, a sufficently even

distribution of energy density in the frequency range of human hearing (16 Hz to 16 kHz) is attained if the duration of an impulse is less than approximately 25 μs.

A function $x(t)$ can also be analyzed into a series of oscillations at single frequencies (sinusoidal time functions, pure tones). This analysis is carried out by means of the Fourier integral

$$x(t) = \int_{-\infty}^{+\infty} \underline{X}(f)\, e^{j2\pi ft}\, df, \qquad\qquad (1.2)$$

where $\underline{X}(f)$ is the complex Fourier spectrum of the signal under consideration, and the real part of $\exp(j2\pi ft)$ represents a sinusoidal signal of frequency f and amplitude 1. The useful property of a sinusoidal test signal is that the position of its energy on the frequency axis is known exactly; however, there is no specifying its position in time, as a sinusoidal signal by definition is infinitely long. Figure 1.8b shows the time function and spectrum of a sinusoidal signal. Because of the infinite duration of a sinusoidal signal, its energy is infinite and its energy density cannot be defined meaningfully. Instead we show the spectrum of power density, which is defined as the power measured by means of a bandpass filter divided by the bandwidth of the filter (power per bandwidth).

To sum up this discussion, sinusoidal test signals are used when it is desired to concentrate energy or power at one point on the frequency axis, and impulses are used when it is desired to concentrate energy at one point on the time axis.

A function of time may be analyzed into many kinds of more elementary signals. For all of these, the more concentrated the energy is in time, the greater its bandwidth in the frequency domain; conversely, the more concentrated the energy is in the frequency domain, the more indefinite the signal in the time domain. An optimum compromise of these conditions is afforded by the so-called Gaussian tone burst (figure 1.8c), which is therefore often used as a test signal in auditory experiments. The time function and complex Fourier spectrum of a Gaussian tone burst are described in the following expressions:

$$x(t) = Ae^{-\pi[(t - t_0)/\Delta t]^2} \, \mathrm{Re}(e^{j2\pi f_0 t}), \tag{1.3}$$

$$X(f) = \frac{\Delta t \cdot A}{2} \left[e^{-\pi[(f - f_0)/\Delta f]^2} \, e^{-j2\pi(f - f_0)t_0} + e^{-\pi[(f + f_0)/\Delta f]^2} \, e^{-j2\pi(f + f_0)t_0} \right].$$

$$\tag{1.4}$$

Here A is the maximum amplitude of the burst signal, and Δt is the width of a rectangle of the same amplitude whose area is equal to that under the envelope of the signal. The equation $\Delta t \, \Delta f = 1$ applies to these expressions.

When a broadband excitation of a system is desired (e.g., with an input signal covering the entire range of human hearing), it is possible, as previously described, to apply a short impulse. However, the energy such an impulse can introduce into the system is limited. The limitation exists because a definite maximum sound pressure cannot be exceeded without risking damage to the sound transmitter and the human auditory system. This difficulty can be avoided by substituting a series of short impulses for the single impulse. The series of impulses may be of any convenient duration, with the temporal spacing between each pair of impulses and the mathematical sign (positive or negative) of each impulse being random; that is, any spacing, and either sign, must be equally probable. The result is what is called "white noise." There is no limit to the energy in white noise, since it may have any desired duration. Its power density is the same at all frequencies. The probability of any particular instantaneous value of a white noise signal follows a Gaussian distribution (figure 1.9).

By means of linear filtering, random functions of any desired bandwidth and power density spectrum may be derived from white noise. Such signals are used to ensure that the system into which they are introduced is not set into a steady-state oscillation at its resonant frequencies—for example, that standing waves do not build up in a room. Filtered noise is therefore often used to simulate speech and music, at least with regard to their power density spectra. Typical power density spectra of speech and music are shown in figure 1.10.

Power density spectra, and under certain conditions energy density spectra as well, may be measured by means of tunable bandpass filters. In acoustics, two types of filters are customarily used for this type of measurement. In one, the bandwidth remains constant regardless of

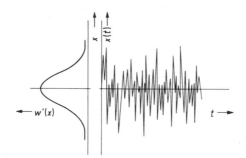

Figure 1.9
Probability density $w'(x)$ of the instantaneous value $x(t)$ of white noise.

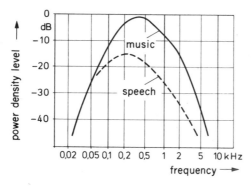

Figure 1.10
Typical power density spectra of speech and music (after Skudrzyk 1954).

changes in the filter's center frequency (Δf = constant, so that the filter has a constant absolute bandwidth, as in a heterodyne-tuned filter). In the other type, the ratio of the bandwidth to the center frequency is constant ($\Delta f/f_0$ = constant, so that the filter has a constant relative bandwidth, as in a 1/3-octave or octave filter). If the power level at the output of the filter is plotted against the filter's center frequency, a different curve results depending upon the type of filter used. For example, in figure 1.11, the measured power level at the output of the filter is shown for both white noise and so-called pink noise, for both types of filter. For white noise, the power is constant with constant absolute bandwidth; for pink noise, the power is constant if the ratio of bandwidth to the filter's center frequency remains constant. Since, roughly speaking, the human auditory system analyzes sound signals

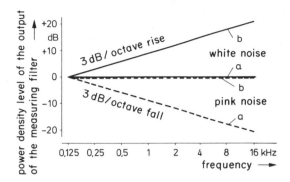

Figure 1.11
Power density spectra of white and pink noise represented two different ways. a:
Power for constant absolute bandwidth (here 60 Hz). b: Power for constant relative
bandwidth (here 1/3 octave).

in terms of constant relative bandwidth, pink noise has considerable
importance as a test signal in auditory experiments.

In certain phenomena related to spatial hearing, the envelopes of
signals play a role. Band-limited time functions (at least those without
a constant term — a condition that always holds for common sound
signals) may in most cases be transformed according to the equation

$$x(t) = A(t) \, \mathrm{Re}(e^{j\varphi(t)}), \tag{1.5}$$

$\varphi(t)$ being a monotonically increasing time function. For information
about the algorithm by which this transformation is carried out, see,
for example, Voelcker (1966). In the most general case, $x(t)$ represents
an oscillation whose amplitude and frequency change constantly with
respect to time. Figure 1.12 shows such a signal. Here $A(t)$ is the envelope;
its plot is the dashed line.

Sound fields may be analyzed into elementary fields according to
laws that are to some extent analogous to those by which time functions
are analyzed into elementary signals. One possible mode of analysis is
based on a principle of Huygens and Fresnel according to which every
point in any system of waves propagating in space can be regarded as
the source of a spherical, or elementary, wave. By the superposition of
such elementary waves, the wave field at any point within the system
may be determined.

A spherical wave is a point-symmetric wave, that is, a wave whose
parameters depend only on the distance from its origin and not on the

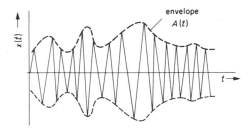

Figure 1.12
The envelope of a signal.

direction of propagation. Sound sources that radiate spherical waves
are called spherical radiators of the zeroth order, elementary radiators,
or pulsating spheres. The term "pulsating sphere" arises from the following considerations: A sound source that radiates only spherical waves
must itself be spherical in shape. Also, all points of its surface must,
as seen from its center, move inwards and outwards radially in phase;
hence "pulsating."

The sound field generated by a pulsating sphere is described by the
two equations

$$p(t, r) = \text{Re}\left\{\text{const} \cdot \frac{j2\pi f\rho_0}{r} e^{j2\pi ft} e^{-j2\pi r/\lambda}\right\}, \tag{1.6}$$

$$v(t, r) = \text{Re}\left\{\text{const} \cdot \left(\frac{j2\pi/\lambda}{r} + \frac{1}{r^2}\right) e^{j2\pi ft} e^{-j2\pi r/\lambda}\right\}, \tag{1.7}$$

where ρ_0 represents the density of the medium. Recognizable in these
equations is the decrease in sound pressure with increasing distance
from the center of the sphere, becoming half as great with every doubling
of this distance r. Figure 1.13 plots this decrease on a log-log grid. The
amplitude of the sound (particle) velocity at large distances from the
sphere ($r \gg 2\pi r/\lambda$) also falls off as $1/r$, but nearer the sphere ($r \ll
2\pi r/\lambda$) it falls off as $1/r^2$. At large distances, pressure and velocity
oscillations are in phase. The ratio $p(t)/v(t)$ then represents a purely
resistive impedance and takes on the value of the specific impedance
of the medium, $z_0 = \rho_0 c$.

Under certain conditions, the equations for fields generated by pulsating spheres are very nearly correct also for pulsating radiators of

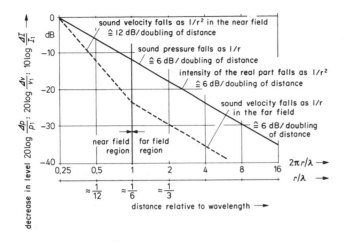

Figure 1.13
Pressure, velocity, and intensity of the sound field near to and distant from a spherical radiator of the zeroth order.

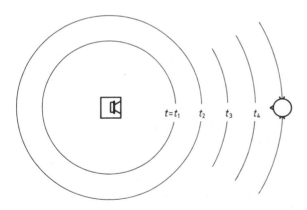

Figure 1.14
Any pulsating sound source that is small compared with the wavelength generates spherical waves at a moderate distance. As the distance is increased, the spherical waves become more and more plane.

other shapes, and even for radiators only parts of whose surfaces oscillate (figure 1.14). The equations are nearly correct if the point of measurement is far enough away from the radiator and if the radiator is small in comparison with the wavelengths of the sounds. The first condition can be fulfilled without any special considerations as to the design of equipment; the second is more difficult to fulfill. As an example, a loudspeaker in a sealed box of normal dimensions (the longest edge approximately 30 cm) can be considered to be a spherical radiator only for frequencies up to approximately 100 Hz. At higher frequencies, it no longer radiates equally in all directions. Nonetheless, pulsating spheres may be approximated at higher frequencies by a device such as a hose or pipe, one end of which opens into a pressure chamber transducer. The free end of the hose or pipe then behaves as a pulsating radiator whose dimensions are approximately determined by the hose diameter. This method of approximating small pulsating spherical sound sources was used, for example, by Mills (1958) and by Shaw and Teranishi (1968).

With increasing distance from any radiator, the sound field becomes more and more similar to a plane wave. Pressure and velocity are in phase for all practical purposes, and, with respect to any object of reasonable size, the curvature of the wavefront becomes less and less noticeable. At a distance of 3 m from loudspeakers in rooms of the usual size, a level difference of less than 1 dB is measured if a microphone is displaced perpendicularly to the axis of the loudspeaker over a distance approximating the dimensions of the human head (± 9 cm). Hence the microphone is, for all practical purposes, being displaced in a plane of equal sound pressure. The curvature of the wavefront is no longer significant, and the sound field is nearly planar.

The sound field of a source located in front of a planar reflecting wall may be represented simply as a superposition of the original sound field upon that of its virtual mirror image (figure 1.15). This description is especially useful in explaining the processes of spatial hearing in enclosed spaces. In chapter 3 it will be shown that the first wavefronts that reach the ears in an enclosed space are particularly important. The propagation of these first wavefronts may easily be traced by constructing mirror-image sound sources.

Headphones are a special type of sound source often used in auditory experiments. They are particularly useful when it is desired for exper-

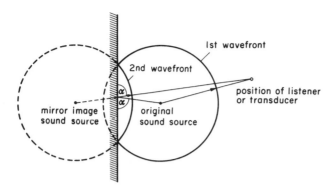

Figure 1.15
Representation of a reflected wavefront as if generated by a mirror-image sound
source.

imental purposes to eliminate the dispersion, shadowing, and resonance
effects of the external ears or the acoustical coupling between the two
ears that occurs in free sound fields. Headphones are distinguished as
intraaural, circumaural, and supraaural, according to their construction.
Intraaural headphones are tightly plugged into the ear canals; circumaural headphones surround the pinna, often making an airtight seal
to the head; and supraaural headphones rest on the pinna.

It has often been assumed that sound pressure is the same everywhere
inside the volume enclosed by each headphone, as if this volume were
a pressure chamber. The assumption, in this generalized form, is incorrect. This error has been an important reason why some of the
characteristics of spatial hearing have long gone without explanation.
If the dimensions of the volume enclosed by the headphone are examined carefully, it becomes clear that, with some variation according
to the type of headphone, the sound inside this volume must be regarded
as a wave phenomenon for frequencies above about 1 kHz (see, e.g.,
Villchur 1969). It is precisely the frequency range above 1 kHz that is
especially important for some effects relevant to spatial hearing.

1.3.3 Probe microphones

The most relevant acoustical inputs for the subject are the sound signals
at the eardrums. Special transducers are needed to measure these signals,
or signals at a nearby location inside the ear canal. These transducers
must fulfill the following conditions, among others:

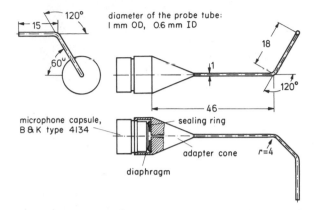

Figure 1.16
Dimensions (mm) of a probe microphone used to measure sound pressure in the auditory canal.

1. They must not appreciably disturb the sound field in the ear canal, pinna, or anywhere near the head.
2. They must allow the measurement of a defined signal parameter throughout the entire range of human hearing.
3. They must not be hazardous to the subject.

So-called probe microphones fulfill these conditions. These usually consist of a condenser microphone (dielectric microphone) coupled by means of the smallest possible chamber to a thin hose or pipe. This construction fulfills the conditions for a sound pressure–dependent microphone, that is, one at whose output a voltage appears that is proportional to the sound pressure at the opening of the tube. The proportionality may, however, vary strongly with frequency due to resonances and attenuation inside the tube. A probe microphone has a spherical directionality characteristic; in other words, it is equally sensitive to sound from all directions. This characteristic is easily understood according to the principle of reciprocity: If the microphone were used as a sound generator—as is, in fact, possible with dielectric microphones—then the opening of the tube, being small in proportion to the wavelength, would approximate a pulsating sphere or radiator of the zeroth order.

For measurements inside the ear canal, probe microphones with tubes 1–2 mm in diameter are used. Often a length of soft plastic hose

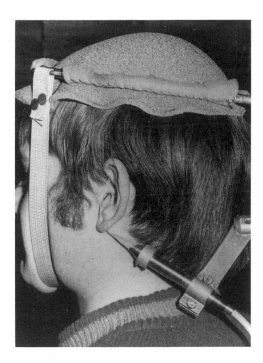

Figure 1.17
The probe microphone in use.

is added to the end of the tube for measurements near the eardrum. It can be shown that the sound field is not appreciably distorted by introducing a second probe into the ear canal while observing the changes in output of the first microphone. The resonances in the tube can be damped by packing mineral wool or metal wool lightly into the tube, or they can be compensated electrically.

Section 2.2 surveys measurements using probes described in the literature. Here, by way of example, we shall describe one particular microphone developed by Laws (1972), which the author has used in a series of measurements. The dimensions of this microphone are shown in figure 1.16. The essential parts of the microphone come from a kit manufactured by Brüel and Kjaer of Copenhagen. The probe tube is bent so that sound pressure measurements can be made 0.5 cm inside the ear canal (at the entrance to the bony part of the ear canal), even when the subject is wearing headphones. Figure 1.17 shows the microphone in use and also shows how the subject's head is immobilized.

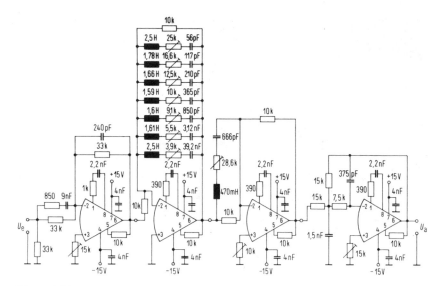

Figure 1.18
Circuit of the equalizing amplifier. R in ohms, L in henries, and C in farads. Operational amplifiers are Motorola type MC 1439.

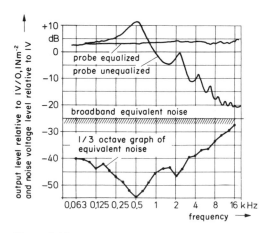

Figure 1.19
Magnitude response of the equalized and unequalized probe microphone, and a 1/3-octave level graph of equivalent noise.

One special feature of this microphone is that, by means of a matched equalizing amplifier (figure 1.18), its output is corrected so that its sensitivity varies no more than 1 dB throughout the range of human hearing. Figure 1.19 shows the frequency response curve with and without the equalizing amplifier. Also shown are the noise levels at the end of the system of microphone, cathode follower, preamplifier, and equalizing amplifier. These noise levels were measured using 1/3-octave filters. The noise is equivalent to a loudness level of 50–55 phon at the input to the microphone.* Such a signal-to-noise ratio is clearly too low for high-quality reproduction of music, but it is nonetheless high enough for many purposes having to do with measurement in spatial hearing, especially when sinusoidal test signals are used.

---

*Three definitions of pressure or intensity level will be used in this book. First there is sound pressure level L in dB: $L = 20 \log(p/p_0)$, where $p_0 = 20 \ \mu\mathrm{Nm}^{-2}$; additional tags such as dBA or dBB indicate that the measurement has been made through a special weighting filter. Second is sound pressure level L in dBSL, where SL stands for "sensation level": $L = 20 \log(p/p_s)$, where p_s is the threshold of audibility of the sound event to be measured. Third is the loudness level in phon: $\Lambda = 20 \log(p_{1kHz}/p_0)$, where $p_0 = 20 \ \mu\mathrm{Nm}^{-2}$ and p_{1kHz} is the sound pressure level of a 1 kHz sinusoidal signal at the position of the subject that gives rise to an auditory event equally as loud as the event induced by the sound to be measured. For further details see DIN 1318 (1970).

2 Spatial Hearing with One Sound Source

An appropriate place to begin a systematic investigation of the physical and psychological phenomena that play a role in spatial hearing is with instances in which there is only one sound source. From the standpoint of physics, these instances represent an elementary case for analysis. If the physical factors resulting in a given sound signal at the eardrums are known for all positions of the sound source relative to the subject, then it is possible to determine the ear input signals not only for the case in which there is one source, but also by superposition for any combination of sound sources. This result follows from the linearity of the equations for sound fields.

From the psychophysical standpoint, the situation is more complicated, since the (nervous) system that evaluates the signals presented to the ears and that determines the position of the auditory events cannot be regarded as linear. Still, the psychophysical relationships developed for spatial hearing with one sound source are also important for spatial hearing with multiple sound sources. There are, however, additional laws and rules that apply only to the latter case.

In this book the phrase "one sound source" will always be taken to mean a sound source in a free sound field, that is, in an anechoic environment. Reflected sound, which may be conceived of as generated by mirror-image sound sources, will be discussed in chapter 3. A free sound field is not necessarily an artificial phenomenon. The peak of a mountain or an open field with high grass or deep snow approaches free-field conditions. In the laboratory free sound fields are approximated with sufficient accuracy in an anechoic chamber.

Many studies of spatial hearing have employed headphones. The results of such studies that relate to spatial hearing with one sound source will be discussed in this chapter (see especially sections 2.3.2–2.4.3).

2.1 Localization and Localization Blur

The following sections will investigate spatial hearing analytically. An attempt will be made to examine the properties and functions of individual physical and psychophysical auditory-system elements separately, so as to make clear their relative roles and importance as parts of the total system. Before discussing details, however, it seems reasonable to begin with an overview of the capabilities of the total system. Before examining the role of the pinna in spatial hearing, for example, we should ask the larger question: How "well" does a human being actually hear spatially?

First, we offer two definitions. "Localization" is the law or rule by which the location of an auditory event (e.g., its direction or distance) is related to a specific attribute or attributes of a sound event, or of another event that is in some way correlated with the auditory event. Examples include the relation of the position of the auditory event to the position of the sound source; the relation of the direction of the auditory event to the interaural sound level difference of the ear input signals; and the relation of the direction of the auditory event to the amplitude of head motion. "Localization blur" is the smallest change in a specific attribute or in specific attributes of a sound event or of another event correlated to an auditory event that is sufficient to produce a change in the location of the auditory event (e.g., direction or distance again). Localization blur is a property of localization. Examples include localization blur of the direction of the auditory event when the sound source is displaced laterally and localization blur of the distance of the auditory event for specific spectral changes in the sound signals at the ears.

If we restrict ourselves at this point to the case of only one sound source, these two definitions lead to two questions that may serve to summarize our discussion:

1. Where does the auditory event appear, given a specific position of the sound source? (A question relating to localization.)
2. What is the smallest possible change of position of the sound source that produces a just-noticeable change of position of the auditory event? (A question relating to localization blur.)

The meaning of the word "localization," as applied to these two questions, is the mathematical function relating the points of the physical (sound-source) space and those of the auditory space. These two spaces are by no means identical in the sense that the auditory event always appears at the position of the sound source. Both the position of the sound source and the type of signal it radiates can affect localization; previous events can also affect it. Under certain conditions localization can be ambiguous; in other words, different auditory events can sometimes occur simultaneously at different positions even when there is only one sound source. Furthermore, localization varies within certain limits from one subject to another and undergoes nondeterminable variations over time.

The concept of "localization blur" reflects the fact that auditory space is less differentiated than the space in which sound sources exist. The auditory system possesses less spatial resolution than is achievable using physical measuring techniques. A point sound source produces an auditory event that is spread out to a certain degree in space. The above-mentioned nondeterminable variations of localization over time also contribute to localization blur.

In the following discussion localization blur will be taken as the amount of displacement of the position of the sound source that is recognized by 50 percent of experimental subjects as a change in the position of the auditory event (see section 1.3.1). This definition reflects the usual practice in psychophysics. Data from the literature based on other definitions of thresholds will, as far as possible, be recalculated under the assumption that measured values follow a normal distribution.

The first question to ask here is just how accurate spatial hearing is, or, more precisely: What is the minimum value of localization blur under optimum conditions? Research has shown that the region of most precise spatial hearing lies in, or close to, the forward direction and that, within this region, a lateral displacement of the sound source most easily leads to a change in the position of the auditory event. In the majority of relevant works the localization blur for changes in the azimuth of the sound source near the forward direction is consequently taken to represent the maximum spatial resolution of the auditory system. A survey of measured results is given in table 2.1. The absolute lower limit for the localization blur is, as shown, about 1°. The spatial resolution limit of the auditory system is, then, about two orders of

Table 2.1
A survey of measurements of localization blur $\Delta(\varphi = 0)_{min}$, i.e., for horizontal displacement of the sound source away from the forward direction. Because different measuring techniques were used, reference is made to the original works, where the techniques are described in detail.

Reference	Type of signal	Localization blur (approximate)
Klemm (1920)	Impulses (clicks)	0.75°–2°
King and Laird (1930)	Impulse (click) train	1.6°
Stevens and Newman (1936)	Sinusoids	4.4°
Schmidt et al. (1953)	Sinusoids	>1°
Sandel et al. (1955)	Sinusoids	1.1°–4.0°
Mills (1958)	Sinusoids	1.0°–3.1°
Stiller (1960)	Narrow-band noise, cos² tone bursts	1.4°–2.8°
Boerger (1965a)	Gaussian tone bursts	0.8°–3.3°
Gardner (1968a)	Speech	0.9°
Perrott (1969)	Tone bursts with differing onset and decay times and frequencies	1.8°–11.8°
Blauert (1970b)	Speech	1.5°
Haustein and Schirmer (1970)	Broadband noise	3.2°

magnitude less than that of the visual system, which is capable of distinguishing changes of angle of less than one minute of arc.

The table shows a considerable range of values of localization blur for narrow-band signals such as sinusoids and Gaussian tone bursts. A closer look at the data reveals a specific relationship to the frequency of the signal. Figure 2.1 shows measured results that delineate this relationship. These results were derived using a measurement procedure in which the subject must choose between two possible answers (two-interval forced choice). In each experimental run a signal from directly ahead was presented to the subject, followed by one from a position to one side that could be changed between runs. In each run the subject was required to state whether the second auditory event lay to the right or to the left of the first. A lateral displacement of the second auditory event is accepted, according to this procedure, when 75 percent of the answers are in agreement. This is the halfway point between 50 percent of either answer (i.e., the assumption that no subject perceives a lateral

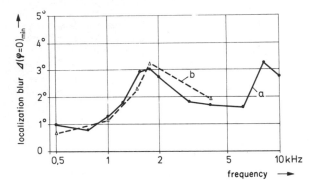

Figure 2.1
Localization blur $\Delta(\varphi = 0)_{min}$ for lateral displacement of the sound source away from the forward direction as a function of frequency. a: Sinusoidal signals (Mills 1958; 3 subjects, 50 dB sound pressure level, head immobilized). b: Gaussian tone bursts of critical bandwidth (about 1/3 octave) (Boerger 1965a,b; 4–7 subjects, 50–60 phon, no head movement).

displacement and that all are guessing randomly) and 100 percent of a single answer (i.e., the assumption that all subjects perceive a lateral displacement).

The remainder of this section will deal with three items that will be of particular interest in connection with the later analytical treatment of spatial hearing:

1. Localization and localization blur of the azimuths of auditory events relative to the directions of sound incidence in the horizontal plane ("directional hearing in the horizontal plane").
2. Localization and localization blur of the angles of elevation of auditory events relative to the direction of sound incidence in the median plane ("directional hearing in the median plane").
3. Localization and localization blur of the distance of auditory events relative to the distance of sound sources ("distance hearing").

For directional hearing in the horizontal plane the minimum localization blur occurs in the forward direction (see table 2.1 and figure 2.1). With increasing displacement from the forward direction toward the right or left, the localization blur increases. At right angles to the direction in which the subject is facing, the localization blur attains between three and ten times its value for the forward direction (Politzer

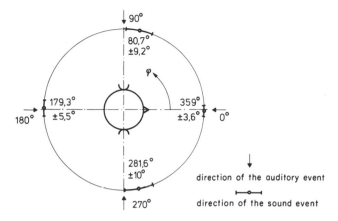

Figure 2.2
Localization blur $\Delta\varphi_{min}$ and localization in the horizontal plane (after Preibisch-Effen-berger 1966a and Haustein and Schirmer 1970; 600–900 subjects, white-noise pulses of 100 ms duration, approximately 70 phon, head immobilized).

1876, Bloch 1893, Perakalin 1930, van Gilse and Roelofs 1937, Stevens and Newman 1936, Tonning 1970). Behind the subject the localization blur decreases once more, to approximately twice its value for the forward direction.

Figure 2.2 shows the results of a large-scale experiment described by Preibisch-Effenberger (1966a) and by Haustein and Schirmer (1970), using respectively 600 and 900 untrained subjects. Localization and localization blur were measured in the horizontal plane. The subjects were asked to bring a movable loudspeaker into alignment with a fixed one (an "acoustical pointer") and, in a separate experimental run, to displace the loudspeaker so that, in their opinion, it was positioned exactly forward, to the left, to the right, or behind. In the latter series of measurements deviations of the direction of incidence of sound from $\varphi = 0°$, 90°, 180°, and 270° were observed. It is still an open question whether these deviations result entirely or in part from systematic errors in the subjects' judgments about direction or whether they actually reflect auditory localization. Similar deviations were, however, observed by van de Veer (1957) and by Wilkens (1972).

In the experiments whose results are shown in figure 2.2, 100 ms white noise pulses were used. Signals of different duration or having a different spectral content can lead to other measured results. Zerlin

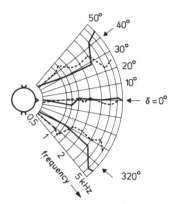

Figure 2.3
Direction of incidence of sound for sinusoids and Gaussian tone bursts of critical
bandwidth so that the same direction of the auditory event is achieved as with broadband noise from the directions $\varphi = 0°$, 40°, 320°. Solid lines: sinusoidal signals (after
Sandel et al. 1955; sound pressure level 35 dB, 5 subjects, head immobilized). Dashed
lines: Gaussian tone bursts (after Boerger 1965a,b; 50–60 phon, 4–7 subjects, no head
movement).

(1959), Tobias and Zerlin (1959), and Houtgast and Plomp (1968),
among others, hypothesize that increases in signal duration in the range
up to 700 ms lead to decreases in localization blur (see figure 2.77
below). Dubrovsky and Chernyak (1971) could, however, confirm this
hypothesis only with reservations.

It is true for pure sinusoids, just as for broadband signals, that localization blur increases with displacement of the sound source away
from the forward direction (Schmidt et al. 1953). Furthermore, there
is a strong dependence on the frequency of the signal, and additional
relative minima of localization blur can appear in various directions
to the sides (Galginaitis 1956, Mills 1958).

The localization of pure sinusoids and of other narrow-band signals
differs from that of broadband signals. Figure 2.3 shows how one loudspeaker radiating pure sinusoids or Gaussian tone bursts must be displaced with relation to another loudspeaker radiating broadband noise
in order to make the directions of the auditory events coincide. Three
cases are shown in which the azimuth φ of the loudspeaker radiating
broadband noise is 320°, 0°, and 40°. It is plausible, based on these
results, to suggest that several simultaneous or successive auditory events
in different directions might appear in connection with signals consisting

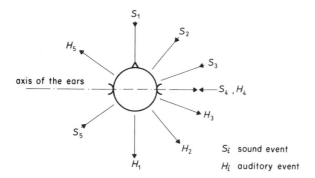

Figure 2.4
Examples of a special type of localization that is most common with narrow-band signals. The auditory event lies in a direction symmetric to the direction of incidence of the sound, with respect to a line through the two ears.

of multiple narrow-band components (e.g., in connection with a series of tone bursts or musical chords). Von Hornbostel (1926) reported that the song of a bird constantly changes position, though the bird may not. As another example, consider a sinusoidal voltage driving a loudspeaker at a level that produces slight distortion, so that higher harmonics are generated. If the frequency of the input signal is altered, several auditory events may be heard, following different paths. The individual auditory events have pitches that correlate either with the frequency of the fundamental tone or with the frequencies of the higher harmonics of the signal at the loudspeaker.

Another seeming anomaly of localization, especially common with relatively narrow-band signals, is for the auditory events to appear not in the direction of incidence of the sound, or even close to it, but systematically in a direction more or less axially symmetric with respect to the axis of the ears (a line passing through both ears) (see, e.g., Rayleigh 1877, Perekalin 1930, Stevens and Newman 1936, Fisher and Freedman 1968). In the horizontal plane an incidence angle of φ = 30° might correspond to an auditory event at 150° (figure 2.4). It will be shown below that the auditory system obtains the information to differentiate between two such directions from the spectra of the ear input signals. With narrow-band signals, this information is absent; with "unnaturally" altered signals, it is deceptive.

If the subject can move his or her head freely, and signal duration is long enough to allow exploratory head movements, effects like those

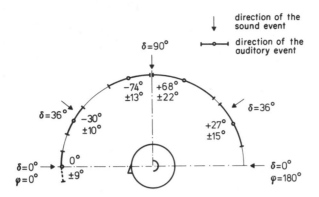

Figure 2.5
Localization and localization blur in the median plane for continuous speech by a familiar person (after Damaske and Wagener 1969; 7 subjects, 65 phon, head immobilized). Note that the view is different from that in figure 2.2.

just described almost never occur. After sufficient head movements, the auditory event always appears in the direction of the sound source (for more on this subject see section 2.5.1). In all cases in which localization is at first imprecise or anomalous, exploratory head movements take on great importance.

Directional hearing in the median plane is fundamentally different from that in the horizontal plane. When the sound source is in the median plane, the signals at both ears are identical to a first approximation; interaural signal differences are therefore rarely available to aid in interpretation of the signals. The localization blur $\Delta(\delta = 0)_{min}$ for changes in the elevation angle δ of the sound source in the forward direction is approximately 17° for continuous speech by an unfamiliar person (20 subjects, 35 phon; see Blauert 1970b), about 9° for continuous speech by a familiar person (7 subjects, 65 phon; see Damaske and Wagener 1969); and 4° for white noise (2 subjects, 60 phon; see Wettschurek 1971). Damaske and Wagener's study also gives the localization and the localization blur for continuous speech by a familiar person at several other incidence angles in the median plane. A glance at these results is given in figure 2.5 (see also Röser 1969).

Plenge and Brunschen (1971) indicate that there is a trend with very brief signals having impulse content (e.g., logatomes) for the auditory event to shift to the rear sector of the median plane. When these signals have been presented to the subject a short time before the actual ex-

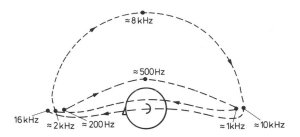

Figure 2.6
Path of the direction of the auditory event as a function of the center frequency of
narrow-band noise from any direction in the median plane (1 subject, head immobilized, simplified depiction).

periment, this effect does not occur. Familiarity with the signal therefore
plays a role in directional hearing in the median plane.

For signals having a bandwidth less than about 2/3 octave, neither
localization nor localization blur with respect to the position of the
sound source can be determined in the median plane. The direction of
the auditory event depends not on the direction of the sound source,
but only on the frequency of the signal (Blauert 1968b). There is no
rule that correlates the direction of the sound source with that of the
auditory event. Figure 2.6 shows the path described by the auditory
event. The sound source is a loudspeaker that can be positioned in any
direction in the median plane and that radiates a narrow-band noise
signal whose center frequency is variable.

All directions in the median plane are symmetrical with respect to
the axis of the ears. As mentioned earlier, the directions of the auditory
event and of the sound source do not coincide for certain signals in
the horizontal plane; instead, they are symmetrical with respect to the
axis of the ears. The same phenomenon occurs in the median plane,
where it can be studied, so to speak, in its pure form.

We now offer a few general remarks about "distance hearing." Familiarity of the experimental subject with the signal plays an important
role in localization between the distance of the sound source and that
of the auditory event. For familiar signals such as human speech at its
normal loudness, the distance of the auditory event corresponds quite
well to that of the sound source. Discrepancies arise, however, even
for unusual types of speech at their normal loudness. As an example,
figure 2.7 shows localization in the range of distance from 0.9 to 9 m

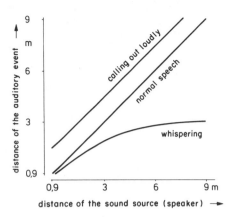

Figure 2.7
Localization between the distance of the speaker and that of the auditory event for
different types of speech from the forward direction (Gardner 1969a; 10 subjects).

with a human speaker whispering, speaking normally, and calling out
loudly (Gardner 1969a).

For impulse sounds Haustein (1969) obtained a correlation between
the distances of the sound source and of the auditory event approximately as good as the one Gardner obtained for normal speech. As a
prerequisite, though, the test signal had to be demonstrated thoroughly
to the subject before the actual auditory experiment, from different
distances. Haustein's results also allow a conclusion about localization
blur, although only as a collective average value for the group of experimental subjects since values for individual subjects are not available
(figure 2.8). Also, it must be noted that in Haustein's experiments
subjects were not asked to identify the distance of their auditory events,
but rather to estimate the distances of the sound sources. This procedure
sets a further restriction on the results.

For unfamiliar sounds localization with respect to the distance of the
sound source is largely undefined. The auditory event is, to be sure,
precisely spatially located, but for sound sources more than 3 m away—
and, with narrow-band sounds, for closer sources as well—the auditory
event's distance depends on the loudness and not on the distance of
the sound source. Only for broadband signals is a trend demonstrable
with unfamiliar sounds whose source is less than 3 m away for the
auditory event to be shifted into the vicinity of the head, or into the

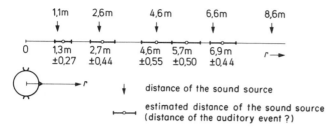

Figure 2.8
Localization blur Δr_{min} and localization between the distances of the sound source and the auditory event in the forward direction (after Haustein 1969; impulse sound, approximately 70 phon, from a distance of 4 m, 20 subjects, head immobilized).

head. Specific questions about distance hearing are dealt with in section 2.3.2.

Adaptation and learning are observed in studies of directional hearing in the median plane and particularly in studies of distance hearing. This means that localization may change as a function of time. At this point another time-dependent characteristic of spatial hearing should be described, namely, its persistence (or inertia). In connection with spatial hearing, the term "persistence" refers to the fact that the position of the auditory event can only change with limited rapidity. Under appropriate conditions the position of the auditory event exhibits a time lag with respect to a change in position of the sound source. Persistence must always be taken into consideration when using sound sources that change position rapidly.

Aschoff (1963) described an experiment in which subjects sat at the center of a circle of 18 loudspeakers. At any one time one of the loudspeakers radiated a noise signal. The noise signal was constantly shifted from one loudspeaker to another around the circle by means of a bank of electrical switches. When the switching speed was slow, the subjects heard the noise circling around their heads. As the switching speed increased, the noise was heard to oscillate between the left and right sides; finally, as the switching speed was increased further, a diffusely spatially located, spatially constant auditory event was heard, approximately in the middle of the head.

Supplementing these experiments, Blauert (1968a) and Plath et al. (1970) have shown that persistence is shorter when the sound source alternates from left to right than when it alternates from front to rear.

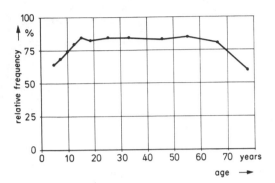

Figure 2.9
Localization blur $\Delta\varphi_{min}$ in the frontal section of the horizontal plane as a function of age. Shown is the relative number of cases in which the directions of the auditory event and the sound source differ by no more than 7.5° (after Röser 1965; white noise, approximately 70 phon, 428 subjects).

In the first case (i.e., left-right alternation), a full cycle must take, on average, 172 ms, and in the second case (front-rear alternation), 233 ms, if the auditory event is to follow the sound source accurately (white noise, approximately 50–60 phon, 10 subjects). The greater persistence for front-to-rear alternation may be attributed to the nearly identical sound signals at the ears in this case, which exclude the evaluation of interaural signal differences.

Diseases of the auditory system, particularly hearing loss, may be related to changes in spatial hearing. Ear, nose, and throat specialists often seek to measure these changes and interpret them diagnostically. Recent studies include Röser (1965, 1966a,b), Preibisch-Effenberger (1966a,b), Steinberg (1967), Plath, Blauert, and Klepper (1970). Further notes on the literature of this subject may be found in Röser (1965) and Preibisch-Effenberger (1966a). Matzker must also be named as one of the more important originators of a battery of audiological tests used in the differential diagnosis of hearing disorders originating in the central nervous system (see, e.g., Matzker 1964, 1965). These tests are based on the observation that many central hearing disorders show, as a symptom, specific impairments of the right-to-left balance of spatial hearing. Few of the measurement and evaluative techniques using spatial hearing have yet achieved widespread application in medical diagnosis. This situation may change when more sophisticated electronic test equipment becomes available. We shall note here only two clinical

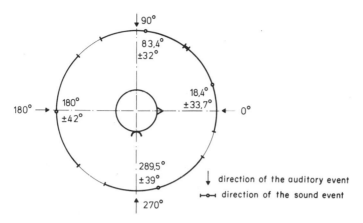

Figure 2.10
Localization blur $\Delta\varphi_{min}$ and localization in the horizontal plane with total deafness in the left ear and normal hearing in the right ear (Preibisch-Effenberger 1966a; white-noise pulses of 100 ms duration, approximately 70 phon, 32 subjects, head immobilized).

findings that provide interesting insights into normal spatial hearing. Both have been applied only to spatial hearing in the horizontal plane.

First, symmetrical hearing loss of peripheral origin of as much as 30–40 dB has almost no noticeable effect on localization or on localization blur. In particular, age-related hearing loss hardly detracts from spatial hearing, or, to be more precise, from directional hearing in the horizontal plane. Figure 2.9 shows changes in one index of localization blur as a function of age.

Second, with asymmetrical hearing loss, localization blur is greater than with normal hearing, and localization is altered. Even with total deafness in one ear, however, measurable localization and a finite value of localization blur still exist (see, e.g., Bloch 1893, Angell and Fite 1901a, Klemm 1913, Allers and Bénésy 1922, Rauch 1922, Brunzlow 1925, 1939, van Gilse 1928, Veits 1936, Güttich 1937, Meyer zum Gottesberge 1940, Klensch 1949, Jongkees and van de Veer 1958, Batteau 1967).

Figure 2.10 shows the results of a measurement involving 32 subjects. Angell and Fite (1901b), Röser (1965), Perrott and Elfner (1968), and others show, furthermore, that in cases of asymmetrical hearing loss and of total deafness in one ear, localization blur decreases with ex-

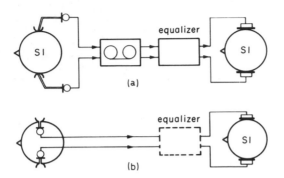

Figure 2.11
Electroacoustical system for accurate transmission of the direction and distance of auditory events. a: Transducers in a subject's ear canals. b: Transducers in a dummy head.

perience and localization becomes more normal; with time the direction of the auditory event coincides better and better with that of the sound source. For further bibliographical notes on this subject see Güttich (1937) and Lehnhardt (1960).

Spatial hearing with total deafness in one ear is of interest in the study of normal spatial hearing, since it presents a case in which no interaural signal differences are available for evaluation. The interpretive phenomena are related to those of normal spatial hearing in the median plane.

2.2 The Sound Field at the Two Ears

Figure 2.11a shows an electroacoustical communications chain. Probe microphones are introduced into the external ears of a subject S1. The microphones respond to sound pressure at the entrances to the ear canals, and the consequent electrical signals are stored on magnetic tape. The signals are then played back to the same subject through headphones. An electrical equalizer corrects the amplitude and phase of the signals, so that the sound pressure at the outer ends of the ear canals corresponds very accurately to that during recording. There is no movement of the subject's head either during recording or during reproduction. The room in which the experiment takes place is darkened.

This system allows reproduced auditory events whose position (direction and distance) and spatial extent correspond exactly to those that occur during recording. This is true despite the relatively high noise voltage of most probe microphones, which may lead to audible interfering noise in large regions of the subject's auditory space.

Figure 2.11 shows a system in which recording is performed by means of two microphones contained in what is called a "dummy head" (Kunstkopf). There is a large literature on dummy heads, which can imitate more or less accurately the acoustical characteristics of natural heads (examples include Firestone 1930, de Boer and Vermeulen 1939, de Boer 1946, Kock 1950, Niese 1956/57, Wendt 1963, Nordlund and Liden 1963, Harris 1964, Mertens 1965, Schirmer 1966a,b,c, Torick et al. 1968, Damaske and Wagener 1969, Kürer, Plenge, and Wilkens 1969, Damaske 1971a, Wilkens 1971a,b, 1972, Mellert 1972). Reproduction, as noted earlier, is by headphones, and an equalizer is used in some cases. Loudspeakers may be used for reproduction instead of headphones, though in this case a compensating circuit is necessary to eliminate crosstalk between the two channels as they are reproduced (Bauer 1961b, Atal and Schroeder 1966). A technical procedure to accomplish this compensation (Damaske and Mellert 1969/70, 1971; Damaske 1971b,c), called the TRADIS procedure, will be described briefly in section 3.3.

It has been shown that the reproduction of the original auditory space (i.e., the auditory space that would be perceived by a subject at the position of the dummy head) has been imperfect for all systems using dummy heads up to 1972. Imperfections in reproduction are smallest for dummy heads in which an attempt is made to duplicate the acoustical effects not only of the shape of the head but also of the pinnae, the auditory canals, and the eardrums.

Two conclusions may be drawn from what has just been said:

1. The sound signals in the ear canals (ear input signals) are the most important input signals to the subject for spatial hearing.
2. Even slight alterations to these signals can lead to noticeable alterations in spatial hearing.

Clearly, then, precise information about the ear input signals is necessary in order to gain an understanding of spatial hearing. The ear input signals when there is one sound source, and their dependence on the position of that sound source, are the subject of the present section. But first we shall offer a few notes about the anatomy of the ear (see

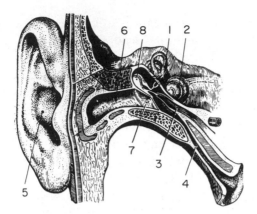

Figure 2.12
A cross section of the ear (adapted from Möricke and Mergenthaler 1959). 1: Semi-circular canals. 2: Cochlea. 3: Eardrum-tensioning muscles. 4: Eustachian tube. 5: Ca-vum conchae. 6: External auditory canal. 7: Eardrum. 8: Hammer.

also Berger 1952, Sobotta and Becker 1963, HNO-Handbuch 1965, Möricke and Mergenthaler 1959, Plath 1969, Klinke 1972).

Human beings have two ears located at the same height on the right and left sides of the head. Distinctions are made between the external ear (auris externa), the middle ear (auris media), and the inner ear (auris interna). The external ear consists of the pinna, or auricula, and the external ear canal (meatus acusticus externus). The middle ear consists of the eardrum (membrana tympani), the tympanic cavity (cavum tympani), and the ossicles within the cavity known as the hammer, anvil, and stirrup (malleus, incus, and stapes); also, associated muscles and ligaments, as well as the eustachian tube (tuba auditiva), which leads to the back of the throat. The inner ear (labyrinth) includes the organ of Corti, which lies within the cochlea and contains the receptors for the sense of hearing, and also the vestibular organs, which contain the receptors for the sense of balance. The vestibular organs are the statolithic organ (utriculus and sacculus), which lies within the vestibule (vestibulum), and the ampullar organs, which lie within the three semicircular canals (ductus semicirculares).

Figure 2.12 is a diagrammatic representation of an ear. In the present context we are interested mostly in the sound field in the external ear, as far inward as the eardrum. We shall therefore examine in somewhat more detail the parts that are important in this context.

The pinna lies at the side of the head, between the articulation of the jawbone and the mastoid process of the temporal bone. It surrounds the entrance to the ear canal and stands out at an angle of between 25° and 45° to the surface of the head. The pinna consists of a framework of cartilage, covered with skin. It has a characteristic bas-relief form, with features that differ distinctly from one individual to another. For a long time textbooks indicated that the pinna had no particular importance for hearing and noted only its protective function (see, e.g., Henneberg 1941). Today it is known that the pinna performs an essential function in spatial hearing and that it also serves to quiet wind noises (Feldmann and Steimann 1968). Details of the form of the pinna will be discussed later.

The external ear canal is a slightly curved tube, entirely lined with skin. It leads from the central hollow of the pinna (cavum conchae) to the eardrum. The outer third of the ear canal (cartilaginous ear canal) passes through cartilage and connective tissue; farther toward the inside (bony ear canal) its lining of skin lies directly upon bone. On average, the ear canal is 25 mm long. The lengths of its individual walls differ (front wall 27 mm, rear wall 22 mm, upper 21 mm, lower 26 mm). Its average diameter is 7–8 mm, with sometimes a round, sometimes a slightly oval cross section. The opening of 5–7 mm diameter at the entrance is followed by a slight widening in the cartilaginous part, to 9–11 mm, and then by a narrowing in the bony part to 7–9 mm.

The external ear canal is terminated by the eardrum. This is a nearly circular, or slightly elliptical, thin, cutaneous diaphragm. Its width on its long axis is 10–11 mm, and on its short axis 8.5–9 mm; its thickness is approximately 0.1 mm. The eardrum lies at an angle of approximately 40°–50° to the axis of the ear canal. Motions of the eardrum occur when there are variations of pressure (such as sound signals) in the ear canal. These motions are transmitted by way of the linkage of the ossicles to the inner ear. The surface area of the eardrum that is coupled to the ossicles—the effective area—is approximately 0.55 cm^2, at low frequencies, according to von Békésy (1941). The eardrum is, then, acoustically loaded by the ossicles and the inner ear. It also rests on and is loaded by the cushion of air in the tympanic cavity and adjoining cavities. Static air pressure in the tympanic cavity is regularly and repeatedly equalized to the exterior air pressure by brief opening of the eustachian tube, generally during the processes of yawning and swallowing. Normally, however, the eustachian tube forms an airtight closure, and the volume of air in the middle ear is sealed in. When high sound pressures—more than approximately 80–90 dB—occur at the eardrum, a reflexive contraction of middle ear muscles is elicited. Known as the "acoustical reflex," this effect leads to a decrease in the sensitivity of hearing; it will be discussed later in more detail.

2.2.1 Propagation in the ear canal

The external ear canal is terminated by the eardrum. Sound in the ear canal leads to oscillations of the eardrum that are transmitted to the middle ear and inner ear; thus the eardrum is the receiver of sound. The other possibility for reception of sound in the external ear canal is excitation of the lining of the canal, the sound being transmitted through the temporal bone to the inner ear. This process, called "bone conduction," is of secondary importance for spatial hearing under normal conditions.

The eardrum is a diaphragm. In order to set it into oscillation, a force must be exerted against it. This force results from the difference in pressure between the two sides of the diaphragm and is, for all frequencies,

$$F = S_{eff}(f)(p_{Tr} - p'_{Tr}), \tag{2.1}$$

where $S_{eff}(f)$ is the effective area of the diaphragm, which varies as a function of frequency. In the case of the eardrum, sound pressure behind the diaphragm is coupled to the external sound field only by way of the sound pressure at the front of the diaphragm. As long as the eustachian tube is closed, as it normally is, this represents the only coupling of the volume of air in the middle ear to the exterior sound field. Consequently, in equation 2.1, which defines F, only p_{Tr} is an independent variable. Therefore, for all practical purposes,

$$F \sim p_{Tr}. \tag{2.2}$$

A receiver of sound in which the force on the diaphragm depends only on the sound pressure on one side of the diaphragm is called a pressure-sensitive receiver (Reichardt 1968, Aschoff 1968, Cremer 1971). By this definition the eardrum is a pressure-sensitive receiver. The input, and thus the adequate stimulus for the ear in receiving sound transmitted through the air, is the sound pressure $p_{Tr}(t)$ on the eardrum.

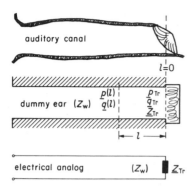

Figure 2.13
The auditory canal, a dummy ear canal, and an analogous electrical transmission line.

The external ear canal is interposed into the auditory system ahead of the eardrum. If the external ear canal is approximated as a tube of constant width—an approximation valid up to about 2 kHz—with walls of high acoustical impedance, then the propagation of sound within the canal can be conveniently described by one-dimensional waveguide or transmission-line equations. For a slightly lossy waveguide excited with a sinusoidal input, these take the form

$$\underline{p}(l) = \underline{p}_{Tr} \cosh \gamma l + \frac{\underline{Z}_{w}}{\underline{Z}_{Tr}} \underline{p}_{Tr} \sinh \gamma l, \tag{2.3}$$

$$\underline{q}(l) = \underline{q}_{Tr} \cosh \gamma l + \frac{\underline{Z}_{Tr}}{\underline{Z}_{w}} \underline{q}_{Tr} \sinh \gamma l. \tag{2.4}$$

Here $\underline{p}_{Tr}$ and $\underline{q}_{Tr}$ are sound pressure and volume velocity at the termination of the waveguide, that is, in a reference plane approximating the position of the eardrum (figure 2.13). Because of the angle of the eardrum, this plane can only be determined to within approximately ±2 mm. The acoustical impedance of the waveguide, $\underline{Z}_{w}$, is derived from the field impedance z_0 of air and the cross-sectional area of the waveguide according to the formula

$$\underline{Z}_{w} \approx Z_{w} = \frac{z_0}{S}. \tag{2.5}$$

$\underline{Z}_{Tr}$ is the acoustical impedance of the termination; it is often called the "eardrum impedance" since it describes the acoustic effect of the termination at a cross-sectional reference plane intersecting or close to the eardrum. This impedance is given by

$$Z_{Tr} = \frac{p_{Tr}}{q_{Tr}} = \frac{p_{Tr}}{v_{Tr} \, S}.$$ (2.6)

Waveguide equations in the one-dimensional form given here are valid when only a plane wave can propagate in the tube, along its l-axis. According to Skudrzyk (1954, p. 146), the upper frequency limit for which this condition holds is 23 kHz, given that the diameter of the tube is 8 mm. The limiting frequency thus lies above the frequency range of interest. A further prerequisite for this statement is, however, that the walls of the tube in fact have a high acoustical impedance. According to von Békésy (1932; see also Metz 1946), the acoustical impedance of skin over bone is approximately the same as that of the surface of water. More recent measurements confirm this finding (Krückel 1972). It follows that the coefficient of reflection of the walls of the ear canal is nearly unity. There are, generally, no pronounced propagation losses in the ear canal (as might be expected because of the hairs inside it). Such greater losses could not be described by equations 2.3 and 2.4.

The waveguide equations 2.3 and 2.4 show that the relative distribution of sound pressure and velocity in a given tubular one-dimensional waveguide depends only on its termination. It follows that we can calculate the transfer function for sound pressure between a point along the waveguide and the eardrum as

$$A(f) = \frac{p_{Tr}}{p(l)} = \frac{1}{\cosh \gamma l + (Z_w/Z_{Tr})\sinh \gamma l}.$$ (2.7)

Conversely, if $A(f)$ is known, it is possible to calculate the eardrum impedance. If to a further approximation lossless transmission is assumed, then equation 2.7 simplifies to

$$A(f) = \frac{p_{Tr}}{p(l)} = \frac{1}{\cos \beta l + j(Z_w/Z_{Tr})\sin \beta l},$$ (2.8)

where the phase coefficient $\beta = 2\pi/\lambda$ substitutes for the complex propagation coefficient γ.

If the eardrum impedance were known, then the sound pressure transfer function between the entrance to the ear canal and the eardrum could be calculated according to equation 2.8. Furthermore, the input impedance of the ear canal (i.e., the impedance of the acoustical termination at the pinna) could also be calculated. The impedance in both of these cases is given by

$$Z(l) = \frac{Z_{Tr} + jZ_w \tan \beta l}{1 + j(Z_{Tr}/Z_w)\tan \beta l},$$ (2.9)

which, more generally, defines the impedance at any point along a lossless waveguide.

Many measurements of the eardrum impedance have been described in the literature (see, e.g., Tröger 1930, Geffcken 1934, Waetzmann and Keibs 1936b, Keibs 1936, von Békésy 1936a, Metz 1946, 1951, Morton and Jones 1956, Zwislocki 1957a,b, Møller 1959, 1960, Onchi 1961, Zwislocki 1962, Fischler et al. 1966). The strong interest in the impedance of the eardrum is due to the conclusions it allows about the functioning of the middle ear, which is coupled to it. These conclusions can be useful in medical diagnosis of hearing problems as well as in other applications. Measured results in the literature are limited to the lower frequency range, up to about 3 kHz. Two exceptions are the results given by Onchi and by Fischler et al. These include frequencies up to 10 kHz; however, they were made using cadaver ears. Laws (1972) and Blauert (1972a) have made a few measurements on living subjects that supplement those of Onchi and of Fischler et al.

Before describing measured results in detail, it is appropriate to take a look at a few of the techniques used for measuring ear impedances. Some of these techniques are also useful in measuring the impedance that loads a headphone resting against the external ear. For a survey of the literature on this latter topic, which is not discussed in the present monograph, see Delany (1964).

The most direct way to measure the impedance of the eardrum is to measure sound pressure and sound velocity at its surface. Sound pressure can be measured easily using a probe microphone, as was first done by Kuhl (1939). The measurement of velocity is difficult; but it is possible to measure displacement instead and then to calculate velocity by differentiating with respect to time. Capacitative probes (von Békésy 1941, Fischler et al. 1966), small optical mirrors cemented to the eardrum (von Békésy 1936a), and more recent techniques using the Möss-

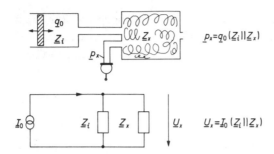

$$p_x = q_0 (Z_i \| Z_x)$$

$$U_x = I_0 (Z_i \| Z_x)$$

Figure 2.14
Measurement of acoustical impedance with the aid of a source whose parameters are known.

bauer effect (Gilad et al. 1967) or a laser interferometer (Tonndorf and Khanna 1970) all may be used to measure the displacement of the eardrum.

Another class of techniques measures the impedance of the eardrum as the termination of a measuring tube (Kundt's tube). One such technique is to determine the positions of the maxima and minima of sound pressure along the tube (Tröger 1930). This technique requires the use of a tube several wavelengths long, though, and there are difficulties in coupling such a device to the ear. Furthermore, this technique only allows the impedance of the eardrum to be determined at individual points in the frequency spectrum. Another possibility is to measure the sound-pressure transfer function between two given points along the tube by measuring the amplitude and phase at these points. The impedance of the termination can then be determined according to equation 2.8.

It is also possible to measure an acoustic impedance by using it as the termination of a sound source with a known volume velocity $q_0 = v_0 S_0$ and internal impedance Z_i and then measuring the sound pressure at the termination (Zwislocki 1957a, Møller 1959, 1960). The impedance is given by

$$Z_x = \frac{p_x Z_i}{q_0 Z_i - p_x}. \tag{2.10}$$

Figure 2.14 gives a more detailed description of this procedure. An acoustical circuit and its electrical analog are shown. If Z_i is very high

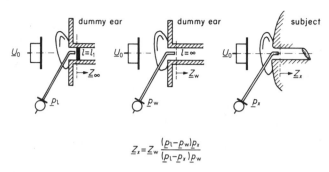

$$Z_x = Z_w \frac{(p_1 - p_w)p_x}{(p_1 - p_x)p_w}$$

Figure 2.15
A substitution procedure for measuring the input impedance of the auditory canal.

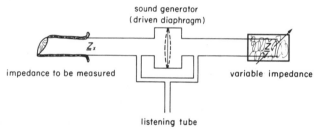

Figure 2.16
The principle of the acoustical bridge (after Schuster 1936).

compared with the terminating impedance, the source has constant volume velocity. Then $Z_x = p_x/q_0$. The q_0 and Z_i of an unknown sound source can be determined by measuring p_x for two known impedances. Two equations are obtained, from which q_0 and Z_x can be determined. Figure 2.15 shows a procedure used by Laws (1972), and by the present author. Onchi (1961) used a related procedure. He placed a constant sound-pressure source in series with a known and an unknown impedance. The unknown impedance can be determined from the sound pressure against it.

Another procedure, used by von Békésy (1936b) and Metz (1946, 1951), uses the acoustical bridge described by Schuster (1936). The principle of such a bridge is shown in figure 2.16. One branch of the bridge circuit is terminated by the impedance to be measured, and another by an adjustable impedance. The diaphragm excites each of the two branches with signals of opposite phase. When the impedance being measured is equal to the test impedance, the signal in the listening tube cancels out. The practical applicability of this technique depends in great measure on the quality of the adjustable test impedance. It is possible to avoid the difficulties involved in achieving an acoustical comparison by measuring the sound pressure in the vicinity of both the test impedance and the impedance to be measured, using microphones. The voltages at the outputs of the two microphones can be compared electrically in an "electroacoustical bridge."

With some of the techniques described, it is possible to measure only the input impedance of the ear canal and not the eardrum impedance itself; or it may be simpler to measure the input impedance of the ear canal. But this measurement, along with equation 2.9, permits an estimate of the eardrum impedance. Often, waveguide equations are not even used in arriving at the estimate; rather, the volume of air between the measuring instrument's transducer and the eardrum is accounted for in the calculation as an acoustical spring (Gran 1966). The limit frequency for which this simple method may be used in each individual case depends on the position of the transducer in the ear canal and the allowable estimation error.

Figure 2.17a shows measured values of the eardrum impedance given by various authors. The values given by Zwislocki (1962) are representative of those given by a number of authors (Tröger 1930, Geffcken 1934, Waetzmann and Keibs 1936a,b, von Békésy 1936a, Metz 1946, Møller 1960, Morton and Jones 1956). They are based on measurements on a total of more than 120 living subjects. The point of measurement was either at the entrance to the ear canal or somewhat inward of the entrance. The curves from Onchi (1961), on the other hand, were obtained using cadaver ears. Measuring probes were placed directly on either side of the eardrum. Discrepancies between Zwislocki's and Onchi's measurements have been interpreted differently by the two authors. The maxima and minima of Onchi's curves at higher frequencies were confirmed by Fischler et al. (1966), who, however, measured only the amplitude of the impedance of the eardrum. Like Onchi, they used cadaver ears.

Figure 2.17b shows the results of exploratory measurments (Laws 1972) using the technique illustrated in figure 2.15. The values shown are averages for 11 persons; a few typical standard deviations are shown.

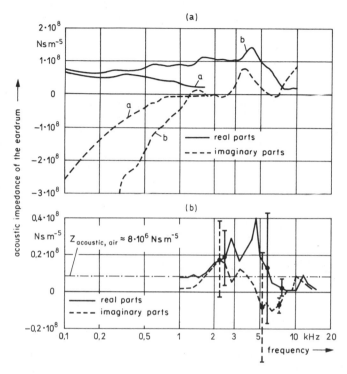

Figure 2.17
Measured results for the impedance of the eardrum. a: After Zwislocki (1962) and
Onchi (1961). b: Results of Laws (1972), using the method shown in figure 2.15.

These measured values are almost an order of magnitude smaller than
Onchi's. I have also reexamined and confirmed the order of magnitude
of these values using the impulse method on five subjects. It consequently seems quite safe to say that the impedance of the living eardrum
cannot be assumed equal to that of the cadaver eardrum. Further measurements will be needed to determine the average impedance curve
for living ears in the frequency range above 1 kHz. Still, the curves
shown in figure 2.17b are quite similar in some ways to curves that
Zwislocki (1936) obtained by measurements of an electrical analog of
the middle ear.

In figure 2.18, finally, are shown measured results for the sound
pressure transfer function relating a point of measurement near the
entrance to the ear canal to a point near the eardrum. Shown are the

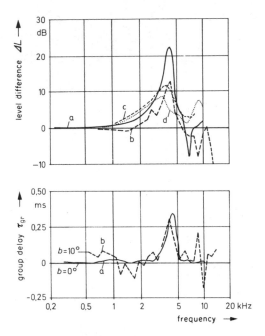

Figure 2.18
Transfer function $p_{\mathrm{Tr}}/p\,(l) = A(f)$ between sound pressure close to the outer surface of the eardrum and that at the entrance to the auditory canal (4 mm inside the canal). a: Calculated by Onchi (1961). b: Calculated from Blauert's measurements (11 subjects). c: Measured by Wiener and Ross (1946; 6 subjects). d: Measured by Jahn (1960; 6 subjects).

sound-pressure level difference $20 \log |A(f)|$ and the group delay $\tau_{\mathrm{gr}} = \mathrm{d}b/\mathrm{d}2\pi f$. (For an explanation of the meaning of these symbols see figure 2.75. Figure 2.18 shows results of direct measurements using probe microphones and also results calculated from measured values of the eardrum impedance, given that the distance between the eardrum and the point of measurement is 21 mm. The trend of the measurements is in basic agreement and also agrees with the prediction made by von Békésy (1932).

Some additional detail is needed about a phenomenon that has already been mentioned: the acoustical reflex. This reflex brings about a contraction of the muscles of the middle ear, after a certain reflex time lag. The contraction leads to a stiffening of the linkage that transmits sound in the middle ear, and consequently to a decrease in the sensitivity of the ear. An increase in the impedance of the eardrum of up to 100 percent in the low-frequency range occurs in connection with the acoustic reflex. (For more detail see Metz 1951, Møller 1962, Feldman and Zwislocki 1965, Ross 1968, Müller 1970.) The acoustic reflex is elicited when the sound pressure level reaches 80–90 dB (measured with sinusoidal signals or noise in a free sound field) and acquires its full effect when the sound pressure level is more than approximately 100 dB. The change in the eardrum impedance that occurs with the onset of the acoustic reflex leads to corresponding changes in the input impedance of the auditory canal and the termination at the pinna, as described in equation 2.3.

2.2.2 The pinna and the effect of the head

The open end of the external ear canal leads into the largest hollow in the pinna, the cavum conchae. The pinna, then, is interposed into the auditory system directly before the ear canal, and it is terminated by the ear canal's acoustical impedance. Acoustically the pinna functions as a linear filter whose transfer function depends on the direction and distance of the sound source. By distorting incident sound signals linearly, and differently depending on their direction and distance, the pinna codes spatial attributes of the sound field into temporal and spectral attributes. Therein lies its importance for spatial hearing.

The acoustical effect of the pinna is based on various physical phenomena such as reflection, shadowing, dispersion, diffraction, interference, and resonance. In connection with the study of these phenomena, it can be stated at the outset that, just as inside the ear canal, the field impedance of the surfaces of the pinna is very high compared with that of air.

The first attempts to explain the function of the pinna involved its "sound-gathering" effect. Schelhammer (1684) took the ear of an animal as an example and hypothesized a series of reflections that led the sound to the auditory canal. He believed that it was possible to describe the path of the sound by means of geometric constructions using rays, as is done in the study of optical systems (see also Steinhauser 1877, 1879). More recently, Petri (1932) espoused this point of view, even with regard to the human ear. Such constructions suggest, however, that rays of sound that do not fall upon the open side of the pinna do not reach the ear canal but are instead shadowed. This incorrect conclusion is based upon the unacceptable approximation of the incident and reflected parts of the sound field by rays. For this approximation to be useful, the reflecting surfaces must be large in comparison with the wavelength. This is not the case with the human pinna. Instead of the reflection and shadowing of rays, dispersion and diffraction processes occur. Because of the irregular shape of the pinna and its variation from one individual to another, it has not yet been possible to give a detailed mathematical description of these phenomena.

A point of view opposite to that using ray models, but equally false, was until recently quite widespread, especially in the field of otology (see, e.g., Röser 1965, HNO-Handbuch 1965). It had been recognized that the dimensions of the pinna in the midfrequency range—the range of speech—are small in comparison with the wavelength. The conclusion followed that the pinna had no importance beyond its mechanical function in protecting the ear canal. It was not considered that the human pinna had cavities in which a "guided" propagation of sound waves takes place. Resonances can occur in these cavities when their width is as small as a quarter-wavelength.

The description of the pinna as a sound reflector was recently taken up in revised form by Batteau (1967, 1968), who takes into account interference between direct sound and sound reflected from the pinna. According to his explanation, the dependence of the transfer function of the pinna on distance and direction of the sound source is due to differences in path length between direct and reflected sound. He regards reflections as occurring at the convex, projecting parts of the pinna, and he attempts to assign individual functions to the different parts. Figure 2.19a shows his classification diagrammatically. For a sound source in the horizontal plane there would be two reflections, as shown in figure 2.19a. The analogous electrical circuit is shown in figure 2.19b. The impulse response of the pinna would, according to Batteau's description, take the form

$$h(t) = \delta(t) + a_1\delta(t - \tau_1) + a_2\delta(t - \tau_2) \tag{2.11}$$

and the transfer function would be

$$\underline{A}(f) = 1 + a_1 e^{-2\pi f \tau_1} + a_2 e^{-2\pi f \tau_2}. \tag{2.12}$$

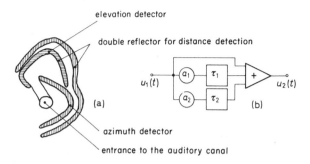

Figure 2.19
a: An analytical model intended to explain the effect of the pinna (after Batteau 1967).
b: An electrical analog of part a for one particular position of the sound source in the horizontal plane.

In order to prove Batteau's hypothesis, it would be necessary to find a_1, a_2, τ_1, and τ_2 such that $A(f)$ would agree with the measured transfer function of the natural ear.

The same objection applies to Batteau's model as to all models of the pinna based on reflection, namely, that the reflecting surfaces are small in comparison with the wavelength. Besides (or instead of) reflection, dispersion occurs; in other words, additional delays occur besides the two Batteau describes. In the final analysis dispersion can produce an indefinite number of delays. Batteau himself was aware of this difficulty and came to hypothesize a system with an infinite number of parallel delays as a model for calculating the transfer function, according to the equation

$$A(f) = \int_{-\infty}^{+\infty} h(\tau)e^{-j2\pi f\tau}\, d\tau. \tag{2.13}$$

This is, however, only the complex Fourier transform of the impulse response, a relationship that holds true generally for linear systems. (Batteau used the Laplace transform instead of the Fourier transform.) Any linear system can be represented as a branched network with an infinite number of parallel delays. Batteau's attempt to describe the function of the pinna in a simple way in terms of its impulse response (i.e., in the time domain) has been of only limited success.

Another way of analyzing the processing of sound in the pinna is to investigate its behavior in the frequency domain. Shaw and Teranishi

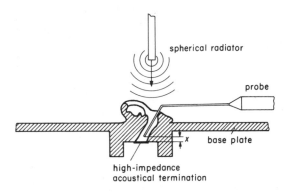

Figure 2.20
Experimental apparatus used in investigations of sound processing in the pinna (after
Shaw and Teranishi 1968).

(1968) undertook a most thorough investigation in this domain using
a model of the external ear as well as natural ears. Using probe microphones, they measured the sound pressure transfer function under a
wide variety of conditions of incident sound. They were successful in
determining the precise conditions responsible for the most important
peaks and dips in the plot of the magnitude of the transfer function
against frequency, at least for sound incidence along the axis of the
ears.

Figure 2.20 shows the experimental apparatus as it was arranged for
some of the measurements taken using a model. An imitation pinna
made of rubber is attached to a backing plate that also contains an
imitation of the external ear canal. Interchangeable acoustical terminations are provided for the ear canal; in the case shown in the figure,
the termination has a high acoustical impedance. Sound pressure anywhere in the ear canal and in the pinna can be measured by means of
a probe microphone. The sound source is the open end of a tube 1 cm
in diameter that might, for example, lie 8 cm from the entrance to the
ear canal. The tube is attached to a sound transducer at its far end.
The input to the transducer is adjusted so that sound pressure at the
end of the tube is equal at all frequencies.

Shaw and Teranishi's most significant result was to identify a number
of resonance frequencies (eigenfrequencies) using their model. The first
five of these resonances are shown in figure 2.21. The resonances co-

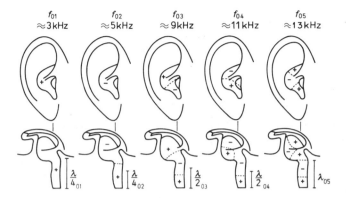

Figure 2.21
Distribution of sound pressure for several natural resonances of a model of the external ear with a high-impedance termination. The dotted lines denote nodal planes of sound pressure (after Shaw and Teranishi 1968).

incide with maxima in the frequency plot of the sound-pressure transfer function between the entrance to the ear canal, or the eardrum, and the sound source. These maxima may thus be identified as eigenfrequencies of the system.

The first resonance of the system, at $f_{01} \approx 3$ kHz, is apparently a $\lambda/4$ resonance of a tube closed at one end. The effective length of the tube is approximately 30 mm, approximately 33 percent longer than the dummy ear canal used in the experiment. The pinna thus functions as a prolongation of the ear canal. This effect is supplemented by an aperture effect.

The second resonance is at $f_{02} \approx 5$ kHz. A pressure maximum fills the entire cavum conchae. The pressure distribution is very similar to what would be obtained if the auditory canal were plugged. Shaw and Teranishi therefore describe this resonance as a $\lambda/4$ "deep" resonance of the cavum conchae, in which the aperture effect contributes approximately half of the effective depth of the cavum conchae. They note that oscillations of the same phase occur over the entire surface facing the sound field. This first cavum conchae resonance is thus damped by a high radiation resistance, which leads to a relatively broad resonance curve. The present author has been able to confirm that the peak of the transfer function around 5 kHz can be attributed to the cavum conchae and also that a dip can be produced in the same frequency range by filling the cavum conchae with putty. Yamagushi and Sushi (1956) give further confirmation.

Longitudinal standing waves are the essential features of the higher resonances $f_{03} \approx 9$ kHz, $f_{04} \approx 11$ kHz, and $f_{05} \approx 13$ kHz. Nodes of sound pressure arise, and these divide the cavum conchae into different regions. The higher resonances have relatively higher Q than the f_{02} resonance—a fact explained by a weaker coupling to the sound field and by the consequently smaller radiation losses.

In addition to their research using the model, Shaw and Teranishi took measurements on six natural ears and were able to confirm the first two resonances f_{01} and f_{02}. In the natural ear the resonances f_{03}, f_{04}, and possibly f_{05} evidently combine into a single, relatively broad rise in the plot of the transfer function.

Some of the resonances occur at different positions along the frequency axis in the natural ear, but this fact is easily explained. Differing geometry and a different acoustical termination at the plane of the eardrum are responsible.

It has been shown, then, using sound incident from a point on the axis of the ears, that the ear has resonances corresponding to peaks in its transfer function. But the question still remains: How does the dependence of the transfer function of the pinna on the position of the sound source come about? Shaw and Teranishi measured this dependence, but they give no explanation of it, with one exception relating to a sharp dip in the plot of the transfer function around 8 kHz, which depends on the angle of elevation of the sound source. They regard this dip as the result of an interference phenomenon. The dispersion and diffraction effects mentioned previously are, however, certainly also of importance.

Results of experiments conducted by the present author in 1967 provide some further clues to the details of these effects. The experimental apparatus was nearly identical to that of Shaw and Teranishi, except for the length of the dummy ear canal. These experiments examined how the direction of sound incidence in the horizontal plane affected the transfer function of the pinna. The following relationship was observed in connection with the f_{02} resonance of the cavum conchae: the peak of the transfer function that is correlated to this resonance maintains a constant height for incidence angles between $\varphi = 0°$ and $\varphi = 90°$. The response falls by 15–20 dB between $\varphi = 90°$ and $\varphi =$

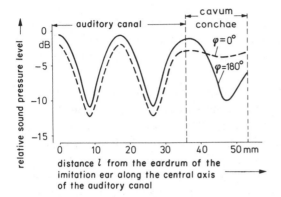

Figure 2.22
The distribution of sound pressure in one dummy outer ear with a high-impedance termination (frequency 10 kHz, incidence angles $\varphi = 0°$ and $\varphi = 180°$).

110°, remaining at the lower level through $\varphi = 180°$. Sound incident from ahead of the axis of the ears thus excites this resonance more strongly than does sound from behind the axis of the ears. Furthermore, it has been observed at some frequencies that the pattern of standing waves of sound pressure in the region of the pinna depends on the direction of sound incidence, but that this is not the case inside the ear canal. Figure 2.22 shows an example of such relationships at 10 kHz, in the range of the resonances f_{03} and f_{04}. With sound incident from $\varphi = 0°$, no standing waves were observable in the cavum conchae at this frequency. With sound incident from $\varphi = 180°$, on the other hand, marked standing waves were observed. This result, too, points to differences in the acoustic excitation of the cavum conchae that depend on the direction of sound incidence.

The attempt to understand the acoustical properties of the pinna based on its behavior in the frequency domain leads to the following, simplified analytical model: *The pinna, along with the ear canal, forms a system of acoustical resonators. The degree to which individual resonances of this system are excited depends on the direction and distance of the sound source.* More precise investigations remain to be undertaken.

We have so far been studying the system of the ear canal and the pinna. But these elements of the hearing apparatus do not exist as isolated objects in space; rather, they are located on both sides of an acoustically rigid object, the human head. We have not yet studied the effects of the head, which clearly represents a considerable obstacle to the free propagation of sound. The disturbance of the sound field by the head has significant influence on the sound signals in the pinna and the ear canal.

In studying the influence of the head on the sound field, common practice is to approximate it by a sphere of similar dimensions (Hartley and Fry 1921, Firestone 1930, Kietz 1953, Woodworth and Schlosberg 1954, Mertens 1960, Aschoff 1963, Wendt 1963, Röser 1965). The first precise mathematical description of the sound field at the surface of a rigid sphere was given by Lord Rayleigh (1904). Stewart (1911, 1914, 1916), Ballantine (1928), Stenzel (1938), and Schwarz (1943) made further contributions to the study of this problem. A brief description of the mathematical procedure follows. Suppose that a point sound source radiates a sinusoidal signal at a distance sufficiently far from a sphere that the sound field in the neighborhood of the sphere is approximately planar. Then the sound pressure at a point on the fictional surface of the sphere, when the sphere is not actually present, is

$$p_0(t) = \text{Re}(\hat{p}_0 \, e^{j2\pi ft}).   \tag{2.14}$$

This equation describes plane, undisturbed sound waves.

Since diffraction is a linear process, the sound pressure at the same point when the sphere is present is given by

$$p(t) = \text{Re}(\hat{p} \, e^{j(2\pi ft + \Phi)}).   \tag{2.15}$$

which represents plane, disturbed sound waves. The expression

$$\frac{p}{p_0} = \frac{\hat{p}}{\hat{p}_0} \, e^{j\Phi} = \frac{\hat{p}}{\hat{p}_0} \, e^{-jb}   \tag{2.16}$$

represents the so-called diffraction ratio, whose coefficients are $\hat{p}/\hat{p}_0$ and Φ or b. The calculation of the diffraction coefficients starts with the assignment of boundary conditions. The disturbed sound field must fulfill the following conditions:

1. At great distances from the sphere it behaves as a plane, undisturbed wave.
2. At the surface of the sphere the normal component of the velocity vector must be zero.

The solution to the problem makes use of the principle of Huygens and Fresnel, according to which any field of waves may be dissected into spherical waves. As expressed in the form used by Morse (1948), the solution is:

$$\frac{p}{p_0} = \left(\frac{\lambda}{2\pi r}\right)^2 \sum_{m=0}^{\infty} \frac{2m + 1}{D_m} L_m(-\cos \varphi)\, e^{j(\vartheta_m - m\pi/2)}, \qquad (2.17)$$

where ϑ_m and D_m can be determined according to

$$(2m + 1)D_m \cos \vartheta_m = \left(\frac{\lambda}{4r}\right)^{1/2} \left[mN_{m-1/2}\left(\frac{2\pi r}{\lambda}\right) + (m + 1)N_{m+3/2}\left(\frac{2\pi r}{\lambda}\right) \right]$$

$$(2.18)$$

and

$$(2m + 1)D_m \sin \vartheta_m = \left(\frac{\lambda}{4r}\right)^{1/2} \left[(m + 1)I_{m+2}\left(\frac{2\pi r}{\lambda}\right) - mI_m\left(\frac{2\pi r}{\lambda}\right) \right].$$

$$(2.19)$$

In these equations $L_m(Z)$, $I_m(Z)$, and $N_m(Z)$ are Legendre, Bessel, and Neumann functions of order m. Since this complex series converges slowly, its evaluation is time-consuming. A series of tables of values is given by Schwarz (1943).

Results for several cases are given in figures 2.23–2.26. The head is approximated by a rigid sphere 17.5 cm in diameter. The ears are represented as two points on the surface of the sphere in the horizontal plane at azimuth angles of 100° and 260°.

Figure 2.23 shows the difference between the sound pressure level in an undisturbed plane wave and at the position of the left ear of the model sphere for sound incidence at angles in the range $100° \leq \varphi \leq 280°$ in the horizontal plane. Note that sound pressure can be higher when the ear is opposite the direction of sound incidence than when it is in the free sound field. Though the sphere is positioned directly between the ear and the sound source, it has, in this case, an amplifying rather than an attenuating effect. This is a well-known phenomenon in diffraction.

The differences between sound signals at the two ears are of special interest in the study of spatial hearing. These differences are represented by the relationship

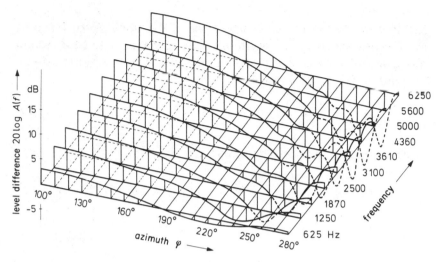

Figure 2.23
Sound pressure as a function of sound incidence angle at the left-ear point (see text),
compared to sound pressure with the sphere removed, at the point where the center
of the sphere would be (diameter of the sphere 17.5 cm, left-ear point at $\varphi = 100°$,
$\delta = 0°$).

$$(\hat{p}_{\text{right}}/\hat{p}_{\text{left}})e^{j\Phi} = (\hat{p}_{\text{right}}/\hat{p}_{\text{left}})e^{-jb}. \tag{2.20}$$

The corresponding relationships, using the model sphere, are represented
in figures 2.24–2.26. The left ear is the one turned toward the sound
source. Figure 2.24 shows the interaural difference in sound pressure
level, figure 2.25 the interaural phase delay $b/2\pi f$, and figure 2.26 the
interaural group delay $db/d2\pi f$. In every case, except when $\varphi = 0°$ or
180°, sound reaches the ear on the far side later and is weaker there.
At sound incidence angles around 90° the interaural attenuation shows
an interference dip. It is to be expected that this dip is less marked
with the natural head than with an isolated sphere, since the head rests
upon the neck.

The relationship between the sound signals at the two ears changes
considerably when a point sound source is brought close enough that
the wavefronts in the region of the head are no longer plane. The
dependence of the diffraction coefficients of a model sphere on the
distance of the sound source was calculated by Steward (1914) and was
evaluated by Hartley and Fry (1921) with respect to interaural sound

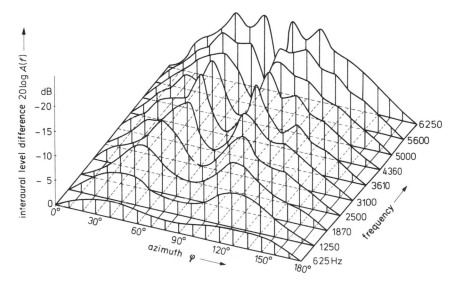

Figure 2.24
Interaural difference in sound pressure level as a function of sound incidence angle, calculated for a sphere 17.5 cm in diameter with the ears represented by points on its surface at the positions $\varphi = 100°$ and $\varphi = 260°$ with $\delta = 0°$.

level and phase differences. An example is shown in figure 2.27 for frequencies up to 1.86 kHz. Hartley and Fry showed that the interaural sound level difference depends heavily on the distance of the sound source, but that the interaural phase difference or delay shows little or no such dependence.

We have so far shown that the sound-pressure transfer function between the sound source and the eardrum is assembled from terms that represent the influence of the eardrum, the ear canal, the pinna, and the head. All of these influences must be considered in any attempt to arrive at a precise mathematical representation of this transfer function. However, a number of simplified mathematical formulas have appeared in the literature. Most of these are formulas for the calculation of interaural signal differences. For the sake of completeness, they will be mentioned briefly here.

The simplest formula is that of von Hornbostel and Wertheimer (1920). The two ears are regarded as points in free space separated by 21 cm. The head is not taken into consideration. For simultaneous sound incidence on both ears, the difference in path length between

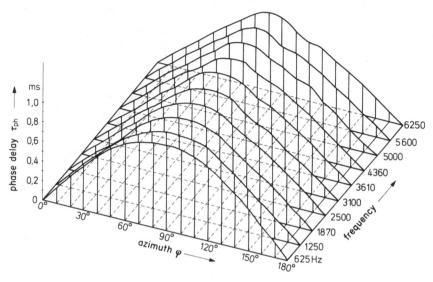

Figure 2.25
Interaural phase delay (sphere as in figure 2.24).

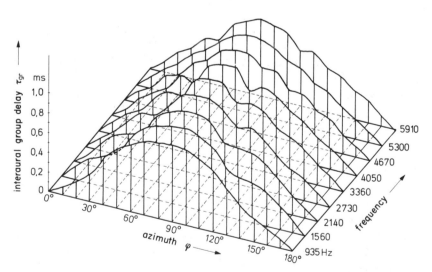

Figure 2.26
Interaural group delay (sphere as in figure 2.24).

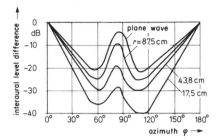

Figure 2.27
Dependence of the interaural sound pressure level difference on distance at 1,860 Hz, calculated for a sphere similar to that in figure 2.24 (after data of Hartley and Fry 1921).

the two ears is given as Δs, and the corresponding difference in arrival times follows the simple law

$$\Delta s = \kappa \sin \varphi \quad \text{with} \quad \kappa = 21 \text{ cm.} \tag{2.21}$$

This "sine law" for spatial hearing played an important role in the literature around the year 1920. The value $\kappa = 21$ cm does not represent the actual distance between the ears, and this formula ignores the effect of shadowing by the head. Consequently, the empirical correction

$$\Delta s = D\kappa' \sin \varphi \tag{2.22}$$

was later introduced, where D is the distance between the ears and $\kappa' = 1.2\text{–}1.3$.

Improved formulas that account for the curved path of sound around the head have been devised by de Boer (1940a), Kietz (1953), Woodworth and Schlosberg (1954), Wendt (1963), and Röser (1965, 1966c). Woodworth and Schlosberg and Röser consider the cases of a point sound source near the head and of plane waves. For these cases the following formulas may be used. For parallel sound incidence, that is, for $r \gg D/2$ (figure 2.28a):

$$\Delta s = \frac{D}{2}(\varphi + \sin \varphi). \tag{2.23}$$

For point sources near the head with sound reaching both ears by indirect paths, that is, for $\sin \varphi \le D/2r$ (figure 2.28c):

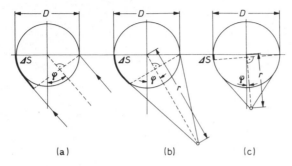

Figure 2.28
Simplified formulas for the calculation of interaural signal differences. a: Parallel
sound incidence. b, c: Point radiators near the head.

$$\Delta s = D \cdot \varphi. \tag{2.24}$$

For point sources near the head with sound reaching one ear by a direct
path, that is, for $\sin \varphi > D/2r$ (figure 2.28b):

$$\Delta s = D\left[\left(n + \frac{1}{2}\right)\cos \epsilon + \frac{1}{2}(\varphi + \epsilon)\right.$$

$$\left. - \sqrt{n^2 + n + \frac{1}{2} - \left(n + \frac{1}{2}\right)\sin \varphi}\right]$$

with $\quad n = \dfrac{r - D/2}{D} \quad$ and $\quad \epsilon = \arcsin\left(\dfrac{D}{2r}\right) = \arcsin\left(\dfrac{1}{1 + 2n}\right).$

$$\tag{2.25}$$

The dependence of the interaural path length on the azimuth angle
may be calculated using these formulas. They can accommodate any
distance of the sound source. Some calculated results are shown in
figure 2.29. In some situations simple approximations of the type just
described can lead to results that agree reasonably well with experimental
results. Figure 2.30 shows the interaural delay $\Delta s/c$, where c is the speed
of sound, and the results of two authors who measured the difference
in arrival time of the onset of the ear input signals, which is approximately equivalent to an average value of interaural group delay. Similar
results were obtained by Nordlund (1962).

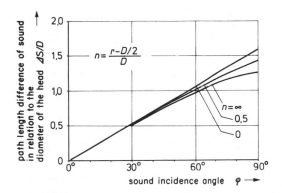

Figure 2.29
Dependence of the path length difference for sound at the two ears on the distance of the sound source (after Röser 1965, 1966; calculated according to equations 2.24 and 2.25).

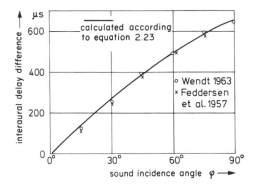

Figure 2.30
Interaural delay difference for the rising slopes of brief, rectangular pulses as a function of the sound incidence angle. Measured results are compared with results calculated according to equation 2.23.

2.2.3 Transfer functions of the external ear

The two preceding sections investigated the influence of the head and of the individual elements of the external ear on sound signals received by the auditory system. The present section will deal with the same matters in a more general way. Inquiries will no longer be made about the influence of the individual elements; instead, the general question will be: What alterations does a sound signal undergo on its path to the eardrum, and how do these distortions depend on the direction and distance of the sound source?

The alterations a variable undergoes in a linear system—so-called linear distortions—can be described by the system's transfer function, defined as the complex ratio of the Fourier spectrum of the output variable to that of the input variable. In connection with the external ear, three types of transfer functions are commonly defined:

1. The *free-field transfer function* relates sound pressure at a point of measurement in the auditory canal of the experimental subject—preferably at the eardrum—to the sound pressure that would be measured, using the same sound source, at a point corresponding to the center of the head (i.e., at the origin of the coordinate system) while the subject is not present.
2. The *monaural transfer function* relates sound pressure at a point of measurement in the ear canal for any given direction and distance of the sound source to sound pressure measured at the same point but with the sound source at a reference angle and distance. (As a rule, a plane wave from the direction $\varphi = 0°$, $\delta = 0°$ is used as a reference.)
3. The *interaural transfer function* relates sound pressures at corresponding points of measurement in the two ear canals. The reference sound pressure is that at the ear facing the sound source.

All three definitions may be written in the form

$$A(f) = \frac{\hat{p}(f)e^{j[2\pi ft + \Phi(f)]}}{\hat{p}_0(f)e^{j[2\pi ft + \Phi_0(f)]}} = |A(f)| e^{-jb}, \qquad (2.26)$$

where $\hat{p}_0(f)$ and $\Phi_0(f)$ are the parameters of the reference sound pressure, namely the amplitude and phase of its Fourier spectrum. In any specific case one must indicate which transfer function is being applied; one must also indicate the type, distance, and direction of the sound source being used and which, if any, reference sound is being used. In what follows the level difference $\Delta L = 20 \log |A(f)|$ and the group delay $\tau_{gr}(f) = db(f)/d2\pi f$ will for the most part replace $|A(f)|$ and the parameter $b(f)$. τ_{gr} contains the same information as $b(f)$, with the exception of a constant of integration that can be determined if the phase coefficient is given for any one frequency (see equation 2.32). Another variable that is sometimes used is the phase delay $\tau_{ph} = b(f)/2\pi f$.

In order to measure the free-field transfer function, one must generally take measurements directly in front of the subject's eardrum. Procedures for taking such measurements are well known and are safe if carried out correctly. The assistance of an otologist is helpful in placing the tip of the probe microphone in the ear canal before the eardrum, since in general only an otologist is practiced in the technique of visual inspection of the ear canal, using a special mirror. Because the sound-pressure transfer function of the ear canal is independent of the sound source and of its position, a point of measurement near the entrance to the ear canal may also be chosen. This should be at least 5 mm inward of the entrance. The transfer function for a point of measurement at the eardrum is then obtained by multiplying the transfer function of the ear canal by the measured transfer function. If these functions are expressed logarithmically, in terms of level difference and phase coefficient, group delay, or phase delay, they are added instead of multiplied (see the values given in figure 2.18). When measurements are taken at the entrance to the ear canal, reproducibility of the point of measurement is of great importance (Jahn 1958, Jahn and Vogelsang 1959).

For measuring the monaural transfer function, a point of measurement at the entrance to the ear canal is as good as any other, since the reference sound also passes through the ear canal. If one is interested only in the amplitude of the transfer function or the level difference, then one can use auditory experiments for purposes of measurement instead of taking measurements with the probe microphone. As Jahn (1958) showed, the same sound pressure at the eardrum always leads to the same loudness of the auditory event. One exception is the case in which the acoustical reflex comes into play; in practice, the sound pressure level must be kept below 80–90 dB. Two psychometric methods are possible. In one the threshold of perceptibility is determined as a function of frequency for the different conditions of sound incidence

under examination. This is called the "threshold of audibility method."
In the other a point of equal loudness is determined between the sound
to be measured and a standard sound, as a function of frequency. This
is called the "loudness-comparison method." The amplitude of the
monaural transfer function or the corresponding level difference is determined from the difference between the plot made under the conditions
of sound incidence being examined and a plot made under reference
conditions. In the first method these are plots of thresholds of audibility;
in the second, plots of points of equal loudness.

For auditory experiments of this type, the method of oscillating adjustment described by von Békésy (1947) has proven useful (see also
Zwicker and Feldtkeller 1967). In this method the level of the sound
whose auditory event is to be judged is constantly raised by an automatic
control device, until the subject presses a button. Then the level decreases automatically until the subject presses the button again. Then
it rises again, and so forth. If a threshold of audibility is to be determined,
the subject presses the button whenever the auditory event has just
appeared or disappeared. To make a comparison of loudness, the subject
presses the button whenever the auditory event has just become louder
or quieter than a reference auditory event. The level of the sound
presented to the subject oscillates continually around the threshold to
be determined. As the frequency is gradually changed, this oscillation
can be plotted automatically by means of a level recorder. It is possible
to read the average values of the threshold directly off the plot.

Finally we consider measurement of the interaural transfer function.
A theoretically correct technique requires simultaneous measurements
in both ear canals. When a large number of subjects has been used,
though, it has often been assumed that, on average, their heads are
symmetrical. If this assumption is made, then the interaural transfer
function can be calculated from the free-field transfer function or the
monaural transfer function. The interaural transfer function is calculated
as the reciprocal of the ratio of the transfer function of the ear facing
the sound source to the transfer function of the same ear when the
sound source is in a position on the far side symmetrical with respect
to the median plane; for example,

$$A(f)_{\text{interaural},\varphi=30^\circ} = \frac{A(f)_{\text{monaural},\varphi=330^\circ}}{A(f)_{\text{monaural},\varphi=30^\circ}}. \tag{2.27}$$

Table. 2.2
Survey of measurements of the transfer function of the external ear, to 1972. (For work published after 1972, see chapter 4.)

Reference	Description	Test signal	Frequencies measured (kHz)	Number of subjects
Tröger (1930)	One ear, horizontal plane, $0° \leq \varphi \leq 360°$, auditory loudness comparison relative to $\varphi = 0°$, measured outdoors in far field of sound source	Sinusoids	0.2, 0.4, 0.6, 0.8, 1.0, 2.5, 5	1
Sivian and White (1933)	One ear, horizontal plane, $0° \leq \varphi \leq 360°$, auditory threshold measured relative to $\varphi = 0°$, loudspeaker 1 m away in acoustically treated room	Sinusoids	0.3, 0.5, 1.1, 2.2, 3.2, 4.2, 5, 6.4, 7.6, 10, 12, 15	3
Wiener and Ross (1946)	One ear, probe microphone at various positions in the auditory canal, magnitude of sound pressure relative to free field, horizontal plane, $\varphi = 0°$, 45°, 90°, anechoic chamber, distance of sound source not given	Sinusoids	continuous, 0.2–8	6–12
Wiener (1947)	One ear, probe microphone at entrance to ear canal, magnitude of sound pressure relative to free field, horizontal plane, $\varphi = 0°$, 45°, 90°, 135°, 180°, 225°, 270°, 315°, anechoic chamber, distance of sound source 140 cm	Sinusoids	continuous 0.2–6	6
Feddersen et al. (1957)	Two ears, probe microphone at entrance to auditory canal, interaural sound pressure level difference and interaural "impulse delay" (figure 2.30), horizontal plane, $0° \leq \varphi \leq 180°$, loudspeaker distance c. 2 m, no information about space in which measurements were made	Sinusoids and brief impulses	0.2, 0.5, 1, 1.8, 2.5, 3, 4, 5, 6 broadband	5

Table. 2.2 (continued)

Reference	Description	Test signal	Frequencies measured (kHz)	Number of subjects
Jahn and Vogelsang (1959), based on Jahn (1958)	One ear, probe microphone before eardrum, amplitude of sound pressure relative to $\varphi = 0°$, $\delta = 0°$ for $0° \leq \varphi \leq 360°$ and $\delta = 0°$, 30°, 60°, 90°, anechoic chamber, plane wave	1/3-octave noise	0.9–1.14, 2–2.56, 4–5, 7.1–9	2
Robinson and Whittle (1960)	One ear, probe measurements in cavum conchae, horizontal, median and frontal plane in 10° steps of φ or δ, magnitude of sound pressure relative to $\varphi = 0°$, $\delta = 0°$, anechoic chamber, loudspeaker distance c. 1 m	Narrow-band noise	1.6, 2.5, 4, 6.4, 8, 10	16–20
Schirmer (1963)	One ear, probe microphone at eardrum, magnitude of sound pressure relative to $\varphi = 0°$, $\delta = 0°$, for $0° \leq \varphi \leq 360°$, $\delta = 15°$, 30°, 45°, 60°, 90°, $-15°$, $-30°$, $-60°$, anechoic chamber, loudspeaker distance 1.5 m	1/3-octave noise	0.7, 3.5, 5, 7	20
Shaw (1966)	One ear, probe microphone at entrance to auditory canal, magnitude of sound pressure relative to free-field sound pressure, horizontal plane, $\varphi = 0°$, 45°, 90°, 180°, 270°, 315°, anechoic chamber, loudspeaker distance 1 m	Sinusoids	Continuous 0.2–15, partially only up to 8	10

Table. 2.2 (continued)

Reference	Description	Test signal	Frequencies measured (kHz)	Number of subjects
Blauert (1969a)	One ear, probe microphone at entrance to auditory canal, horizontal plane, $\varphi = 0°$, 180°, magnitude of sound pressure at $\varphi = 180°$ relative to that at $\varphi = 0°$, anechoic chamber, plane wave. Similarly in the median plane: magnitude of sound pressure at $\delta = 90°$ relative to that at $\delta = 0°$	1/3-octave noise	0.125–16 in 1/3-octave steps	10 in hor. plane, 2 in median plane
Harrison and Downey (1970)	Two ears, probe microphone at entrance to auditory canal, interaural sound pressure level difference, $-90° \leq \varphi \leq +90°$, loudspeaker distance 90 cm with a reflective horizontal plane 60 cm below the loudspeaker, no information about space in which measurements were taken	Sinusoid	4	3
Wilkens (1971a, 1972)	One ear, auditory loudness comparison relative to $\varphi = 0°$, horizontal plane, $0° \leq \varphi \leq 360°$ in 30° steps and $\varphi = 45°$, anechoic chamber, distance 2 m. Also probe microphone at eardrum, $\varphi = 0°$, $\delta = 0°$, otherwise as above	Narrow-band noise, 100 Hz wide	0.25, 0.5, 0.7, 1, 2, 2.5, 3, 3.5, 4, 5, 6, 7, 8.2, 10, 12, 14	2
		Sinusoids	0.2–15	1
Blauert, Hartmann, and Laws (1971)	Two ears, probe microphone at entrance to auditory canal, magnitude of sound pressure and group delay for $\varphi = 0°$ with 25 cm loudspeaker distance relative to $\varphi = 0°$ and 3 m distance. Also interaural sound pressure level differences and group delays, 3 m, $\varphi = 0°$, 30°, 60°, 90°, 120°, 150°, anechoic chamber	Sinusoids	0.1–16, τ_{gr} 0.5–10 only	5–12

Table. 2.2 (continued)

Reference	Description	Test signal	Frequencies measured (kHz)	Number of subjects
Laws (1972)	One ear, auditory threshold, differences relative to $\varphi = 0°$ and 3 m loudspeaker distance for $\varphi = 0°$ and distances of 25 cm, 1 m, 2 m. Also probe microphone at entrance to ear canal, sound pressure level and group delay relative to $\varphi = 0°$ and 3 m for $\varphi = 0°$ and distances of 25 cm, 50 cm, 1 m, 2 m (group delay not measured for 50 cm or 1 m), anechoic chamber	Sinusoids	Auditory experiments: 0.2–16, continuous. Probe measurements: 0.1–16, τ_{gr} 0.5–10 only	3–12 12
Mellert (1972)	One ear, auditory threshold measurements, free-field transfer function with $\varphi = 90°$, $\delta = 0°$	Sinusoids	0.5–10	17
This work (1972)	One ear, probe microphone in auditory canal, horizontal plane, sound pressure level, group delay, and phase delay relative to $\varphi = 0°$ for $\varphi = 30°$, 60°, 90°, 120°, 150°, 180°, 210°, 240°, 270°, 300°, 330°, anechoic chamber, loudspeaker distance 2 m	Impulses	0.5–16	25

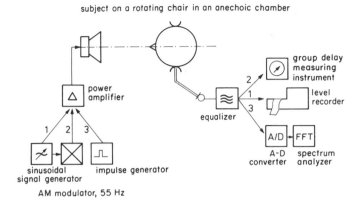

Figure 2.31
Apparatus for the measurement of transfer functions of the external ear using probe
microphones.

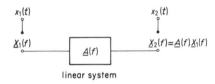

Figure 2.32
An explanation of the impulse method.

Detailed information about the transfer function of the external ear
and its dependence on the direction and distance of the sound source
is of interest not only in the study of spatial hearing, but also in other
fields—for example, in examining how loudness and annoyance of noise
depend on the position of the sound source. For this reason there are
a large number of investigations of this matter in the literature. Table
2.2 surveys the ones this author has been able to obtain. It gives a brief
description of the measuring procedures and the results for each investigation. Qualitative information about the directional characteristics
of the external ear are also to be found in Kessel (1882), Brunzlow
(1925), and Klensch (1948, 1949).

Figure 2.31 shows an apparatus this author has used to measure the
monaural and interaural transfer functions of the external ear. The
subjects sat on a rotating chair in an anechoic chamber. Both the head

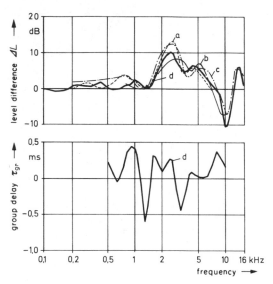

Figure 2.33
Free-field transfer function for a point of measurement about 5 mm inside the entrance to the ear canal, with sound incident from the front ($\varphi = 0°$, $\delta = 0°$), plane wave, anechoic chamber, conventional measuring techniques. a: Wiener (1947), 6 subjects. b: Jahn (1960), 6 subjects. c: Shaw (1966), 10 subjects. d: Blauert's measurements, 12 subjects.

and the upper body were immobilized, as has proven necessary during measurements of group delay (Laws 1972). The sound source was a loudspeaker at 3 m, a distance sufficient to produce a good approximation of a plane wave. Two measurement procedures were used at different times:

1. A conventional procedure: Level differences were recorded, using a sine-wave generator and a level recorder. Group delays were measured using an instrument built by Laws according to the principles described by Nyquist and Brand (1930).
2. A computer-aided impulse technique: A brief impulse of sound pressure was presented to the subjects. The impulse as received was sampled at a rate of 40 kHz and stored in a core memory. Subsequently the transfer function was calculated.

A few notes should be added about the impulse technique. It is possible to use test signals of impulse form to determine the transfer

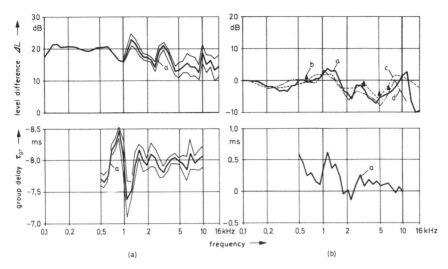

Figure 2.34
Monaural transfer function. a: Sound incident from the front ($\varphi = 0°$, $\delta = 0°$), 25 cm loudspeaker distance. b: Sound incident from the rear ($\varphi = 180°$, $\delta = 0°$), 3 m loudspeaker distance. Both taken relative to sound incident from the front from a distance of 3 m, 12 subjects, anechoic chamber, conventional measuring techniques. Confidence intervals for $\gamma = 95°$ are included in part a (after Laws 1972). The "a" curves incorporate measurements by Blauert and by Laws (1972). Points b are from Schirmer (1963; 20 subjects). Curve c shows results of Shaw (1966; 10 subjects), and curve d those of Blauert (1968b; 10 subjects).

function $A(f)$ of a linear system. Figure 2.32 sketches the relevant relationships. It is important to choose time functions at the input that contain energy at all points in the frequency range of interest; the transfer function is not defined at a null of the Fourier spectrum of the input signal. Rectangular pulses with widths of 25 μs or less are suitable test signals, since their Fourier spectrum comes sufficiently close to having a constant magnitude in the range from 0 to 16 kHz. (For 25 μs pulses, the magnitude is down 2.4 dB at 16 kHz.)

The results of measurements of the transfer functions of the external ear with one sound source under various conditions are assembled in figures 2.33–2.38. It should be noted that these results represent average values and describe groups of experimental subjects collectively. They may not be valid for individuals. The curves registered by individual subjects differ from the averaged curves especially in that they show more marked—higher and lower—maxima and minima. Comparisons

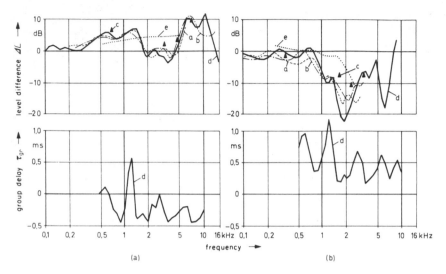

Figure 2.35
Monaural transfer functions of the left ear. a: Sound incident from $\varphi = 90°$, $\delta = 0°$, 3 m loudspeaker distance. b: Sound incident from $\varphi = 270°$, $\delta = 0°$, 3 m loudspeaker distance. Both taken relative to sound incident from the front with 3 m loudspeaker distance, anechoic chamber, conventional measuring techniques. Curve a shows results of Wiener (1947; 6 subjects); curves b, Shaw (1966; 10 subjects); points c, Schirmer (1963; 20 subjects); curves d, Blauert (5 subjects); curves e were calculated for a sphere as shown in figure 2.24.

of measured values for individuals against average values are given, for example, in Shaw (1966).

The curves in figures 2.33–2.36 were obtained in the following way. The level difference curve and the group delay curve were derived for each individual subject. Then an average level difference curve was determined by averaging the individual level difference curves, and an average group delay curve by averaging the individual group delay curves. This represents the type of averaging commonly used in acoustical laboratories.

An alternative procedure would be to average the input and output impulses of the system in the time domain and then take the Fourier transform of the averaged time functions. The corresponding procedure in the frequency domain would be to average the real and imaginary parts of the individuals' transfer functions separately, and to calculate the average curves for level differences and group delays from the

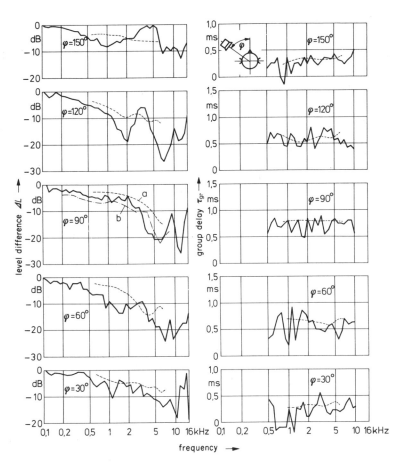

Figure 2.36
Interaural transfer functions for several directions of sound incidence in the horizontal plane, anechoic chamber, conventional measuring techniques, 3 m loudspeaker distance, 5 subjects. Also included are values calculated for a sphere as shown in figure 2.24 (curves a), and measured values obtained by Shaw (1966; 10 subjects) (curves b).

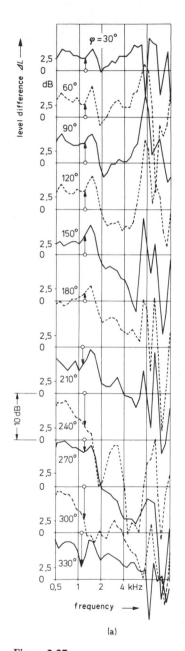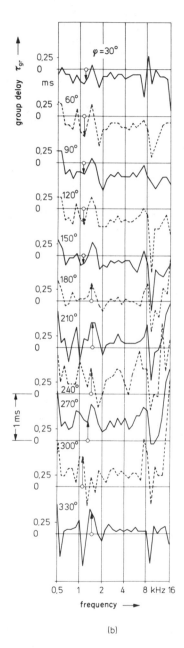

Figure 2.37
Monaural transfer functions of the left ear for several directions in the horizontal plane, relative to sound incident from the front ($\varphi = 0°$, $\delta = 0°$), anechoic chamber, 2 m loudspeaker distance. Impulse technique, 25 subjects, complex averaging.

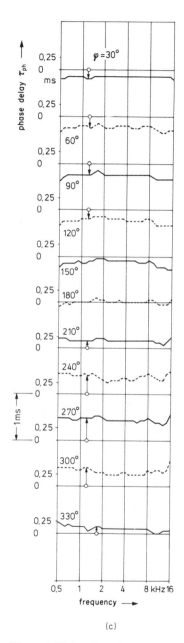

(c)

Figure 2.37 (continued)

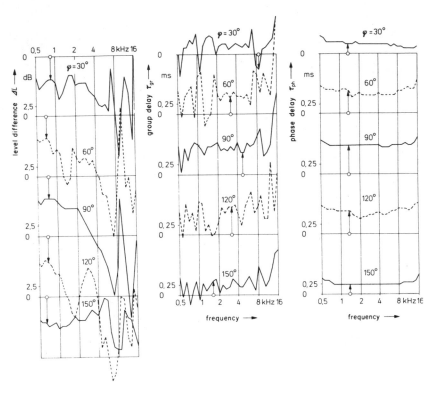

Figure 2.38
Interaural transfer function calculated from figure 2.37 (25 subjects, impulse technique, complex averaging).

averaged real and imaginary parts. The plots in figures 2.37 and 2.38 have been derived by means of this kind of "complex averaging." The ultimate answer as to which averaging algorithm is best can only be given with respect to a specific problem.

2.3   Evaluating Identical Ear Input Signals

We have now shown that sound signals on the way to the eardrum undergo linear distortions that depend in a characteristic way on the position of the sound source. It had previously been established that the sound signals at the eardrums are the most important inputs for forming the location of the auditory event, and also that the positions of the auditory event and of the sound source coincide more or less exactly in the majority of cases. Clearly the ear input signals contain attributes indicative of the position of the sound source, and the auditory system evaluates these attributes in the process of forming the location of the auditory event.

Spatial coincidence of the sound source and the auditory event is certainly a common situation, but it is by no means the only possible one. It also occurs—and not infrequently—that the auditory event appears in a position different from that of the sound source. The goal of this and the following section will be to describe in detail the conditions under which either situation occurs.

A normal human being has two functioning ears. In considering the input signals to the two ears, two classes of attributes may be distinguished:

1. Attributes that, in principle, require only one ear for sensitivity. Even a person who is deaf in one ear is sensitive to these attributes, to which the descriptive though slightly inaccurate term "monaural" is often applied.
2. Attributes of the difference between or ratio of the input signals to the two ears. Sensitivity to these attributes, which are called "interaural," clearly requires two ears.

Monaural and interaural attributes of the ear input signals must be separated if we are to investigate their importance for spatial hearing independently. In experiments with either of these sets of attributes, the other set must be held constant. The separate investigation of interaural attributes is impossible with sound sources that radiate freely into the space around the subject, since a change in the position of the sound source cannot change the interaural attributes alone: it must always change the monaural attributes too. For this reason the technique of dichotic presentation of signals over headphones is used for experiments investigating interaural attributes of ear input signals.* The application of this technique will be described in section 2.4.

The presentation of signals over headphones is also used for experiments with monaural attributes of the ear input signals. Diotic presentation is particularly appropriate in these cases, because it assures with great accuracy that the signals at both ears will be identical; in other words, that interaural signal differences will be absent. There is, however, one particular case in which sound in free space at least approximates the diotic condition. This is the case in which the sound source lies in the median plane. If it is assumed that the head is symmetrical, then identical signals are to be expected at both ears. If the position of the sound source in the median plane is changed, then, according ot this assumption, only monaural attributes of the signals are changed; interaural attributes remain constant at zero.

If the sound source is located in the median plane, or if identical signals are present at both ears, the auditory event generally also appears in the median plane. If the hearing apparatus is to determine the position of the auditory event on the basis of the attributes of the ear input signals, then these must be monaural attributes. Spatial hearing in the median plane or with identical ear input signals thus proves to be an important special case for use in experimentation, since it is possible to draw from this case general conclusions about the evaluation of monaural signal attributes in spatial hearing.

Before we analyze this case, however, we should add a few more notes about the prerequisites for the generation of identical ear input signals by means of a sound source in the median plane. One prerequisite is for the head to be symmetrical, so that there are no interaural signal differences. Results of measurements carried out to test whether such differences exist are shown in figure 2.39. The figure shows the standard

*Stumpf (1905) distinguished the following three categories of signal presentation using headphones: monotic presentation, in which a signal is present in only one headphone; diotic presentation, in which the same signal is present in both headphones; and dichotic presentation, in which a different signal is present in each headphone.

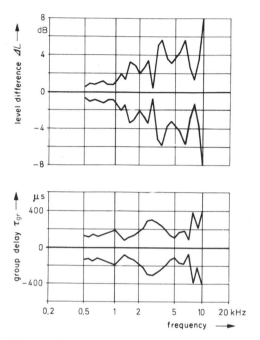

Figure 2.39
Standard deviations of the interaural level difference and group delay difference from the ideal value (0) with sound incident exactly from the front ($\varphi = 0°$, $\delta = 0°$), 10 subjects.

deviation for 10 experimental subjects of the interaural level difference and of interaural group delay from the theoretical value of zero. A comparison with tables 2.3 and 2.4 below shows that all of the values shown in the figure lie above the threshold of perceptibility. It is therefore only an approximation to state that identical ear input signals result when the sound source lies in the median plane.

A second prerequisite for the use of sound originating in the median plane in the study of spatial hearing is that the subject's head not move appreciably during the presentation of the signal. This condition is fulfilled automatically for signals that have a duration of less than 200–300 ms; von Wilmowsky (1960) showed that head motion elicited by a signal begins only after an interval of, on average, 350 ms. Woodworth and Schlosberg (1954) give typical motor times of approximately 250 ms; Thurlow and Mergener (1970) could find no difference in

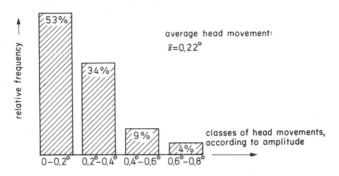

Figure 2.40
Histogram of the relative statistical frequency of different amplitude classes of head rotation when noise is presented from the front and from the rear (10 subjects per direction, 20 measurements each, head voluntarily held still but not immobilized).

localization blur using signals of 300 ms duration whether or not the head was mechanically immobilized.

When signal duration is greater, the possibility of head movement must be taken into consideration. There have been two investigations of involuntary head movements by subjects who were instructed to hold their heads absolutely still (König and Sussmann 1965, Blauert 1969a). The same measuring technique was used in both cases. A small mirror attached to the head of the subject reflected a parallel beam of light from a projector onto a measuring grid. The head movement, measured in degrees of arc, was calculated from the movement of the point of light on the grid. During measurement, the subject's eyes were closed. König and Sussmann reported small movements, of up to 5 minutes of arc, at the rate of the heartbeat. They also reported larger movements of up to 5°, occurring at irregular intervals of up to several seconds.

Blauert (1969a) presented noise signals of exactly 1 s duration to the subjects precisely from the front or from the rear. The maximum head movement (magnitude) occurring during the presentation of the impulse was registered without regard for the direction of the movement. Results are shown in figure 2.40. A statistical evaluation shows that the probability of head movements of more than 1° of arc is less than 5 percent. One degree is, it will be noted, approximately the minimum localization blur of the human auditory system.

The following conclusion can be drawn from these investigations. When the duration of the sound is short—1 s or less—there is no particular advantage in immobilizing the subject's head. The instruction to hold the head still is sufficient in experimental investigations of spatial hearing in the median plane. If the duration of the signal is longer, or if it is inconvenient to realign the head for each one of a series of experimental runs, a simple support for the head is sufficient. There is, as a rule, no need to position the head with great precision, for example by means of a clamp or bite board.

2.3.1 Directional hearing in the median plane

The concept of directional hearing in the median plane embraces the relationship between the directions of auditory events in the median plane and all correlated attributes, especially those of sound events. Discussion in this section will be limited to relationships of the direction of the auditory event to the position of the sound source and to the attributes of the ear input signals. Relationships with other correlated attributes will be dealt with in section 2.5.

Earlier hypotheses and measured results on the matter of the present section are to be found in Preyer (1887), Urbantschitsch (1889), von Kries (1890), Bloch (1893), Seashore (1899), Pierce (1901), Myers (1914), Hecht (1922b), Carsten and Salinger (1922), and von Hornbostel (1926). In that period it was understood that directional hearing in the median plane represents a special case in which interaural ear input signal differences are only slightly available, if at all, for use as attributes to be evaluated. Furthermore, experiments with directional hearing using sound sources in the median plane had led to the discovery that the direction of the auditory event often does not coincide with that of the sound source. The frequency of occurrence of this "error of localization" proved to be dependent on the type of sound signal used. It was evident that the discrepancy between the direction of the sound source and that of the auditory event was not random; there were consistent tendencies for specific "errors" to occur with specific types of signals (von Kries). With broadband test signals, especially those of long duration or those repeated several times, a quite good agreement between the direction of the sound source and that of the auditory event was usually observed. Localization blur when the direction of the sound source was changed proved quite large, sometimes on the order of three times as large as in the horizontal plane. Using signals produced by tuning forks and presented diotically by means of a T-shaped double listening tube (stethoscope), Urbantschitsch observed that the position of the "subjective auditory field" was dependent on frequency, but he did not note the relationship of this phenomenon to directional hearing in the median plane.

It was already well understood that distortions of the sound signals by the head and pinnae were relevant to the direction of the auditory event. In this connection it was found, for example, that loud auditory events appear in the forward half of the median plane more often than do quiet ones. By varying the intensity of the higher harmonics of a sound consisting of four harmonic components, Myers succeeded in showing that the direction of the auditory event depends on the spectrum of the ear input signals. Bloch and Carsten and Salinger mention the following experiment. A broadband sound source is placed in front of the subject. If both hands are cupped over the ears so as to form cavities that open toward the rear, the auditory event will jump to the rear, away from its normal position at the front. The opposite is also true: With the sound source behind the subject and hands cupped toward the rear, the auditory event jumps to the front.

Great credence was given to the idea that the effects of learning play an especially important role in directional hearing in the median plane. For example, it is possible to train a subject to report the position of a sound source in the median plane with a higher assurance of correctness if the sound source radiates a constant broadband signal. It is, however, unclear whether the subject reaches a decision about the position of the sound source on the basis of the position of the auditory event or on the basis of the tone color. A less than rigorous cognitive analysis leads to the conclusion, frequently expressed in this context, that the position of the auditory event in the median plane is determined on the basis of its tone color. For example, von Hornbostel (1926) regards directional hearing in the median plane as based on "indirect" and, in his opinion, inferior experiential criteria: With repeated experience it is learned step by step how the sound appears "with respect to tone color as it comes from one direction or another." He in no way takes into consideration the position of the auditory event.

In that past era further progress in the study of directional hearing in the median plane was frustrated by the lack of any sound source that could produce signals with precisely controllable characteristics. It remained an unanswered question whether it would be possible "to determine the outcome of localization at will according to the nature of the sounds chosen" (von Kries); in other words, to generate an auditory event in any predetermined direction in the median plane by a choice of ear input signals corresponding to that direction.

In dealing with works written since approximately 1930 on the problem of directional hearing in the median plane, it is helpful to distinguish the following subdivisions of this problem:

1. The role of specific linear distortions of the sound signals introduced as they pass the head and external ears.
2. The question of which types of sound signals are associated with coinciding positions of the auditory event and the sound source, and which types are associated with discrepancies between them.
3. The role of experience, adaptation, familiarity with the signals, and other similar phenomena; and so, more generally, the question of the degree to which localization between the sound source and the auditory event depends on previous occurrences.
4. The question of which specific attributes of the ear input signals are correlated with the direction of the auditory event; in other words, which specific attributes are evaluated by the auditory system.

The understanding that distortions introduced by the head and the pinnae are of central importance gained confirmation with time. Perekalin (1930), for example, undertook auditory experiments in which the effect of the pinnae was eliminated by the use of short rubber hoses inserted into the auditory canals. He compared the localization between the directions of the sound source and auditory event under these conditions with localization under normal conditions. He established that the directions of the sound source and auditory event coincided much more rarely when the hoses were used than when they were not. He obtained similar results by bending the pinnae forward so that they stood at an angle of 90° to the temporal bone. In this latter case reversal of directions occurred frequently, with the sound source at the front and the auditory event at the rear or vice versa.

Similar experiments were carried out by Kietz (1952, 1953) and Tarnóczy (1958). These authors, however, used only sound sources in front of and behind the subjects, and allowed the subjects, in judging

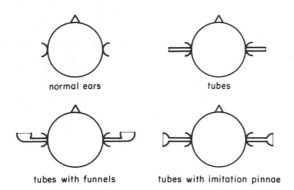

Figure 2.41
Modifications of the pinna used in auditory experiments involving the front–back impression (Kietz 1952, 1953, Tarnóczy 1958).

the direction of the auditory events, only the answers "ahead" and "behind." In this way they limited the scope of their investigation to what is called the "front–back impression." The experimental setup was as follows. In an anechoic chamber (Kietz) or outdoors (Tarnóczy), broadband noise was generated randomly either from the direction $\varphi = 0°$ or from the direction $\varphi = 180°$, with $\delta = 0$ in both cases. For different experimental runs the pinnae of the subjects were modified as follows (figure 2.41): (1) no modification; (2) short, 3 cm long brass tubes in both auditory canals; (3) brass tubes opening at the outer ends into small funnels, which had approximately the shape of hands cupped to the front; (4) imitation pinnae of gypsum (Kietz) or putty (Tarnóczy) affixed to the outer ends of the brass tubes (Tarnóczy constructed these in such a way that they could face either forwards, as in the normal ear, or backwards). With normal, unmodified pinnae, the adjudged direction of the auditory event generally coincided with that of the sound source even when the noise used as test signal was unfamiliar. When the brass tubes were inserted—with or without funnels at the outer ends—the auditory event usually appeared at the rear for most subjects, regardless of the direction of sound incidence. This result was reconfirmed by Blauert (1969a). If imitation pinnae replaced the funnels at the ends of the tubes, and, as normal, faced forward, then the normal relationship between the direction of the sound source and that of the auditory event was restored. If the imitation pinnae faced the rear, then the auditory event generally appeared in the opposite direction from the sound source.

Blauert (1969a, 1969/70) carried out a further variation of these experiments that in theory avoids all the possible failures of simulation in Kietz's and Tarnóczy's experiments. To avoid the use of imitation pinnae, the subject's own pinnae were used as filters. The experimental arrangement was similar to that in figure 2.11. Test signals including noise, speech, and music were presented to the subject from the front and from the rear. The resulting signals at the entrances to the ear canals were collected using probe microphones and stored on magnetic tape. Subsequently these signals were played back to the subject. The playback apparatus was equalized in such a way that exactly the same signal was reproduced at the entrance to the ear canal as had been present during recording. Although the loudspeaker arrangement used for playback was not the same as that used during recording, the subjects' auditory events appeared in the same directions as during recording. This experiment was carried out on 10 subjects and succeeded for all of them spontaneously and without error.

Having confirmed the role of distortions introduced by the head and external ears, we can now systematically take up the question of which types of signals are most clearly associated with coincidence of the positions of the sound source and the auditory event. Specifically, the filtering effect of the head and the external ear canals can affect only the level of narrow-band signals; with broadband signals this filtering effect can alter both the amplitude as a function of frequency and the relative phase angle of individual spectral components, and consequently the relative arrival time of these components at the eardrums. It may therefore be hypothesized that broadband ear input signals can contain more information about the position of the sound source than can narrow-band signals. Coincidence of the directions of the sound source and the auditory event should therefore occur most frequently with broadband signals. There is a long list of works confirming this hypothesis.

Stevens and Newman (1936) established that a large number of front–back reversals occurred with sinusoidal signals, especially when the signal level was varied constantly. Burger (1958) investigated the front–back impression using noise pulses of one-octave bandwidth and, with 15 subjects, confirmed a high proportion (about 35 percent) of reversals of direction. He found that the direction of the auditory event did not depend on the signal level. Franssen (1960) showed that the directions of the auditory event and the sound source coincide approximately 85 percent of the time when the signal is a square-wave-modulated sinusoid. Evidently the broadband rising and falling slopes of such a signal are of special importance to this result. Toole (1969) also mentions a dependence of the direction of the auditory event on the bandwidth.

Thorough investigations with various types of signals are described by Roffler and Butler (1968a,b) relative to angle of elevation and by Blauert (1969a) relative to the front and rear directions. These authors found that, in the median plane, the directions of sound incidence and of the auditory event coincide, as a rule, when the signals fulfill the following conditions: Relative to angle of elevation (Roffler and Butler), they must be broadband and include components above 7 kHz; if this is the case, localization blur with changes in the direction of the sound source falls to 4° (see the results in section 2.1). Relative to the front and rear directions (Blauert), the signals must be broadband, for example high-pass filtered noise with a low-frequency cutoff between 2 and 8 kHz.

With low-pass filtered noise, however, reversals of direction occur which depend systematically on the high-frequency cutoff. With very brief signals, for example 0.5 ms impulse sounds, reversals of direction are frequent. Evidently the duration of these signals is not sufficient to allow evaluation by the auditory system.

Proceeding to the next part of our examination of spatial hearing in the median plane, we deal with the question of the effect of previous occurrences in establishing the direction of the auditory event. In order to avoid an overly facile interpretation of experimental results, though, we should, before reporting them, undertake a cognitive analysis of the problem. Either of two tasks may be asked of a subject in an auditory experiment: to report the direction of the auditory event ("Where is what you hear?"), or to report the direction of the sound source ("Where is the sound source?"). The information given by the subject in the first case relates exclusively to judgment about the location of the auditory event; in the second case it is possible that entirely different criteria are judged, including above all the tone color rather than the location of the auditory event.

In the first case dependence on previous occurrences might mean a possible change in the direction of the auditory event corresponding to a particular signal from a particular direction. Localization itself could vary with time, for example during the course of an adaptation or learning process; it might, in some cases, become more precise (localization blur might get smaller). In the second case adaptation or learning would mean only that the subject came to associate particular auditory events with a particular direction of the sound source, and to call upon this association. In the literature the two cases are, as a rule, not differentiated with sufficient rigor. Consequently a definitive treatment of the meaning of previous occurrences for directional hearing in the median plane is not yet possible. Nonetheless some assertions can be made with confidence.

Coincidence of the directions of the sound source and auditory event definitely does not depend on a prior familiarity with the signal for all types of signals. Kietz (1952) reports, for example, that his subjects' auditory events in the front–back experiment spontaneously appeared in the direction of incidence of sound, even though he used a great number of different noises—impacts of various objects on wood or metal—that had not been presented to the subjects previously. The present author has more recently carried out the same experiment on more than 140 subjects, using pulses of white or pink noise. Approximately 90 percent of the subjects had precisely spatially located auditory events in the direction of the sound source.

On the other hand, it is also definitely true with many types of signals that the subjects evaluate the position of the sound source with greater accuracy if they are familiar with the test signal. Batteau (1967) and Plenge and Brunschen (1971) give quantitative information on this relationship. Batteau made use of an imitation external ear that had a microphone in place of the eardrum. The signal from the microphone was presented monotically to the subjects, by means of a distortion-free intra-aural headphone, and the subjects were asked to report the position of the sound source in relation to the imitation ear. White noise pulses were used as test signals. After experimental runs in each of which 36 judgments were required, the average number of "errors" by the six subjects had already decreased significantly. This result is consistent with the observation that the ability of persons deafened in

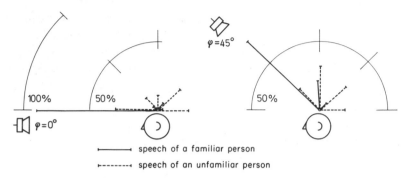

>———————< speech of a familiar person

>--------< speech of an unfamiliar person

Figure 2.42
Directional hearing in the median plane with familiar and unfamiliar human speakers (Plenge and Brunschen 1971, 10–20 subjects, as many as 40 presentations from each direction per subject). Shown are the relative statistical frequencies with which the signal was heard from one of the five loudspeaker directions when it was presented from a given direction.

one ear to report the direction of the sound source correctly improves with time (see section 2.1).

Plenge and Brunschen spaced five loudspeakers around the upper half of the median plane. Over these loudspeakers they presented short speech fragments (logatomes) pronounced by familiar and unfamiliar persons. Additionally, the familiar speakers' speech fragments were presented to the subjects several times from all five directions before the auditory experiment, with the direction identified each time. The unfamiliar signals, which were not presented in advance, consisted of speech fragments by a number of speakers in random sequence. The subjects' task was to report from which of the five directions they heard the signal. Some of the results are shown in figure 2.42. Clearly the agreement between the actual direction of the signal and the reported one is far better for the familiar signals than for the unfamiliar ones. There is a trend to report the unfamiliar signals more often as coming from the rear. It can be added that many authors report that the judgment "behind" predominates when the subject is uncertain (Wallach 1938, Tarnóczy 1958, and others).

Von Békésy (1930a) observed, using headphones, that with the same signal, the auditory event could be made to appear by choice at the front or rear depending on the state of mind of the subject, that is, depending on the subject's expectations or will. In connection with this

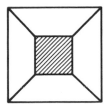

Figure 2.43
An optical analog of the ability to reverse the direction of auditory events in the median plane at will (von Békésy 1930a). The figure may appear either as a truncated pyramid or as a hollow basin.

phenomenon it is to be borne in mind that the filtering effect of the pinnae is lost when the signal is presented by means of headphones; the ear input signals then usually contain no information about the location of the sound source. Von Békésy suggests that the optical analog shown in figure 2.43 is comparable with the shifting of the auditory event to the front or rear at will (see also Klensch 1949). He regards the ability to reverse the direction as based on the human ability to concentrate at any one time on particular attributes of a signal and to suppress others; in the final analysis he regards it as an adaptive effect.

Present understanding is approximately as follows. When the sound source is in the median plane, and with many types of signals, the auditory event appears spontaneously in the direction of the sound source, even if the subject is unfamiliar with the signal. But with other signals, particularly ones that contain insufficient or contradictory information about the position of the sound source, the location of the auditory event depends on familiarity with the signal, on expectations, on habit, on the will of the subject, and on other possible factors. In such cases the congruence of the actual and the evaluated directions of the sound source, and possibly also of the auditory event, can sometimes be improved by adaptation or learning. To see how this improvement might occur, suppose that the ear input signals include attributes that suggest contradictory positions of the auditory event; then the subject might, in the course of time, come to pay attention only to attributes that allow a plausible correlation of the auditory event with the total situation.

This hypothesis leads directly to the final part of our examination of spatial hearing in the median plane: the question of which specific

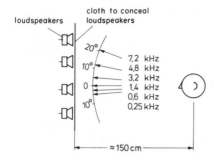

Figure 2.44
The experimental apparatus used by Roffler and Butler (1968a,b). When pulsed sinusoidal signals at various frequencies were presented, the auditory events appeared approximately in the directions shown, regardless of the direction of sound incidence.

characteristics of the ear input signals are actually correlated with the
direction of the auditory event. We have already made reference to a
paper by Urbantschitsch in which he describes, among other phenomena, how, when sinusoidal signals are presented diotically, the location
of the auditory event changes with the frequency of the sound event.
The same effect, or a similar one, was observed by Pratt (1930), confirmed by Trimble (1934), and thoroughly investigated by Roffler and
Butler (1968a,b). Pratt established that auditory events of high musical
pitch, which he called "high tones," are localized at a higher elevation
angle than are auditory events whose pitch is low, which he called "low
tones." Trimble varied the fundamental frequency of the sound event
continuously. He noted an upward movement of the auditory event
when the frequency was raised and a downward movement when it
was lowered. Roffler and Butler measured the same effect with greater
exactitude, using a larger number of subjects—about 50. The experimental apparatus that they used most frequently is shown in figure
2.44, along with typical results for pulsed sinusoids of various (carrier)
frequencies. In the main series of experiments the array of loudspeakers
was hidden behind a well-lighted, bright-colored strip of cloth. The
position of each loudspeaker was identified by a number that the subjects
could use to help describe the direction of the auditory event. The
subjects did not move their heads. Control experiments were carried
out with different signal levels, with the head free to move, with the
subjects blindfolded, with young children who did not know the meaning

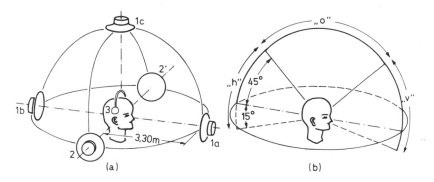

Figure 2.45
a: Different arrays of sound sources that generate identical or nearly identical ear input signals: at the front (1a), at the rear (1b), overhead (1c), right and left simultaneously and in phase (2, 2'), and with diotic headphone presentation (3). b: A scale of measurement relative to the subject for the description of the direction of the auditory event.

of the expressions "higher" and "lower" tones, and with the subjects lying down. In none of these cases were the results substantially different. In every case the elevation angle of the auditory event was described as varying as a function of the frequency of the sound event, as shown in figure 2.44. Frequencies measured were from 250 Hz to 7.2 kHz.

While still unaware of these results, the present author made a similar but more general observation. Sitting before a loudspeaker radiating a sinusoidal signal whose frequency continuously rose from 200 Hz to 16 kHz, I noticed that the auditory event moved back and forth several times on a path from front to rear over the top of my head (figure 2.6). This observation, subsequently verified and confirmed by Mellert (quoted in Damaske 1971a), led to a series of investigations (Blauert 1968b, 1969a, 1969/70) that resulted in important clues as to which attributes of the ear input signals are evaluated by the auditory system in order to establish the direction of the auditory event in the median plane. The two basic parts of these investigations will now be described.

In the first part 1/3-octave noise pulses were presented to subjects in a darkened anechoic chamber. The sound events were presented using the loudspeaker array shown in figure 2.45a. The subjects' heads were immobilized, and they saw in front of them a dim red lamp, which was used as an aid in positioning the head to face directly forward. The duration of the test signals was varied between 200 ms and 1 s, and its level was 30, 40, 50, or 60 dB over 20 μNm^{-2}. Noise was more than 65 dB below the signal level, and nonlinear distortion was less than 2 percent. The signals were presented in a random sequence with respect to frequency, level, and loudspeaker. Five to twenty persons with normal hearing took part in each series of experiments.

It was first established through a series of preliminary experiments that all auditory events appeared in or near the median plane and no more than 15° below the horizontal plane. Then, in order to categorize the auditory events, the scale of measurement shown in figure 2.45b was drawn up. It was decided not to use a finer division of the scale, on the grounds that this would make the experiment too complicated and time-consuming. In figure 2.46 are shown the results obtained with 20 subjects and with sound from the front and rear. In all three groups of curves the relative frequency of the answers h, o, and v (German abbreviations for behind, overhead, and forward, respectively) show a clear dependence on the center frequency of the test signal. A statistical interpretation leads to the conclusion that the relative probability of the answers shows no other significant dependence, such as on the level of the signal or on the direction of incidence of the sound. The other ways of presenting the sound to the listener as shown in figure 2.45a produced no discrepancies in the results. Neither were discrepancies observed when 5 cm long brass tubes were inserted into the auditory canals in order to eliminate the effects of the pinnae.

Figure 2.47 shows the results of a simple nonparametric statistical evaluation of the data from figure 2.46. It can be shown on the basis of this evaluation that more than half of the subjects give one particular answer in certain frequency ranges more often than they give both other possible answers combined. We have given the name "directional bands" to the frequency bands in which this is the case. To test the objectivity of the positions where the directional bands had been found, the standard deviations of the answers given in by one representative subject in 10 auditory experiments were compared with the standard deviations of a group of 10 subjects in one auditory experiment each (figure 2.48). It can be seen from the figure that the limits of the bands vary from one individual to another but that the coincidence between subjects is quite good in the central region of each band. It may be observed, furthermore, that 40 percent of subjects exhibit the same number and type of directional bands as are derived from the averaged

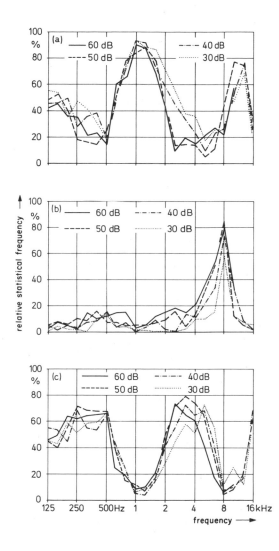

Figure 2.46
a: Relative statistical frequencies of the answer *h* (20 subjects, signal presented once from the front and once from the rear at each 1/3-octave center frequency). b: As in part a, but for the answer *o*. c: As in part a, but for the answer *v*.

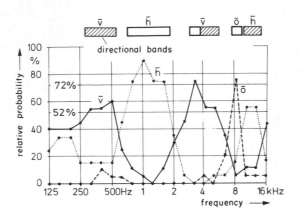

Figure 2.47
Relative statistical frequency of subjects giving one of the answers *h*, *o*, or *v* more often than the other two taken together. At the top the frequency bands are shown in which the absolute majority of a population of subjects gives the same answer more often than it gives the other two possible answers taken together. Bands drawn at a 90 percent confidence level; shaded areas, most probable answers.

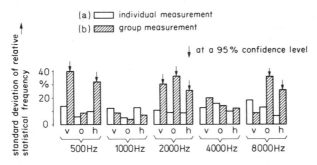

Figure 2.48
Standard deviations of the answers *h*, *o*, and *v*. a: One subject, to whom each of eight signals was presented 10 times per 1/3 octave. b: Ten subjects, to whom each of eight signals was presented once per 1/3 octave.

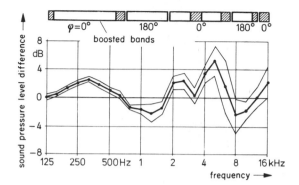

Figure 2.49
Sound pressure level at the eardrum with sound incident from the front minus sound pressure level with sound incident from the rear. Average values and confidence intervals for 10 subjects. At the top of the drawing are shown "boosted bands" in which sound pressure at the eardrum is greater for the absolute majority of a population of subjects with sound from the front than with sound from the rear, or the opposite. Bands drawn at a 95 percent confidence; shaded areas, most probable cases.

representation in figure 2.47, namely, two h, one o, and two v bands. The combination of two h, one o, and three v bands is next most probable, at 15 percent.

The second part of the investigation consisted of physical measurements of the transfer function of the external ear with sound incident from the front and rear. Measurements were taken at the entrance to the ear canal using a conventional technique described in section 2.2.3. Figure 2.49 shows the plot of differences in sound pressure level at the eardrum between sound from the front and sound from the rear, that is, the plot of level difference against frequency for the monaural transfer function $A(f)_{\text{monaural}}$ for $\varphi = 0°$ and $\varphi = 180°$. It can be seen that the averaged sound pressure level at the eardrum is higher in some frequency ranges for sound from the front than it is for sound from the rear. In other frequency ranges the opposite is true. After generalizing these results for an ensemble of subjects, it becomes possible to define the "boosted bands" shown at the top of figure 2.49. Figure 2.50 demonstrates that a marked boosted band appears around 8 kHz when the sound source is overhead (compare Shaw and Teranishi 1968).

What, then, is the relationship between the results of the first and second experiments? In the first part narrow-band noise signals were presented to the subjects. The only influence the head and external

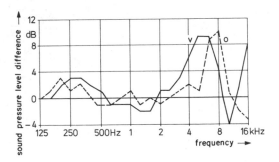

Figure 2.50
Sound pressure level at the eardrum with sound from the front and above, respectively, minus sound pressure level with sound from the rear. Average values of measurements of both ears of two subjects.

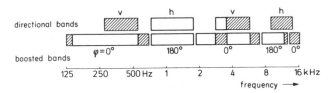

Figure 2.51
Positions of the directional bands and of the boosted bands along the frequency axis.

ears have on these signals is to change their level. There is no change in different parts of the signal spectrum relative to each other. The results of the auditory experiments show that narrow-band signals contain no information about the direction of incidence of the sound that can be used by the human auditory system for evaluation. The auditory system determines the direction of the auditory event on the basis of the center frequency of the ear input signals. Localization can be described in terms of directional bands. In the second part of the experiment the filtering effect of the head and the pinnae was measured. The level difference curves at the eardrums with sound incidence from the front with respect to incidence from the rear exhibit boosted bands, and the same is true when the comparison is reversed. Sound incidence from overhead leads to boosted bands in comparison with sound incidence from both the front and the rear.

In figure 2.51 the positions of the directional bands and the boosted bands along the frequency axis are shown together. It is evident that

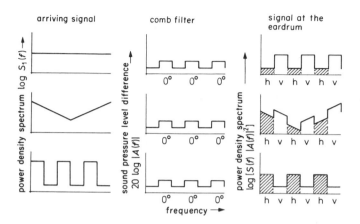

Figure 2.52
Cooperation of the filtering effect of the head and external ears with the mechanism
described by the directional bands. Illustrated in a simplified manner with three special noise signals as examples.

the position of the h directional bands corresponds to that of the $\varphi =$
180° boosted bands. The same is true for the v directional bands and
the $\varphi = 0°$ boosted bands, with the exception that one v directional
band at 16 kHz is missing. However, a glance at figure 2.47 shows that
such a band may well exist and may attain statistical significance in
experiments with larger numbers of subjects. (The o directional band
and the corresponding boosted band are left out here in order to simplify
the discussion.)

The directional bands were discovered in experiments using narrow-
band noise, but their discovery leads to the hypothesis that they influence
localization in the median plane. The direction of the auditory event
might, for example, be established primarily according to the class of
directional bands in which the largest part of the signal power is found.
The way the head and external ear work together with the other parts
of the auditory system could then be explained in the manner illustrated
schematically in figure 2.52. In the first column the power density
spectra $S_1(f)$ of three signals are shown in a simplified form. It is
assumed that their source is to the front of the subject. The head and
external ear operate as a filter, somewhat similar to a comb filter. The
level difference function $20 \log |A(f)|$ of such a filter is shown in the
second column. Signals passing through such a filter become enhanced

in the $\varphi = 0°$ boosted bands relative to the other spectral regions. The resulting power density spectra $S_2(f)$ of the signals at the eardrums are shown in the third column. Assuming that the direction of the auditory event is determined according to which class of directional bands contains the most power, the auditory event that corresponds to the signals in the first and second horizontal rows of the figure will appear in the forward direction. The same will be true for many other signals, as long as their power density spectra are relatively even. This explains why a prior familiarity with the signal is, for many signals, not necessary in order for the auditory event to appear in the direction of sound incidence.

Only with very unusual signals such as that shown in the third row of figure 2.52, or with special band-limited signals, does the hypothetical evaluation mechanism operate "faultily," so that the auditory events appear in directions other than that of sound incidence. Using special predistorted signals, I have been able to demonstrate that this may in fact be the case. Similiar experiments show what happens when there is no clear preponderance of power in any one class of directional bands. If, for example, the v and h bands contain equal power, then the auditory event may appear inside the head (see section 2.3.2) or split into two parts, one at the front and the other at the rear. When a sufficient amount of power falls inside the o band around 8 kHz, the auditory event appears elevated by a certain angle. This helps explain results obtained by Pratt, Trimble, and Roffler and Butler, who used signal frequencies only up to 7.2 kHz and inquired only about the angle of elevation. Their subjects paid no attention to whether the auditory event lay to the front or to the rear but, rather, knew that the only loudspeakers were at the front.

The evaluative mechanism we have assumed so far for directional hearing in the median plan is illustrated once more in figure 2.53 for purposes of summation, in the form of a functional model.

The task of incorporating into the model a possible dependence of the position of the auditory event on past occurrences remains to be undertaken. Two possibilities suggest themselves. First, one might postulate that the position and bandwidth of the directional bands are variable over time (e.g., learned during childhood) and are consequently adaptable to different circumstances. This hypothesis is contradicted by the observation that approximately 10 percent of all subjects show

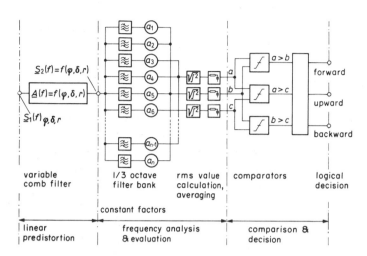

Figure 2.53
Hypothetical model of the evaluation of the ear input signals in the case of directional hearing in the median plane.

no dependence of the position of the auditory event on that of sound incidence in the median plane, even with broadband signals; in a darkened room the auditory event is either always at the front or always at the rear. Tests on a few of these subjects showed that the position of their directional bands does not coincide with the position of their boosted bands. Clearly no matching of the directional bands to the individual characteristics of the pinnae had taken place either by learning or by other time-variant effects. A second way of explaining time-variant processes such as learning and adaptation would be to conceive of the constants a_1 through a_n in the model as variable over time. The weight given to the proportion of signal power falling into particular directional bands would then be variable. Weighting could occur, for example, by efferent inhibition in the inner ear, or it could occur more centrally in the auditory path. Examples of mechanisms of this type are well known in the field of sensory physiology. The actual physiological processes are, however, certainly much more complicated than what we have included in our simple model.

Another essential deficiency of the model should be mentioned. Up to now we have regarded only the power of the signal's spectral regions falling in the various directional bands as the criterion for evaluation.

This way of regarding the power is only applicable to stationary or quasi-stationary processes. With signals of impulse form, the proportions of energy, for example, may replace those of power. Since the energy of an impulse is concentrated in time, the point in time at which it arrives must certainly also be considered. But this will, as a rule, be different for the parts of the energy that fall into the individual directional bands. In some bands the energy will arrive sooner than in others.

Signal theory can describe the implications of this state of affairs, but the description is rather complicated; it will not be repeated here in detail (see Gabor 1946, Mertens 1960, 1965). One possibility is the computation of points of temporal energy concentration from the envelopes of the parts of the signal that fall into the various directional bands. The times at which these points of energy concentration occur with respect to each other are, however, affected by group delay distortions of the signal. The signal does undergo group delay distortions as it arrives at the head and external ears, and these distortions are dependent on the direction of sound incidence. Consequently the arrival times of the points of energy concentration will depend in a characteristic way upon the direction of sound incidence.

The meaning of the group delay distortions to the signal at the eardrums — or the meaning of different arrival times of parts of the signal — has not yet been investigated thoroughly in the context of spatial hearing in the median plane. By means of two simple experiments, the present author has, however, shown that such an influence may exist. In one of these certain parts of a test signal were delayed by means of an allpass filter; in the other the envelopes of two simultaneously presented Gaussian signals were shifted with respect to each other. In both experiments definite changes in the direction of the auditory event were observed when these effects were set at certain levels.

That the auditory system is able to derive information about the spectrum of a signal from the wavefront (i.e., with a very short time available for interpretation) has been shown to be theoretically possible in another context by Patterson and Green (1970) and by Patterson (1971).

2.3.2 Distance hearing and inside-the-head locatedness

Theories of "distance hearing" describe relationships between the distance of the auditory event and attributes of other events correlated with this distance. We here define the distance of the auditory event as the distance from the midpoint of the axis of the ears (see figure 1.4), and we take particular interest in the relationship between this distance and attributes of sound events. "Inside-the-head locatedness" or intracranial locatedness occurs when the distance of the auditory event is smaller than the radius of the head—in other words, when the auditory event occurs inside the head. Problems of inside-the-head locatedness (IHL) are encountered, for example, in the development of electroacoustic systems to reproduce sound by means of headphones; localization of auditory events inside the head often occurs as an undesired side effect when headphones are used to present signals.

A few basic concepts in distance hearing were described in section 2.1; the present section goes into more detail on this subject. The thorough literature reviews of Coleman (1963) and Laws (1972) are also especially recommended. Although a large amount of work is available, our knowledge of distance hearing is deficient compared to our knowledge of directional hearing. This deficiency is due to the extraordinary complexity of the subject.

Investigations of distance hearing and of inside-the-head locatedness have focused mainly on their relationship to monaural attributes of the ear input signals. Many of these investigations have been carried out using sound sources in the median plane or using headphone presentation. It is for this reason that the present section has been placed under the heading "Evaluation of Identical Ear Input Signals." At the end of section 2.4.2 there is a short description of how interaural attributes of ear input signals relate to the distance of the auditory event. The influence on distance hearing of the proportion of direct to reflected sound is described in section 3.3.

Let us assume for now that there is, in the median plane of a subject, a sound source radiating an unchanging broadband signal. Under these conditions, as a rule, the auditory event appears more or less precisely at the position of the sound source. If the distance of the sound source is increased, then the auditory event will also become more distant; and if the sound source is brought closer, the distance of the auditory event will decrease. An explanation of this coincidence of distances proceeds similarly to the earlier explanation of directional hearing in the median plane. It is assumed, on the one hand, that certain attributes of the sound signals in the auditory canals depend on the distance of the sound source and, on the other hand, that the auditory system establishes the distance of the auditory event either completely or partially on the basis of these attributes.

Reflecting briefly on which attributes of the ear input signals depend on the distance from the sound source, we arrive at the following classification scheme:

1. At intermediate distances from the sound source—approximately 3–15 m for point sources—only the sound pressure level of the ear input signals depends on the distance from the source as long as the radiated signal does not change. (This is the rms level, measured broadband.) In a free sound field the sound pressure falls 6 dB for every doubling of the distance (the $1/r$ law: see figure 1.13 and equations 1.6 and 1.7).

2. At greater distances from the sound source—more than approximately 15 m—the air path between the sound source and the subject can no longer be regarded as a distortion-free communications channel. The dependence of the sound pressure level on the distance of the sound source is still present. It is independent of frequency and follows the $1/r$ law. But there is an additional attenuation that depends on the length of the air path and varies with frequency. Higher frequencies are attenuated more than lower ones. Not only does the sound pressure level depend on the distance from the sound source, but the shape of the spectrum also depends on it—or, more precisely, the relative level and phase curves as a function of frequency depend on it.

3. Close to the sound source—at distances less than approximately 3 m for point radiators—the effects of curvature of the wavefronts arriving at the head can no longer be neglected. The linear distortions of the signals due to the head and the external ears vary with distance from the sound source (see figure 2.34). Close to the sound source the sound pressure level changes with distance, and the shape of the spectrum of the ear input signals also changes, though the way the spectrum changes is not the same as at great distances.

4. This fourth point has to do with signals presented over headphones. In this case the normal filtering effect of the pinnae is eliminated. The headphones lie on the axis of the ears very close to the entrances to the auditory canals. It is clear that sound sources in these positions lead to linear distortions of the ear input signals often associated with

inside-the-head locatedness—a phenomenon that occurs most frequently under these conditions.

We proceed now with the case described in point 1: a sound source in the median plane, far enough from the subject so that wavefronts arriving in the region of the subject's head may be regarded as plane. The sound pressure at the ears, p_{rms}, changes at a rate inversely proportional to any change in the distance of the sound source. If $p_{0,\mathrm{rms}}$ is the sound pressure at a reference distance r_0, then

$$\frac{p_{\mathrm{rms}}(r)}{p_{0,\mathrm{rms}}} = \frac{r_0}{r} \quad \text{or} \quad p_{\mathrm{rms}}(r) = \frac{p_{0,\mathrm{rms}}\, r_0}{r} \tag{2.28}$$

or, described in terms of sound pressure level referred to 20 $\mu\mathrm{Nm}^{-2}$,

$$L(r) = 20 \log(p_{0,\mathrm{rms}}/20\ \mu\mathrm{Nm}^{-2}) - 20 \log(r/r_0). \tag{2.29}$$

In order for the level of the ear input signals to indicate the distance of the sound source, two conditions must be fulfilled, as is evident from these formulas. The average radiated power of the sound source must be time-invariant, even if the distance of the source is changed. Also, the level of the ear input signals must be known for some reference distance. These conditions are not often fulfilled. For example, if the sound source is a loudspeaker, its input level might be adjusted so that the signal level at the ears varied while the loudspeaker's distance remained constant, or so that the signal level at the ears remained constant while the distance varied. In both cases the correlation between the level of the ear input signals and the distance of the sound source would no longer be described by the above equations. It should also be borne in mind that the $1/r$ law that is the basis for these equations applies to the propagation of spherical waves in a free sound field. This condition, too, is often not fulfilled for spatial hearing in normal environments.

Due to these physical circumstances alone, it is to be expected that a more or less marked discrepancy from the distance of the sound source would occur if the distance of the auditory event were established only on the basis of the level of the ear input signals. The discrepancy would be greatest for a subject unfamiliar with the sound signal, or when the conditions of sound propagation were unusual.

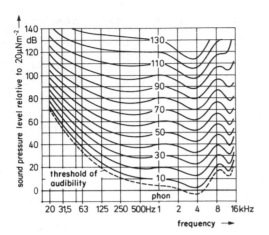

Figure 2.54
Curves of equal loudness level for sinusoids with sound incident from the front (after DIN 45630, sheet 2, 1966).

Before going into detail about measured relationships between the signal level at the ears and the distance of the auditory event, we must note yet another complication—the fact that the sound pressure level of the ear input signals is related not only to the distance of the auditory event but also to its loudness and tone color. Loudness increases with increasing signal level at the ears, and at the same time the tone color becomes darker. The darkening of the tone color may be examined in connection with the well-known curves of equal loudness level (figure 2.54). As the level is increased, the low-frequency components of a broadband signal gain more and more perceptual weight relative to the high-frequency components. As a sound source radiating a broadband signal is brought closer to the subject, the distance of the auditory event decreases, but its loudness increases and its tone color becomes darker.

This effect, which has been known since the time of Mach (1865), creates a problem similar to those encountered in testing directional hearing in the median plane, namely the fact that the subject is aware of changes in various parameters of the auditory event. The subject's judgments depend to an important degree on the experimental task. In the present context, once again, two important modes of inquiry are to be distinguished:

1. Questions may be asked about the distance of the auditory event. Only such questions relate fundamentally to the problem of spatial hearing under investigation.

2. Questions may be asked about the distance of the sound source. In this case the subject may in some circumstances use the loudness and tone color of the auditory event as criteria for identifying a sound source correlated with the auditory event. These criteria are in addition to the distance of the auditory event, so that localization, as we define it, cannot be measured with confidence when such a mode of inquiry is used. Unfortunately, this mode of inquiry has been used in the majority of available works.

The changes in loudness and tone color that occur along with changes in distance of the auditory event have led to numerous investigations. The relationships between loudness and the distance of the auditory event (see on this subject Thompson 1882, von Békésy 1938, Coleman 1963, but also Mohrmann 1939, Warren 1963) or between tone color and the distance of the auditory event (Mach 1865, Klemm 1913) have often been studied in attempts to explain distance hearing. It must be stated with regard to these attempts that distance, loudness, and tone color are all attributes of the auditory event. It is certainly possible to measure the relationships among them, but these relationships do not by themselves contribute to an understanding of the connections between the distance of the auditory event and the attributes of the sound event. At best, loudness and tone color can serve as auxiliary parameters in describing relationships between the signal level at the ears and the distance of the auditory event, and only insofar as their dependence on the signal level at the ears is known in each individual case. Even so, it is important in this context to note that loudness and tone color depend on the shape of the spectrum of the ear input signals, not only on the level.

In discussing the details of measured results, we start with those describing the relationship between the signal level at the ears and the distance of the auditory event. It has often been hypothesized, and has been proven, that the distance of the auditory event decreases with increasing signal level at the ears (Steinhauser 1879, Matsumoto 1897, Gamble 1909, Starch and Crawford 1909, Trimble 1934, Steinberg and Snow 1934, von Békésy 1949, Stevens and Guiaro 1962, Gardner

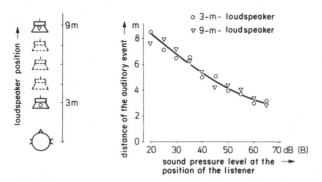

Figure 2.55
A typical curve for the dependence of the distance of the auditory event on the sound
pressure level at the position of the listener (after Gardner 1969a; speech, 5 subjects,
two loudspeakers at 3 m and one at 9 m, 5 loudspeakers visible altogether, anechoic
chamber).

1969a, Haustein 1969, Laws 1972, among others). Figure 2.55 shows
typical results. The dependence of the distance of the auditory event
on the signal level at the position of the listener is shown for two
distances of the sound source. It is clear that the distance of the auditory
event is independent of the distance of the sound source. It is dependent
only on the signal level at the position of the listener, and to a lesser
degree than might be expected. A level reduction of 20 dB, rather than
the expected 6 dB, leads to a doubling of the distance of the auditory
event. This result agrees well with results obtained by von Békésy
(1949) and Laws (1972).

The conclusion to be drawn from these results is inescapable. When
the sound pressure level of the ear input signals is the only attribute
of the sound event available to the auditory system to form the distance
of the auditory event, then a trend exists for this distance to increase
less rapidly than the distance of the sound source. This trend may be
observed in the measured results of a large number of authors (e.g.,
von Békésy 1949, Cochran et al. 1968, Haustein 1969). A localization
curve for the distance of natural speech in an anechoic chamber is
given in figure 2.56. It is clear from this curve that the distance of the
auditory event fails to keep up with that of the sound event. On the
basis of this curve, von Békésy (1949) hypothesized that auditory space
is of limited total extent—in other words, that there is an outer limit
to the distance of auditory events (the "auditory horizon").

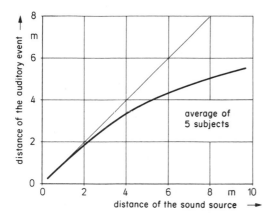

Figure 2.56
Localization between the distance of the auditory event and the sound source with a
human speaker (after von Békésy 1949; anechoic chamber, 5 subjects, blindfolded).

Figure 2.7 also illustrates localization of distance with natural speech.
It shows the relationships between the distance of the auditory event
and that of the sound source in an anechoic chamber for three different
types of speech: "conversational speech," "calling out loudly," and
"whispering." The subject was blindfolded. The trend of the distance
of the auditory event to fall below that of the sound source was significant
only for "whispering." However, the curves show another noteworthy
relationship: Though the signal level at the ears was certainly higher
for "calling out loudly" than for "conversational speech," the auditory
event connected with "calling out loudly" appeared at a greater distance
than that for "conversational speech," and conversely for "whispering."
Clearly there are factors other than the signal level at the ears that
determine the forming of the auditory event; it can, in addition, depend
in a specific way on the type of signal.

It is emphasized by many authors that distance hearing is especially
accurate if the subject is familiar with the signal being presented. It is,
however, not clear whether these authors mean that the distances of
the auditory event and sound source coincide especially well with one
another, or that the subjects are able to evaluate the distance of the
sound source especially well. Work by Coleman (1962) and Haustein
(1969) suggests this second state of affairs, since the subjects' task in
both investigations was to identify the position of the sound source,

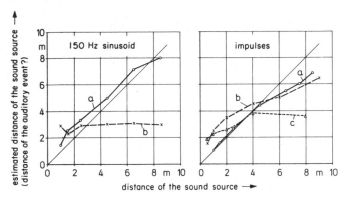

Figure 2.57
The average distance of the sound source evaluated by 20 subjects as a function of
the actual distance for sinusoidal signals and impulses under various experimental
conditions (after Haustein 1969; darkened anechoic chamber, head immobilized).
Curves a: Loudspeaker voltage constant, familiar signal. Curves b: Signal level constant at the ears, familiar signal. Curves c: Signal level constant at the ears, unfamiliar
signal.

not to report the distance of the auditory event. It can certainly be
assumed that the subjects used the position of the auditory event as
an important criterion for evaluating distance. It is, however, not certain
that this was their only criterion.

Coleman (1962) presented broadband noise at a constant power level
to approximately 20 subjects. Fourteen loudspeakers were arrayed at
distances in the range of 3–8 m, visible to the subjects, outdoors. The
ground was covered with snow. The signal was switched at will among
the loudspeakers. The discrepancy between the actual and evaluated
distances of the sound source decreased considerably from the first to
the eleventh presentation.

Figure 2.57 shows the results of Haustein (1969). The curves in the
graph at the left show a relationship between the actual and evaluated
distances of the sound source. The auditory experiments involved click-
free 150 Hz signals, previously presented for long periods from various
distances with the distance of the sound source identified. In one series
of experiments the voltage at the loudspeaker was adjusted so that the
sound pressure level at the position of the listener was 58 dBA. Then
the distance was changed while the voltage at the loudspeakers remained
constant. In another series the voltage at the loudspeakers was adjusted

so that the sound pressure level at the position of the listener remained a constant 58 dBA, though the distance of the sound source changed. The investigations were carried out in a darkened anechoic chamber. It is clear from the results that subjects are able to evaluate the distance of the sound source quite accurately after the signal has been presented previously to them. The relevant attribute of the sound event is the signal level at the ears; if it is held constant when the distance is changed, the evaluated distance of the sound source becomes independent of the actual distance. It is not clear whether the subjects in this experiment had a precisely located auditory event at the evaluated distance of the sound source. They might, for example, have based their conclusions about the distance of the sound source on loudness, though the auditory event was spatially diffuse.

The graph at the right in figure 2.57 shows the results of similar investigations with impulse sounds, which are broadband signals. Experimental conditions were as follows: (a) the loudspeaker voltage was constant, with the sound pressure level at the position of the listener kept at 70 dBA when the sound source was at a distance of 4 m; (b) the level at the position of the listener was kept at a constant 70 dBA, regardless of the distance of the sound source, and the signal was presented before the auditory experiments; (c) the level at the position of the listener was a constant 65 dBA, and the signal was not presented in advance. The curve representing case (a), like the corresponding curve for 150 Hz tones, shows a good agreement between the actual and evaluated distances of the sound source. (Figure 2.8 above, derived from Haustein's experimental results, shows the localization blur of this same relationship.) The curve representing case (b) does not conform entirely to expectations. It might have been hypothesized that the evaluated distance of the sound source would not depend on the actual distance in the range beyond approximately 3 m. Discrepancies seem to result from two features of Haustein's experimental apparatus: The experimental chamber was not totally free of reflected sound, and the loudspeaker did not generate purely spherical waves even in the range beyond 3 m. Curve (c) shows the correlation between the actual and the evaluated distances of the sound source when the signal was not presented previously. This curve shows no dependence between the actual and evaluated distances beyond 4 m.

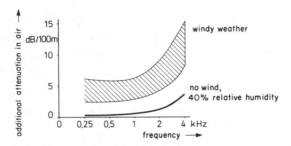

Figure 2.58
The attenuation of sound propagating freely in air (adapted from Ingård 1953). The attenuation caused by the divergence of spherical waves ($1/r$ law) has already been subtracted. Relative humidity, 40 percent.

The last work about distance hearing at intermediate distances that we will mention is an investigation of localization blur by Edwards (1955). The author does not describe the room in which measurements were taken, but it seems not to have been an anechoic chamber. The sound source was behind the subject ($\varphi = 180°, \delta = 0°$), who was asked to judge the smallest displacement Δr_{min} of the sound source that could lead to a noticeable displacement of the auditory event. For the ticking of a metronome, the ratio $\Delta r_{min}/r$ exhibited a nearly constant value of approximately 25 percent when the distance of the sound source was between 3 and 5 m (31 subjects). For quiet ticking of a clock, this ratio decreased steadily with increasing source distance from 55 to 22 percent (1 to 8 m, 50 subjects).

We now extend our discussion to take in greater distances of the sound source. As already mentioned, frequency-dependent attenuation occurs at greater distances as a result of absorption of sound along the air path between the sound source and the subject. This attenuation is in addition to the frequency-independent $1/r$ variation in the signal level at the ears. The additional, frequency-dependent attenuation varies with the moisture content of the air and with wind speed. Some attenuation occurs as a result of turbulence. Typical free-field values of attenuation are shown in figure 2.58; further data may be found in Coleman (1968) and Aschoff (1963). Aschoff also gives typical values of attenuation to be expected in a forest. It should be noted that the effect of air absorption on the spectrum of signals above 10 kHz at the ears can become distinctly audible at distances as short as 15 m.

Aschoff notes the dull, echoing sound of a distant roll of thunder. Coleman presented clicks from various distances over loudspeakers. With a low-pass filter, he truncated the spectrum of the clicks at either 7.7 or 10.6 kHz. The signal at the input to the filter was the same in all cases. The subjects reported a significantly greater distance in connection with the 7.7 kHz band limit. However, the difference in the upper limit frequency changed not only the form of the spectrum but also the overall level of the signals at the ears; the "spectral" effect, therefore, was not studied in isolation.

There is no doubt that subjects associate a dull roll of thunder with the idea of a distant storm. Whether the auditory event of the roll of thunder also appears at a great distance has not yet been investigated. Furthermore, there is still little experimental evidence that the frequency dependence of air attenuation is evaluated in forming the distance of the auditory event. The auditory-horizon hypothesis of von Békésy (1949) deserves to be repeated here, namely that the extent of auditory space, in contrast to that of sound space, is limited.

Our next subject is distance hearing in cases in which the sound source distance is small—in the case of point sound sources, less than approximately 3 m. In this range the sound waves arriving at the head can no longer be regarded as approximately plane; the linear distortions introduced into the sound signal by the head and the external ears are no longer independent of the distance of the sound source. Measured results for one particular case are shown in Figure 2.34. These results were obtained using a particular loudspeaker (Isophon KSB 12/8) at distances of 25 cm and 3 m. The figure shows the differences in level and in group delay of the ear input signals. Up to approximately 600 Hz the measured level difference of approximately 20 dB agrees with the value to be expected according to the $1/r$ law. At higher frequencies there is an additional, frequency-dependent attenuation that rises and falls like that of a comb filter. A difference in group delay of approximately 8 ms is to be expected merely as a result of the difference in distance. The measured difference in group delay shows fluctuations of approximately 0.5 ms around this value.

The dependence of the transfer function of the external ear on distance formed the basis for von Békésy's (1939) attempt to explain distance hearing in the near field. We offer here a short sketch of the considerations that led to this attempt. At frequencies above approximately

1 kHz the impedance of the eardrum approximates the field impedance of air. From this fact von Békésy concluded that the ear is a "velocity-sensitive receiver" in this frequency range. In the distribution of velocity in the sound field of a spherical radiator of the zeroth order (see the sound-field equations 1.6 and 1.7 of a spherical radiator), there is a frequency-independent component that predominates in the near field ($r < \lambda/6$) and a component that depends on frequency as $1/\lambda \sim f$ that predominates in the far field ($r > \lambda/6$). If the sound source radiates a broadband signal, low-frequency spectral components thus show a relative increase in sound velocity in the near field as compared to the far field. Von Békésy assumed that this was evaluated in establishing the distance of the auditory event.

In objection to von Békésy's hypothesis, it may be noted that a receiver exposed to sound only on one side is always a pressure receiver, never a velocity receiver. In this connection the ear may be compared appropriately with a probe microphone. Besides, at frequencies above 1 kHz, the near field of a spherical radiator does not extend more than 5 cm from its surface. When the entrance to the ear canal is this close to the sound source, the ear will certainly disturb the sound field. There have as yet been no investigations of whether the disturbance is noticeable in a way indicative of the effect von Békésy hypothesized, as a relative increase in the level of low-frequency spectral components. Laws (1971), however, includes information about the simulation of the near field of a spherical radiator in the far field of two loudspeakers and its effect on the distance of the auditory event.

Von Békésy supported his assumption with the observation that the tone color of the auditory event becomes darker as a sound source radiating a broadband signal is brought closer to the subject. This phenomenon, which anyone can confirm, has also been described by such authors as Bloch (1893), von Hornbostel (1923), Aschoff (1963), and Haustein (1969). But this effect does not require a relative increase in the level of low-frequency components as the sound source is brought closer. As shown by the curves of equal loudness in figure 2.54, an increase in the level of the ear input signals brings about a change in the tone color of the auditory event without any corresponding change in the shape of the spectrum. The increase in level is proportional to relative changes in the distance of the sound source, so that the increase in level (relative to absolute changes in distance) becomes greater at

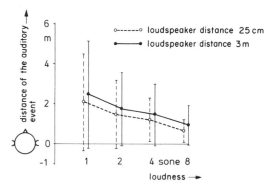

Figure 2.59
Distance of the auditory event as a function of loudness for white noise at two loud-speaker distances. Signal not presented in advance. (After Laws 1972; average values and standard deviations for 27 subjects, darkened anechoic chamber, head immobilized.)

smaller distances. Consequently the change in level also becomes more effective in causing change in the tone color.

Yet another question may be posed. At small distances the transfer function of the external ears does depend markedly on distance; but in forming the distance of the auditory event, does the auditory system make any use of the changes in the ear input signals that result from this dependence? The work of Laws (1972) suggests some answers. Figure 2.59 shows the distance of the auditory event as a function of loudness for two loudspeaker distances. (Loudness was determined through auditory experiments.) It can be seen that, with the same loudness, the auditory event connected with the loudspeaker at 25 cm lies, on average, nearer than that connected with the loudspeaker at 3 m. However, the differences in the distances of the auditory events are considerably smaller than the differences in loudspeaker distance. A doubling of perceived loudness corresponds to an increase in signal level at the ears of approximately 10 dB. It follows that the changes in the shape of the spectra of the ear input signals caused by bringing the loudspeaker closer are equivalent to a level increase of less than 10 dB in their effect on the distance of the auditory event. With the loudspeaker coming as close as 25 cm, the change in the shape of the spectrum does not have a very important effect on the distance of the auditory event. These investigations used the same loudspeaker as was used to generate the results shown in figure 2.34.

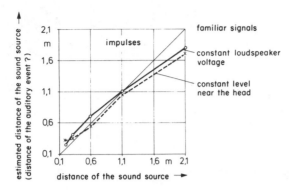

Figure 2.60
The average distance of the sound source as estimated by 20 subjects as a function of
the actual distance for impulses under various experimental conditions (Haustein
1969; darkened anechoic chamber, head immobilized).

Laws (1972) asked subjects to identify the distance of the auditory
event. It would be interesting to compare his results with others in
which the distance of the sound source was evaluated. The results of
Haustein (1969) are available, but they make a poor comparison since
the signals had been presented to the subjects in advance (figure 2.60).
Besides, it was the sound level near the subjects' heads, rather than
loudness, that was kept constant. Nonetheless, Haustein's results show
that subjects can judge the position of the sound source near the head
very accurately even when the sound level is kept constant. However,
objections could be raised to any explanation as to which attributes of
the ear input signals are responsible.

Other authors who have dealt with the problem of distance hearing
with sound source distances under 3 m are von Kries (1890), Bloch
(1893), Shutt (1898), Ikenberry and Shutt (1898), Pierce (1901), Arps
and Klemm (1913), Klemm (1913), and Werner (1922). However,
none of these investigations were carried out in reflection-free surroundings. Furthermore, it is often not clear whether subjects judged
the distance of the auditory event or identified sound sources, and
points of reference for distance measurements are frequently not given.
Most involve two questions:

1. How precise is distance hearing when the distance to the sound
source is short?

2. Are other attributes of the ear input signals besides their level—such as the shape of their spectra—of importance?

In connection with the first question, which concerns localization blur, Pierce's results are of interest. In the distance range from 50 to 150 cm, Pierce measured localization blur $\Delta r_{min}/r$ as 0.13–0.15. He used a wide variety of sounds such as clicks, organ tones, and the ringing of an electric bell. His results agree very well with the average values obtained by Arps and Klemm with an abruptly switched 383 Hz signal. However, in this same range of distances, Werner obtained values of $\Delta r_{min}/r$ nearly twice as high using a sound-generating hammer device. Von Kries's observations, among others, tend to uphold the importance of changes in the shape of the spectrum of the ear input signals. He generated impulse sounds at distances of 35 and 75 cm, using a telephone receiver and varying the sound power level over a wide range. Despite random changes in level, the subjects could always identify the closer and more distant sound sources. The same was true in experiments using abrupt sounds generated by small wooden slats slapping against each other. Bloch's observations using sound-generating hammer devices agree as long as only the sound power and not the type of sound was changed. If the shape of the spectrum was changed, by switching between a metal and a wooden striking-board, confusions occurred in the range beyond 35 cm. Finally, it should be mentioned that Shutt measured greater localization blur with narrow-band signals than with broadband noise. With narrow-band signals there can be no change in the shape of the spectra.

The following conclusions can be drawn about distance hearing when the sound source is close. Clearly the auditory system evaluates distortions of the spectrum of the ear input signals in this distance range, besides evaluating the sound pressure level. At distances greater than approximately 25 cm, however, the influence of these distance-dependent spectral attributes is rather small. It has not yet been determined which specific spectral attributes are evaluated.

Our present discussion would not be complete without a detailed look at the special case of inside-the-head locatedness. It is not an uncommon experience for auditory events to occur intracranially. Examples include auditory events corresponding to one's own voice—for example, the event that occurs when a person hums with mouth closed

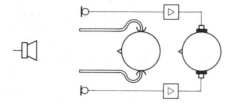

Figure 2.61
Apparatus for the presentation of sound to both a subject's ears. The auditory event generally appears inside the head. The two hearing tubes can also be connected to a common tube by a T-fitting, and the two headphones can be connected in phase to a single microphone. If the headphones are out of phase, inside-the-head locatedness still occurs, but as a rule the auditory event shifts somewhat from the front to the rear inside the head.

and ears plugged. This phenomenon deserves particular attention because it can also occur when the sound source is not inside the head. As Purkyne (1859) seems to have been the first to report (see also Thompson 1877, 1878, Urbantschitsch 1889), the auditory event generally appears inside the head when identical or highly similar sound signals are presented to both ears by means of listening tubes. Headphones may also be used instead of listening tubes (Thompson). Reversing the phase of the input signal to one of the headphones displaces the auditory event inside the head, generally toward the rear (figure 2.61).

After considering all previous work as well as a series of experiments he conducted himself, Schaefer (1890) established that "the closer the evaluated position of the sound sources, taken individually, then, when they act together, the closer to the head will be the acoustical image in the median plane. This image will even appear inside the head when each sound source, considered alone, is heard as being directly before the ear on its side."

More recently inside-the-head locatedness (IHL) has generated renewed interest, especially in the context of binaural (or head-related) stereophonic sound reproduction techniques, in which sound is picked up using a dummy head and reproduced over headphones. In these techniques IHL often occurs as a disturbing error in reproduction. A number of speculations about the cause of this error in headphone presentation of sound were undertaken without review of the older literature. Kietz (1953) attributes IHL to natural resonances of the microphones and headphones; Franssen (1960) to "overmodulation" of the nervous system. Schirmer (1966) assembles a number of further suggestions: invariability of the ear input signals when the head is moved (see section 2.5.1); loading of the eardrum with an impedance different from that of a free sound field; mechanical pressure of the headphone units against the head; no sound presented to the rest of the body besides the ears. He rejects all of these suppositions and puts forward the hypothesis that IHL is due to differences in transfer characteristics between electroacoustic transmission channels. Sone et al. (1968) suggest an unnatural proportion of air-conducted to bone-conducted sound as a cause of IHL.

Reichardt and Haustein (1968) once again illuminated the basis of the IHL problem. First, with two experiments they disposed of Schirmer's hypothesis that differences in the transmission channels lead to auditory events inside the head. They used two listening tubes of equal length and then a communications system of unusually high quality with intra-aural, electrostatic headphones. Differences between the two channels of this system lay below thresholds of perceptibility. In both cases they observed IHL. They also noted cases in which no IHL occurs despite differences between the two ear input signals. (Such differences are normal in spatial hearing, so that this observation is in any case trivial.) For their own part, Reichardt and Haustein suggest that the elimination or alteration of the acoustical effect of the pinnae can lead to IHL; with signal presentation by means of either listening tubes or headphones, the linear distortions caused by the pinnae do not come into play. Furthermore, IHL can be produced when the sound source is a single loudspeaker in an anechoic chamber if the subject covers the pinnae in a particular way with the hands. Some of the authors' own results, however, do not support their hypothesis as well as they expected.

Reichardt and Haustein draw their most important conclusions from the observation that IHL occurs if two loudspeakers, one near each ear, radiate identical or similar signals. On the basis of this observation they are able to establish two prerequisites for IHL:

1. Both ear input signals must be similar (coherent) to such a degree that only one homogeneous auditory event occurs.
2. Each of the two sound sources must be close to the ear, or perceived as being close to the ear when played separately.

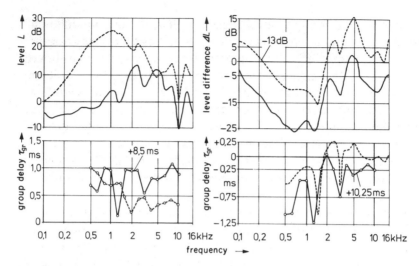

Figure 2.62
Left: Level difference and group delay difference curves of sound pressure at the entrance to the auditory canal, measured electroacoustically. Average of 12 subjects, relative to a constant 2 volts at the input to the electroacoustic transducer. Solid lines: Isophon loudspeaker KSB 12/8 at a distance of 3 m ($\varphi = 0°$, $\delta = 0°$). Dashed lines: Beyer headphones DT 48. Right: Level and delay differences between loudspeaker and headphone presentation. Solid lines: Measurements of 12 subjects. Dashed lines: Electrical simulating network. All measurements taken in an anechoic chamber. Baseline differences between the curves as shown are indicated numerically (after Laws 1972).

This practically repeats the state of affairs described by Schaefer (1890), who assumed condition 1 without stating it openly.

It is reasonable to state condition 2 more generally: Each ear input signal must be so constituted that the auditory event correlated to it appears in the immediate vicinity of the head. This generalization reduces the problem to a consideration of the subject's ear input signals, independent of the type and position of the sound sources. The auditory event's appearance inside the head has been shown, subsequent to Reichardt and Haustein's investigations, to depend entirely or at least principally on attributes of the ear input signals; experimental proof was furnished by Laws (1972).

Figure 2.62 illustrates Laws's experimental procedure. First, the level and group delay of the ear input signals were determined for a group of 12 subjects. Probe microphones were used, and two sets of mea-

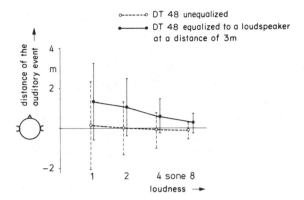

Figure 2.63
The distance of the auditory event as a function of loudness for white noise (signal not presented in advance), over equalized and unequalized headphones (averages and standard deviation for 27 subjects, anechoic chamber, darkened; after Laws 1972).

surements were taken, one with a loudspeaker at a distance of 3 m, the other with headphones. Input voltages to the loudspeaker and the headphones were held constant. In the next stage of the experiment, difference curves were plotted for the spectra of the ear input signals, comparing the two modes of sound presentation against each other as a function of frequency. Then an electrical network was constructed that imitated these difference curves as well as possible. When this network is interposed into the headphone circuit, ear input signals are generated that correspond quite accurately to the ones that would occur with a loudspeaker and with the ears uncovered. In other words, the loudspeaker can be simulated by means of headphones and the equalizing network.

Figure 2.63 shows the results of auditory experiments using this apparatus. The signal is white noise, presented previously to identify any possible relationship between loudness and distance. When the headphones are unequalized, the auditory event lies in the middle of the head regardless of changes in loudness. With the headphones equalized to simulate a loudspeaker, the auditory event lies in the median plane but outside the head, and it comes closer as its loudness is increased. A comparison with figure 2.59 shows, however, that the average distance of the auditory event in the simulation is not as great as with actual loudspeaker presentation. This discrepancy appears to be due to the fact that the equalizing network represents an average of the difference curves for 12 subjects, not those for each individual subject.

It follows from Laws's results that IHL does not occur when the ear input signals are as they would be in a free sound field; this result is independent of the sound source actually used. Attributes other than those of the ear input signals are not necessary in order to generate or to avoid IHL, though they may have a reinforcing effect (see section 2.5). This finding has been confirmed: IHL generally does not occur with some of the more recent head-related sound reproduction systems that use dummy heads with accurate imitations of the outer ears.* However, if headphones are placed on the dummy head, IHL occurs for the human listener!

IHL has been observed along with a number of other types of sound presentation. References to these, and in some cases thorough investigations of them, may be found in Schirmer (1966c), Krumbacher (1969), Toole (1970), and Plenge (1971b, 1972). Arrangements of sound sources with which IHL often or always occurs include several loud-speakers arrayed symmetrically on either side of the median plane and radiating identical signals, or two loudspeakers radiating identical signals out of phase with each other. In these cases, too, it is not wide of the mark to consider attributes of the ear input signals as responsible for IHL. However, measured results are not available for these cases. In connection with phenomena that occur with out-of-phase signals, see also section 3.1.1.

Given that attributes of the ear input signals have been established as being responsible for IHL, the question still remains whether this phenomenon also occurs when narrow-band signals are presented. It has been observed that this is generally the case when the level of the ear input signals is sufficiently high. If it is not, other positions of the auditory event may be observed (Blauert 1969a). Laws (1972) points out that the location of auditory events associated with Gaussian tone bursts is very indefinite with respect to distance, and that judgments of the distance depend largely on the specific concepts the subjects associate with the auditory event. Plenge (1971, 1972) used noise pulses with a 300 Hz bandwidth and 400 Hz center frequency and presented

---

*The present author was able to convince himself of this with the systems developed in Berlin (Kürer, Plenge, and Wilkens 1969, Wilkens 1971a,b, 1972) and in Göttingen (Damaske and Wagener 1969, Damaske 1971a, Mellert 1972).

them either over headphones or by means of loudspeakers. He found that the judgments "inside" or "outside" the head depended not on the type of presentation but on the individual subject. Just as with directional hearing in the median plane, secondary factors—particularly previous occurrences, including familiarity with the signal, expectations, habit, and specific associations—can help determine the distance of the auditory event when definite, determining attributes are not present in the ear input signals.

Plenge (1972) hypothesized that previous occurrences have a far greater importance to IHL than had previously been assumed. To substantiate this hypothesis he carried out experiments such as the following: A sound field corresponding to that of an orchestra in a concert hall was presented to 34 subjects who had experience at judging the distance of auditory events. After a length of time during which the subjects became accustomed to this sound field, an additional signal, such a speech or music with or without reverberation added, was presented over a loudspeaker at a distance of 2 m. The auditory event corresponding to this additional signal almost always appeared inside, or at least close to, the head. From this result Plenge concluded that one situation in which IHL always occurs is when the subject has no information or deficient information about the sound source and the spatial environment, for example, when the subject, so to speak, is surprised by the sound event. Furthermore, he suggests that information about the sound source and spatial environment that the subject uses at any given time is stored in short-term memory, which can be rapidly cleared and reloaded.

2.4   Evaluating Nonidentical Ear Input Signals

Section 2.3 discussed the special case in which the sound source is in the median plane and both ear input signals may, to a first approximation, be assumed to be roughly the same. The auditory event then also occurs in the median plane. We now proceed to the more general case in which the sound source is positioned somewhere in space to the right or left of the median plane. The ear input signals are then no longer identical; they differ in a way characteristic of the direction of the incident sound and the distance of the sound source. As noted in section 2.2, the quotient of the Fourier transforms of the two ear input signals is described by the interaural transfer function

$$A(f) = |A(f)| \, e^{-jb(f)} \, . \tag{2.30}$$

Measured results for $A(f)$ under several sets of conditions are shown in figures 2.36 and 2.38.

It may be assumed that the auditory system obtains the information needed to form auditory events in lateral directions primarily from dissimilarities between the two ear input signals. In this connection it is reasonable to suggest that the system does not evaluate every detail of the complicated interaural signal dissimilarities, but rather derives what information is needed from definite, easily recognizable attributes. Two classes of such attributes may be distinguished:

1. Dissimilarities between the two ear input signals related to the time when the signals occur, or when specific components of them occur— that is, dissimilarities that can be described by the frequency plot of interaural phase difference $b(f)$. These dissimilarities are commonly called interaural time differences.
2. Dissimilarities between the ear input signals related to their average sound pressure level—that is, dissimilarities between signals that might be described by the magnitude of the interaural transfer function $|A(f)|$ or the level difference $20 \log |A(f)|$. These are commonly called interaural level differences.

In order to study these attributes individually and independently of one another, it is necessary to present combinations of ear input signals other than those that occur in normal hearing. One example would be two signals with the same sound pressure level, shifted in time with respect to each other. Sound sources in a free sound field do not lend themselves to this type of presentation. Such investigations rely almost exclusively upon presentation of differing ear input signals to separately driven headphones (dichotic presentation).

We have already noted that the auditory event usually appears in or near the head with headphone presentation. This is also usually the case in investigations using dichotic presentation. For this reason the subject's task is almost always restricted to describing the lateral displacement of the auditory event, specifically as it is projected onto a straight line connecting the entrances to both ear canals (the axis of

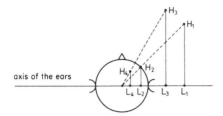

Figure 2.64
The lateral displacement of an auditory event is a function of both its direction and its distance.

the ears). The functional relationship between lateral displacement of the auditory event measured in this way and attributes of the ear input signals is called "lateralization," in contrast to localization as described in section 2.1. As the lateral displacement is only one dimension within the three-dimensional auditory space, there is no generally valid correlation of localization and lateralization such that every point along the axis of the ears corresponds to a specific azimuth of the auditory event (Jeffress and Taylor 1961). Figure 2.64 shows that the lateral displacement of an auditory event is proportional to its distance if its direction is constant.

Despite these restrictions, experiments with lateralization obviously allow conclusions to be drawn about the evaluation of interaural signal differences by the auditory system. On the basis of such experiments, it is possible to suggest various hypotheses about the processes that occur as auditory events are formed in a laterally displaced position. There is some indication that some of these hypotheses may be generalized to spatial hearing in free sound fields. It is for this reason that we examine the details of dichotic investigations at this point.

Techniques for the measurement of the lateral displacement of auditory events correspond in great measure to the techniques already discussed for the measurement of the position of auditory events. A lateral displacement might, for example, be measured in terms of a predefined rating scale, or by comparison with the lateral displacement of a fixed or variable standard auditory event (acoustical pointer). Methods of measuring lateralization blur are similar to those for measuring localization blur, involving a determination of the degree of change in the attribute of the ear input signal that leads to a just-noticeable change in lateral displacement.

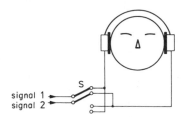

Figure 2.65
Null method of Kikuchi (1957). The center position is reached when the auditory event does not shift laterally after switch S is reversed.

One technique that deserves special note is the null method of Kikuchi (1957). This is often useful when the center position—zero lateral displacement—is to be determined. In this technique the two headphone input signals are repeatedly exchanged with one another: first, signal I to headphone I and signal II to headphone II, then signal I to headphone II and signal II to headphone I, and so forth (figure 2.65). If the position of the auditory event does not change when the signals are switched, then the center position has been reached. The null method, however, demands careful compensation for any asymmetries of the electro-acoustical transmission system or of the two ears of the experimental subject.

2.4.1 Interaural time differences

The following discussion applies to the special case in which the interaural transfer function is of magnitude 1 at all frequencies. In this case the signal at both ears has the same sound pressure level.

All signal differences possible under these conditions can be described by the phase coefficient $b(f)$ as a function of frequency. As noted in section 2.2.3, the phase delay $\tau_{ph}(f) = b(f)/2\pi f$ and the group delay $\tau_{gr}(f) = db(f)/d2\pi f$ may both be substituted for the phase coefficient without loss of information, according to the relationships

$$b(f) = \tau_{ph}(f) \cdot 2\pi f \tag{2.31}$$

and

$$b(f) = \int_{f_0}^{f} \tau_{gr}(\nu) \, 2\pi \, d\nu + b(f_0). \tag{2.32}$$

When equation 2.32 is used, one must also supply the interaural phase difference at some arbitrary frequency f_0.

If an interaural signal difference can be described in terms of an interaural delay or delays, then this difference clearly consists of the temporal displacement of the entire signal, or of parts of it, at one ear relative to the other. This means that there are arrival-time differences between the two ear input signals. The somewhat imprecise term "interaural time differences" is commonly used.

The opinion of the overwhelming majority of authors on this subject is that interaural time differences are the most important attributes of the ear input signals relating to the formation of lateral displacements of auditory events. The first hypotheses on the subject were stated several decades ago. Early exponents of this "time-difference theory of directional hearing" include Rayleigh (1907), Mallock (1908), and Klemm (1914, 1918). Classic studies were done by von Hornbostel and Wertheimer (1920) and von Békésy (1930a).

The plot of the interaural phase coefficient $b(\delta, \varphi, r, f)$ measured as a function of frequency in a free sound field is quite complicated. In lateralization experiments that will be described here, only simplified plots will be used. These are chosen for the ease with which they allow conclusions to be drawn by means of systems theory. Experiments using simplified plots, however, lead to simplified models of the processes under examination. One must use caution in generalizing the results of such experiments to "natural" spatial hearing.

The simplest case of an interaural time difference is for both ear input signals to be identical as a function of time, except that one is shifted in time with respect to the other (figure 2.66a). All components of the later signal must have the same delay compared with the earlier signal. It is thus required of the interaural transfer function that

$$\tau_{ph}(f) = \text{const} \quad \text{and therefore} \quad b(f) = 2\pi f \cdot \text{const.} \tag{2.33}$$

For a signal to be shifted in time without becoming distorted, the phase coefficients must therefore be proportional to frequency.

Figure 2.67 shows the experimental arrangement commonly used for generating two time-shifted, undistorted ear input signals. The signal passes through a delay unit on its way to each of the two ears. The phase delay of each unit is constant with frequency but can be adjusted independently of the phase delay of the other. Acoustical means such

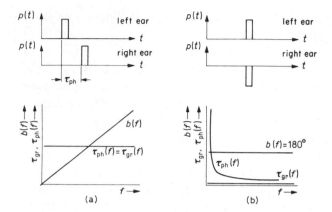

Figure 2.66
Examples of interaural time differences. a: A pure time shift (constant phase delay).
b: Inversion (constant phase difference of 180°).

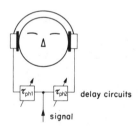

Figure 2.67
An arrangement by means of which a constant interaural phase delay can be
generated.

as tubes, hoses, or free air paths of various lengths may be used to generate delays. Electrical means such as electrical delay lines, magnetic tape devices, shift registers, or core memories can also be used.

If the delay of both units is set to the same value, then the auditory event appears in the median plane of the subject. If the delay is changed at one ear, then the auditory event migrates toward the ear at which the signal appears first. Lateral displacements of the auditory event can thus be achieved in practice by means of interaural time differences.

It is possible to confirm this basic phenomenon of spatial hearing by means of a well-known experiment. The two ends of a rubber hose of suitable diameter and about 1 m in length are inserted into the two ear canals of a subject. If a hard object is then tapped against the hose exactly at its midpoint, the auditory event will appear at the center of the head. If the hose is tapped at a different point, the auditory event migrates toward the ear whose distance along the hose is smaller. The lateral displacement increases approximately linearly until the path difference from the place where the hose is tapped reaches approximately 21 cm. This corresponds to a phase delay of approximately 630 μs. The auditory event will then have reached approximately the position of the entrance to the ear canal at one side. With further increases in the interaural phase delay, until τ_{ph} reaches approximately 0.8–1 ms, the lateral displacement increases at a significantly lower rate; beyond this point it does not increase at all.

In the German literature the 21 cm path difference is often referred to as the "Hornbostel-Wertheimer constant." This is now known, however, not to be a true constant but to depend on the sound pressure level and the type of signal. Its physical significance is that 21 cm corresponds approximately to the maximum path difference for sound signals arriving at the two ears from the side in a free sound field. As shown in section 2.2.3, though, it is not possible to draw the conclusion that the interaural phase delay is 630 μs with 90° sound incidence, regardless of frequency. The actual situation is more complicated.

Recently the lateral displacement of the auditory event has been measured carefully for various types of signals as a function of frequency-invariant interaural phase delay (Teas 1962, Sayers 1964, Sayers and Toole 1964, Toole and Sayers 1965a,b).

A typical curve of lateralization for brief impulse sounds is shown in figure 2.68. This curve agrees with those for other signals with impulse

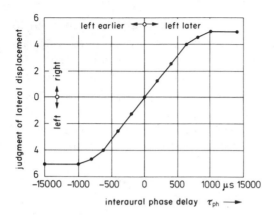

Figure 2.68
Lateral displacement of the auditory event as a function of a pure interaural time shift. Valid for impulses and signals with impulse content. Five subjects, loudness level 30–80 phon (from measured values of Toole and Sayers 1965a).

content, such as noise or speech. The ordinate gives the lateral displacement as rated by the subjects in terms of a linear scale. Here 0 corresponds to the center of the head, and 5 to the average maximum displacement, with the auditory event approximately at the entrance of the ear canal. The linear relationship up to a τ_{ph} of approximately 630 μs is evident.

Clearly the hearing apparatus is able very accurately to determine the arrival time of impulsive components of the ear input signals. In considering how this discrimination might occur, the simplest assumption is that the auditory system is "triggered" when the ear input signal exceeds a particular threshold. Arrival times, according to this assumption, are determimed as this threshold is exceeded on the leading slopes of signals.

This very simple threshold model will be sufficient for our purposes for now, as long as we also note that the inner ear functions as a harmonic analyzer, crudely dissecting the ear input signal into band-passed components. The time of a signal will then be determined not by the time at which the overall signal exceeds the threshold, but by the time at which its spectral components exceed the threshold. A component's relevance depends on its center frequency and power.

It must also be noted that signal slopes corresponding to a reduction in pressure (a rarefaction) at the eardrum are preferably or exclusively

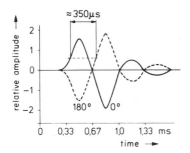

Figure 2.69
The time function of the signal in the inner ear at the point where the strongest excitation occurs (from experiments by Flanagan et al. 1964). The first signal slopes are shifted by approximately 350 μs when the interaural phase shift is 180°.

used in evaluation. This fact was originally established through a study of the physiological workings of the inner ear. It has been supported by auditory experiments, for example, those of Flanagan, David, and Watson (1962, 1964) and Toole and Sayers (1965b). These authors presented out-of-phase impulses to the two ears of their subjects (figure 2.66b). It was shown that the auditory event is localized less precisely under these conditions that when in-phase impulses are presented. A dominant part of the auditory event is recognizable, though it is displaced laterally. If the inner ear responded equally to positive and negative signal slopes, then the position and extent of the auditory event would not be affected by the signals' being presented in or out of phase.

In the experiments of Flanagan, David, and Watson the observed lateral displacement with out-of-phase impulses was the same as with in-phase impulses having an interaural phase delay of approximately 350 μs. A precise look at the time function of the signal in the inner ear revealed that the strongest spectral component with the particular impulses used had a period of approximately 700 μs (figure 2.69). For this component the interaural phase shift of 180° corresponded precisely to 350 μs. The auditory event was displaced toward the side where the first signal slope appeared that corresponded to a rarefaction at the eardrum.

The less definite localization of the auditory event when the ear input signals are 180° out of phase can be explained in terms of the interaural phase delay of a system with a constant phase coefficient (figure 2.66b). Looking at this relationship as a function of frequency, the spectral

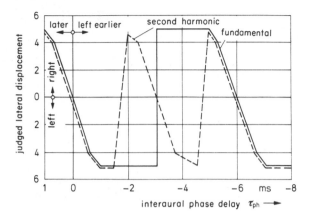

Figure 2.70
Lateralization curves for the fundamental and second harmonic of an impulse train (period 6 ms, frequency 168 Hz; results of Toole and Sayers 1965a).

components of one signal are shifted by different amounts compared with those of the other signal. The auditory event clearly separates into components at different frequencies, displaced laterally by different amounts and creating the appearance that the auditory event has spread out. This easily recognizable apparent spreading of the auditory event has a practical use; it provides an easy way to check the phasing of the loudspeakers in a stereophonic sound reproduction system. (Other effects that occur with out-of-phase loudspeaker signals are discussed in section 3.1.1.)

It is, then, accepted that an auditory event can separate into a series of components adjacent to one another when the interaural phase delay varies with frequency. A prerequisite of this phenomenon is that the auditory system be able to evaluate spectral components of the ear input signals individually with respect to their interaural time differences. That this is true has been convincingly demonstrated by Sayers (1964) and Toole and Sayers (1965a), who presented an impulse train with a fundamental period of 6 ms to both ears of their subjects. The interaural phase delay was independent of frequency and was adjustable. The subjects were able to distinguish a series of simultaneous auditory events, each of which could be correlated with one harmonic component of the ear input signals. The lateral displacement of each of these events could be traced individually as τ_{ph} was varied. Typical lateralization

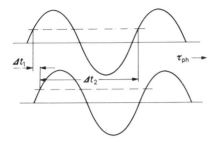

Figure 2.71
The interaural time difference between periodic processes shifted in time with respect
to each other is ambiguous.

curves for the fundamental and the second harmonic are shown in
figure 2.70. Both curves are periodic; the period of the curve corresponding to the second harmonic is half that of the curve corresponding
to the fundamental. How the periodicity of the curves comes about
will be made clear in the following discussion of the lateralization of
sinusoidal signals.

The lateralization of sinusoidal signals (i.e., signals without audible
onset and decay transients) has been dealt with exhaustively in the
literature, though false explanations have often been given, even recently
(see Rayleigh 1907, Lehnhardt 1960, Elphern and Naunton 1964). We
restrict ourselves here to the explanation that is generally accepted
today; this explanation has, to be sure, been known for many years
(see Bowlker 1908, Halverson 1922, von Hornbostel 1923, 1926, among
others).

A simple analytical model has already been put forth according to
which a reaction is elicited in the inner ear whenever the signal exceeds
a certain threshold. According to this model, the trigger point is reached
once during the period of any sinusoidal signal. But the interaural time
differences between the trigger times at the two ears can be defined in
two ways, depending on whether the left or right ear is regarded as the
first one triggered (figure 2.71).

An immediate inference is that the auditory system might register
this ambiguity and might possibly establish two auditory events. This
is, in fact, the case, though with the additional rule that the auditory
event closest to the median plane, which corresponds to the shorter
interaural time difference, dominates with respect to the other one.

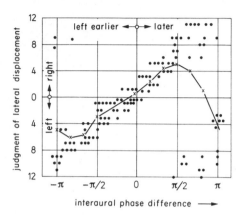

Figure 2.72
Lateralization curve for a 600 Hz sinusoidal signal (after Sayers 1964). The points are
individual judgments; the solid line represents the average value.

Only in the case of an interaural phase shift of approximately half a
period, $T/2 \approx 180°$, do even inexperienced subjects clearly perceive
both auditory events, one on each side. Occasionally, in this case, the
lateral displacement is judged as zero, or the lateral position of only
one of the auditory events is described.

A lateralization curve for a 600 Hz tone clearly shows the details of
this phenomenon (figure 2.72). When the interaural phase shift is approximately 180°, two auditory events appear. An averaged curve of
lateral displacement shows the same periodicity as in figure 2.68. Information about cases in which two auditory events appear is lost
through this type of averaging. This is also the reason why measurements
continue to be published according to which the maximum lateral displacement occurs in connection with a 90° interaural phase shift.

It has already been stated that the full lateral displacement of the
auditory event is attained in connection with an interaural phase delay
of approximately 630 μs and that at any given time the auditory event
corresponding to the shorter time difference is dominant. It follows
that full lateral displacement is only attained with tones whose half-
period is no less than approximately 630 μs, that is, tones whose frequency is no higher than approximately 800 Hz. As the frequency is
raised above 800 Hz, the attainable maximum displacement becomes
smaller and smaller. Also, maximum displacement no longer occurs
when $\tau_{ph} = 630$ μs but, rather, when $\tau_{ph} = T/2$.

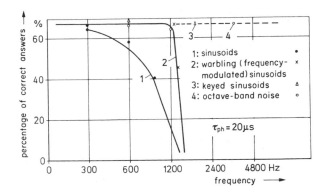

Figure 2.73
Ability to notice an interaural phase delay, shown as a function of frequency for various types of signals (after Scherer 1959; 1 subject).

There is probably an additional effect that makes the fall in maximum lateral displacement even more precipitous. The neurons between the inner ear and the central nervous system are incapable of reacting a second time for approximately 1–2 ms after being triggered (the refractory period). When the signals exceed the threshold at intervals shorter than the refractory period, the number of nerve impulses discharged each time decreases abruptly. According to Stevens and Davis (1938), this phenomenon occurs in the region of 800 Hz and again around 1.6 kHz.

There is widespread agreement in the literature that the lateral displacement of the auditory event attainable for pure tones through interaural phase delay decreases rapidly above 800 Hz. Above 1.5–1.6 kHz, there is as a rule no noticeable lateral displacement. This is proven most simply through use of the phenomenon called "binaural beats," which may have been discovered by Thompson (1877) and which has been treated more recently by Peterson (1916), Stewart (1917), von Hornbostel (1923, 1926), and Perrot and Nelson (1969, 1970). If two tones of only slightly different frequency are presented to the two ears, an auditory event occurs that oscillates inside the head at the rate of the difference between the two frequencies. This phenomenon does not occur for frequencies above approximately 1.6 kHz.

Figure 2.73 shows the results of a measurement by Scherer (1959). His subjects' task was to report the insertion of a 20 μs delay between

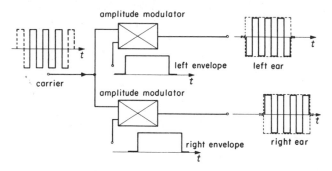

Figure 2.74
Generation of two signals with shifted envelopes but with the carriers in phase.

the two ear input signals. For sinusoidal signals the percentage of correct answers decreases steadily with frequency, just as expected. It falls below 50 percent around 800 Hz. Above 1.6 kHz there are no more correct answers. For frequency-modulated sinusoidal signals with 150 Hz peak-to-peak frequency variation and an 8 Hz sinusoidal modulating signal, results are similar, though the curve does not begin to fall off until approximately 1.2 kHz. Auditory events connected with noise of one-octave bandwidth, or with keyed sine waves, behave in a completely different way. Lateral displacements are just as easily recognizable above 1.6 kHz as below. The auditory system is clearly able to detect interaural delays that are not present in pure sinusoids or frequency-modulated sinusoids. Interaural delays of the envelopes of the signals seem to be the criterion involved.

We now turn to a more detailed discussion of the meaning of interaural temporal displacements of the envelope for spatial hearing. Investigations can, for example, be undertaken using signals whose carriers are in phase but whose envelopes are shifted in time at the two ears. Such signals may be generated by the use of two amplitude modulators (figure 2.74).*

Leakey, Sayers, and Cherry (1958), Boerger (1965a), and Sakai and Inoue (1968) carried out experiments using a signal-generating apparatus of this type. They used sinusoids of various frequencies as carriers and

---

*Amplitude modulators are time-variant systems. Therefore the requirement stated at the beginning of this section that interaural time differences be described only in terms of a phase coefficient $b(f)$ is applicable only in a restricted sense to this case.

sinusoids, narrow-band noise below 1.6 kHz, and Gaussian pulses as envelopes. In all cases in which the carrier was over 1.6 kHz, there was clearly a lateral displacement of the auditory event as a function of the delay between the envelopes. In fact, the lateralization curves were more or less the same as they would have been if the entire signal had been delayed. This experiment provides conclusive proof that, when the signals have no spectral components below 1.6 kHz, the auditory system ignores the interaural time delay of the signals' "fine structure" and evaluates only the envelopes.

Beyond this result, it has been shown that a spatially defined auditory event is produced even when very different signals are presented to both ears, as long as the envelopes of both are similar. Schubert and Wernick (1969), for example, demonstrated that this is the case with two uncorrelated noise signals modulated by a trapezoidal wave. However, if the signals are two sinusoids of different frequencies but modulated by the same envelope, a single auditory event is established only when the frequency difference lies below a certain threshold value (Ebata and Sone 1968, Perrott, Briggs, and Perrott 1970). If the two frequencies are too different, the auditory event dissociates into two parts, one at each ear.

It can therefore be concluded that the envelope of the entire signal is not evaluated. First, the spectrum of the signal is dissected to a degree determined by the finite spectral resolution of the inner ear; then the envelopes of the separate spectral components are evaluated individually. A unified auditory event appears only if the shifts of the envelopes in the different frequency ranges show sufficient similarity to one another.

In a free sound field both the carriers and the envelopes of the two ear input signals are shifted in time with respect to one another, generally by different amounts. For a narrow group of frequencies such as the amplitude-modulated signal shown in figure 2.75, the carrier shift is determined by the phase delay, and the envelope shift is determined by the group delay around the frequency of the carrier.* In general, interaural phase and group delays are not equal.

With ear input signals that have components only above 1.6 kHz, this difference does not lead to conflicts, as lateralization is based on

*See Fettweis (1977) for a detailed analysis of the effect of group delay on bandpass signals.

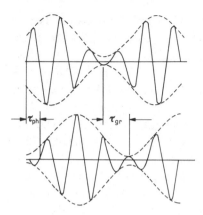

Figure 2.75
Unequal interaural time differences of a carrier and its envelope.

the envelope. The situation is different when the carrier includes only frequencies below 1.6 kHz. In this case some types of envelopes influence lateralization while others do not. Sakai and Inoue (1968) report, for example, that a 500 Hz sinusoid, amplitude-modulated at 200 Hz, leads to three auditory events, correlated with the three spectral components at 300, 500, and 700 Hz; the envelope has no influence. But if the envelope is more pronounced (with steep slopes, step functions, etc.), then envelope time shifts have an influence even with carrier frequencies below 1.6 kHz (Boerger 1965a, Schubert and Wernick 1969). Deather-age (1961) was able to show that the auditory event can dissociate into two parts if the ear input signals include components both above and below 1.6 kHz and the interaural time shifts of the carrier and envelope are different. If the envelope includes any significant components below 3 or 4 Hz, then the auditory event moves in space (Blauert 1970a). Its position at any moment depends on the momentary value of the in-teraural sound pressure level difference.

Measurement of the sensitivity of the auditory system to interaural time differences is useful in comparing the importance of interaural time differences in lateralization with that of other signal parameters. To this end, lateralization blur is measured. This is defined as the smallest change in the interaural phase delay, group delay, or phase coefficient that leads to a lateral displacement of the auditory event. In table 2.3 are assembled several measured results for lateralization

Table 2.3
Survey of measurements of lateralization blur in the median plane for pure interaural time shifts (interaural phase delay independent of frequency); see references for details of the measuring techniques used.

Reference	Signal	Loudness level (phon), approximate	Lateralization blur (μs), approximate
Bowlker (1908)	Sinusoids	Not given	7–14
Klemm (1920)	Clicks	Not given	2–10
Hecht (1922a)	Not given	Not given	c. 30
Klump (1953)	Sinusoids and noise	Optimal	6–12
Klumpp and Eady (1956)	Click		28
	Series of clicks		11
	Noise:		
	broadband		10
	150–1,700 Hz	60–80	9
	425–600 Hz		14
	410–440 Hz		19
	2,400–3,400 Hz		44
	3,056–3,344 Hz		62
Hall (1964)	Clicks	80	20–50
Hershkowitz and Durlach (1969a)	500 Hz sinusoid	50	11.7

blur for auditory events in the median plane, $\Delta(\tau_{ph} = 0)_{min}$, that is, when frequency-independent phase delays (distortion-free time shifts) are applied to one of the ear input signals.

Figure 2.76 illustrates the lateralization blur of sinusoidal signals as a function of frequency, as determined by Klumpp and Eady (1956) and Zwislocki and Feldman (1956). The figure also shows the very significant results of Boerger (1965a) for Gaussian tone bursts whose frequency spectrum spans one critical band. (For a definition of the term "critical band" (Frequenzgruppe) see Zwicker and Feldtkeller 1967.) Either the carrier, the envelope, or the entire signal was shifted in time between the two ears. Carrier shift can no longer be evaluated above about 1.6 kHz, just as in the case of sinusoidal signals. Evaluation of the envelope can already be detected at a carrier frequency of 500 Hz, and it becomes more accurate as the frequency is increased. When the entire signal is shifted as a unit, lateralization is quite sharp throughout the entire frequency range. Kirikae et al. (1970), using a half-octave noise signal, measured an almost linear increase in lateralization blur from approximately 35 μs at 400 Hz to 65 μs at 4 kHz (3 subjects,

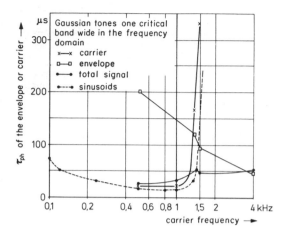

Figure 2.76
Lateralization blur $\Delta(\tau = 0)_{min}$, that is, for interaural differences about 0, for sinusoidal signals and for Gaussian tone bursts whose spectrum is one critical band wide (Zwislocki and Feldman 1956, Klumpp and Eady 1956, Boerger 1965a; 5–6 subjects, approximately 50–60 phon).

approximately 50 phon). With high-pass filtered clicks, Yost, Wightman, and Green (1971) observed that $\Delta(\tau_{ph} = 0)_{min}$ increased when the low-frequency limit of the filter was raised above 800 Hz, that is, when the signals no longer included any low-frequency components (30 subjects, approximately 70 phon).

Elfner and Tomsic (1968) showed that the precision with which the envelope is evaluated in lateralization depends largely on whether it has steep slopes. They presented an in-phase sinusoid to both ears of the subject, and switched it "smoothly," with onset time durations from 10 to 250 ms. The instant of switching for one ear was variable compared to that for the other. Lateralization blur depended on the onset time interval. It varied between 6 and 38 ms for sinusoids between 600 Hz and 6 kHz. With one of the subjects the envelope could not be evaluated at all when the onset time was 250 ms.

If the auditory event is displaced laterally from the median plane by means of interaural time differences, the spatial distinguishability of the auditory event at first glance does not appear to become significantly less definite as long as the interaural time difference is less than 630 μs. Experiments to test this assumption have been carried out by Hershkowitz and Durlach (1969a), using a 500 Hz sinusoid, and by Campbell

(1959), using low-pass filtered noise pulses (f_g = 1.3 kHz). Yet in both cases $\Delta \tau_{ph,min}$ was observed approximately to double when the interaural phase delay was increased from zero to 600 μs.

In connection with interaural time differences, it should be noted that lateralization blur decreases as either the level or the duration of the signal is increased. The first of these properties is illustrated in figure 2.77 as it occurs with a 500 Hz sinusoid. It has also been shown to occur with impulses (Hall 1964). The second property is illustrated in figure 2.78. The work of Klumpp and Eady (1956) also establishes the validity of this relationship (see table 2.3). Attempts to explain these two properties proceed from the observation that increases in both level and signal duration lead to an increase in the number of elicited nerve impulses.

2.4.2 Interaural level differences

This section deals with the effects of attributes of interaural signal difference that can be described in terms of the amplitude of the interaural transfer function $|A(f)|$ or by the sound pressure level difference $20 \log |A(f)|$. We start with a simple experiment in which the same signal is presented to both ears of a subject, with a variable attenuator in the cable leading to each headphone by means of which the amplitude of each signal can be changed individually. We can thus generate two ear input signals that are identical except for their sound pressure level (figure 2.79). We find that if both attentuators are adjusted to produce the same degree of attenuation, the auditory event appears in the subject's median plane; but if the amplitude of one of the ear input signals is varied with respect to that of the other, the auditory event migrates toward the ear to which the stronger signal is being presented. In this way interaural level differences can lead to lateral displacements of the auditory event.

This fact is the basis for the "intensity-difference theory" of directional hearing, which is the oldest theory of directional hearing. Its early exponents (Rayleigh 1877, Steinhauser 1877, 1879, Thompson 1882, Matsumoto 1897, Pierce 1901, Stefanini 1922, Kreidl and Gatscher 1923) assumed that a difference in interaural sound pressure level was the only signal parameter establishing the lateral direction of auditory events, or if not the only parameter, then the most important one by

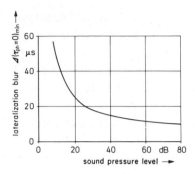

Figure 2.77
Dependence of lateralization blur $\Delta(\tau_{ph} = 0)_{min}$ on the sound pressure level of the test signal for a 500 Hz sinusoid (data from Zwislocki and Feldman 1956, Hershkowitz and Durlach 1969a; 8 subjects).

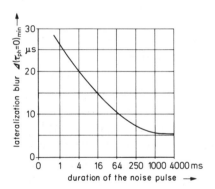

Figure 2.78
Dependence of the lateralization blur $\Delta(\tau_{ph} = 0)_{min}$ on the duration of the test signal. Broadband noise pulses, $f_{max} = 5$ kHz, approximately 65 phon, 5 subjects (after Tobias and Zerlin 1959; see also Houtgast and Plomp 1968).

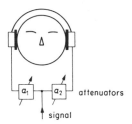

Figure 2.79
Arrangement for generating an interaural sound pressure level difference.

far. This is now known not to be the case, though there is no doubt that interaural level differences do play a role in spatial hearing.

Level differences between the two ear inputs in a free sound field, $\Delta L(\delta, \varphi, r, f)$, depend strongly on frequency. There will be no attempt to imitate ΔL as a function of frequency in the lateralization experiments that will be described here. These experiments have been limited almost exclusively to investigations of the lateral displacement of the auditory event, while the level difference is the same for all frequencies under consideration. This situation can be produced by the apparatus sketched in figure 2.79. This restriction must be considered in generalizing experimental results. Even when we use ear input signals whose level differences are independent of frequency, the excitation of the inner ears is not always identical except for an amplitude difference. This becomes clear if we note that, with weak signals, components of one ear input signal might lie below the threshold of audibility while the same components of the other ear input signal are still perceptible (see figure 2.54).

Kietz (1953) reported that, for signals of any frequency, the auditory event moves "completely to one side" when the interaural level difference is 15–20 dB. When inside-the-head locatedness occurs, the auditory event appears in the approximate position of the ear receiving the stronger stimulus. Pinheiro and Tobin (1969) give approximately 10 dB as a corresponding value for white noise pulses or low-pass filtered noise pulses ($f_g = 1.2$ kHz). Both results must be taken with some caution; almost all authors who have dealt carefully with the subject of lateralization in connection with interaural level differences report that the width of the auditory event—and thus the lateralization

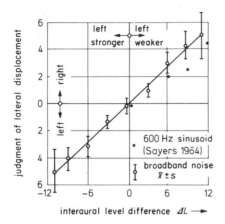

Figure 2.80
Lateral displacement of the auditory event as a function of interaural level difference. Broadband noise and 600 Hz sinusoidal signals, 4 subjects, 30–50 phon.

blur—increases for level differences of more than 8–10 dB. Consequently the limit value "entirely to the side" is especially difficult to measure (von Békésy 1930a, Sayers 1964).

Until full lateral displacement is attained, the displacement depends more or less linearly on the interaural level difference. Figure 2.80 shows, as an example, a few measured results for noise pulses and for a 600 Hz sinusoid. Displacement was evaluated in terms of a linear scale on which 0 corresponds to the middle of the head and 5 to the average maximum displacement (the approximate position of the entrance to the auditory canal).

The lateralization of sinusoidal signals that have a constant interaural level difference depends on their frequency. Feddersen et al. (1957) measured this phenomenon by means of the pointer technique. Their subjects were instructed to make the signals coincide spatially with an acoustical pointer. The signals could be displaced laterally by changing the interaural level difference. The pointer consisted of a noise signal (100 Hz to 3 kHz) that could be displaced laterally by means of an adjustable interaural time difference. Results are shown in figure 2.81. The level difference necessary to bring about a given lateral displacement is smallest around 2 kHz, rising for lower and, to a lesser degree, for higher frequencies.

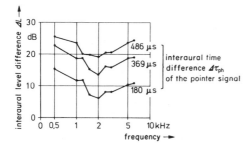

Figure 2.81
Interaural level difference such that the auditory event correlated with a sinusoidal
signal is displaced laterally by the same amount as an acoustic pointer (noise,
100–3,000 Hz), 6 subjects, approximately 60 phon (after Feddersen et al. 1957).

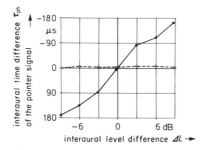

Figure 2.82
Lateral displacement of the two auditory events that occur in connection with a binaurally presented 500 Hz sinusoidal signal. Measured by means of an acoustical
pointer, approximately 50 phon, 1 subject (Whitworth and Jeffress 1961).

Experienced subjects report that not one but two auditory events may be observed in connection with signals that have components below 1.6 kHz. These components seem to unite into a single, broader auditory event only if listened to briefly or casually (Banister 1925, 1926). Whitworth and Jeffress (1961) investigated the lateralization of the two auditory events individually, using a 500 Hz sinusoidal signal. For measurement, they used an acoustical pointer of the same frequency as the test signal. This pointer could be displaced laterally by means of an interaural time difference. It was observed that one of the two auditory events remained in the middle of the head, regardless of the interaural level difference. The other one migrated to the side as the level difference increased (figure 2.82). The interaural difference, then, has an effect on the position of only one of the two auditory events; as long as the interaural time difference is zero, the other one remains centered at the middle of the head.

Multiple auditory events can also appear if the spectral components of the ear input signals have unequal interaural level differences. This has been experimentally proven by Toole and Sayers (1965a) for periodic signals.

In determining the importance of interaural level differences in connection with spatial hearing, the lateralization blur of this parameter is also of interest. The lateralization blur is defined as the smallest change in the interaural sound pressure level difference $\Delta(\Delta L)_{min}$ that leads to a lateral displacement of the auditory event. In table 2.4 are shown several authors' measured results for lateralization blur around an interaural level difference of 0 dB, that is, for auditory events in the median plane. Figure 2.83 gives corresponding results for sinusoidal signals and Gaussian tone bursts as a function of frequency. From a measurement by Scherer (1959) it can be concluded that the values for octave-band noise agree very well with those for sinusoids.

Lateralization blur for laterally displaced auditory events has been investigated by Gage (1935), Chocholle (1957), Rowland and Tobias (1967), Elfner and Perrott (1967), and Babkoff and Sutton (1969). As expected, there is a trend for the lateralization blur to increase as the auditory event becomes broader with increasing lateral displacement. This is especially so for low-frequency sinusoidal signals; the existence of two auditory events correlated with these signals underlies this fact.

Table 2.4
A survey of measurements of lateralization blur in the median plane for interaural
level differences; see references for details of the measuring technique used.

Reference	Signal	Loudness level (phon), approximate	Lateralization blur (dB), approximate
von Békésy (1930b)	Clicks	40	1.5
Upton (1936)	800 Hz sinusoid	40–60	1
Ford (1942)	200 Hz sinusoid	50	1.5
	2,000 Hz sinusoid	50	0.6
Hall (1964)	Clicks	80	1.5
Elfner and Perrot (1967)	1,000 Hz sinusoid	60	2
Rowland and Tobias (1967)	250 Hz sinusoid	50	1.15
	2,000 Hz sinusoid	50	0.72
	6,000 Hz sinusoid	50	0.92
Hershkowitz and Durlach (1969a)	500 Hz sinusoid	40–80	0.8
Babkoff and Sutton (1969)	Clicks	35	1.5

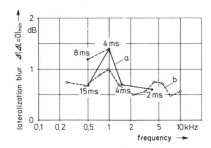

Figure 2.83
Lateralization blur $\Delta(\Delta L = 0)_{min}$, that is, with an interaural level difference about
0 dB. Curve a: Gaussian tone bursts (after Boerger 1965a; durations given, 4 subjects). Curve b: Sinusoidal signals (after Mills 1960; duration 1 s, smoothly switched,
approximately 50–60 phon, 5 subjects).

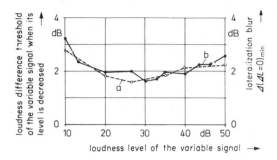

Figure 2.84
Loudness difference thresholds (curve a) and lateralization blur (curve b) are not significantly different if the level of only one ear input signal is varied and level measurement is with reference to the variable signal. Clicks, 2 subjects (after Babkoff and Sutton 1969).

The three last works cited examine a hypothesis made by von Békésy (1930b) that the difference in the levels of the ear input signals necessary to produce a just-noticeable lateral displacement of the auditory event is equal to the monaural loudness difference threshold. Elfner and Perrott's data, and even more so Babkoff and Sutton's (figure 2.84), tend strongly to confirm this hypothesis, but Rowland and Tobias's data do not. All three investigations may be faulted, however, for varying the level of only one of the ear input signals. It is possible that the subjects based their judgments on the variation in loudness that accompanied the displacement of the auditory event.

It seems definitely established that lateralization blur depends on signal levels (Rowland and Tobias 1967, Hershkowitz and Durlach 1969a). Between low and intermediate levels, lateralization blur decreases, then remains constant or increases slightly as the level continues to rise (Upton 1936, Hall 1964, Babkoff and Sutton 1969).

If the auditory system is stimulated for a relatively long period of time, its sensitivity decreases by a certain amount that depends on the type, level, and length of presentation of the signal. The decrease is due to adaptation and fatigue. "Adaptation" refers to the relatively rapid loss in sensitivity that begins after a few seconds and attains its maximum after approximately 3–5 minutes. Readaptation (i.e., a return to the original sensitivity) takes 1–2 minutes. "Fatigue" occurs with signals of higher intensity and longer duration, and the return to normal sensitivity requires a longer rest period. The transition between adaptation and fatigue cannot be easily defined psychoacoustically, although the two phenomena are clearly different from a physiological point of view.

Lateralization in connection with an interaural sound pressure difference is affected to some degree by both phenomena. Since the stimuli to the two ears are signals at different levels, the sensitivity of the more strongly stimulated ear decreases relatively more than that of the less strongly stimulated one. Consequently the lateral displacement of the auditory event decreases while the signal is being presented. The auditory event shifts toward the center (Urbantschitsch 1881, Thompson 1979, von Békésy 1930a).

One way this effect can be used is to measure adaptation (Wright 1960). First, one ear is stimulated with a test signal. After it has adapted itself, the same signal is presented to the other ear. As the second ear is adapting itself, the auditory event migrates toward the median plane. The time from the onset of stimulation of the second ear until the arrival of the auditory event at the median plane is measured.

It must be concluded from an investigation by Elfner and Perrott (1966) that lateralization effects unexplainable in terms of adaptation or fatigue occur when a level difference is presented for a span of time in the range of approximately two hours. In some cases the auditory event was observed to migrate toward the more strongly stimulated ear. The cause of this phenomenon is still unknown.

If the sensitivity of one ear is artificially increased, as may be accomplished by corrective surgery (Betzold 1890, Röser 1965), or by partly plugging the opposite ear (Bauer et al. 1966), subjects first report a systematic shift of all auditory events toward the more sensitive ear. After a period of hours, days, or even weeks this shift can recede, and the subjects react once more in a way normal for persons with symmetrical hearing. Clearly a relearning process is at work, since the time for adjustment can be shortened by appropriate training (Bauer et al. 1966).

It is clear from the descriptions of these phenomena that lateralization in connection with interaural sound pressure differences is a time-variant process. Short-term variations can occur in connection with adaptation and fatigue, and long-term variations occur in connection with learning processes.

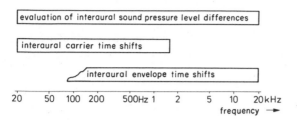

Figure 2.85
Frequency ranges in which different attributes of interaural signal differences are evaluated.

We might expect that the evaluation of interaural sound pressure level differences would be impaired by differences in sensitivity between the two ears. In fact, no significant connection has yet been shown between individual differences in sensitivity (as long as these remain within certain limits) and individual variations in evaluation of level differences (Sandel et al. 1955, Bergmann 1957, Søhoel et al. 1964; but cf. Ferree and Collins 1911). The lack of such a relationship is apparently due to the ability of the mechanism that evaluates level differences to adjust itself to the individual sensitivity curves of the ears through learning processes.

2.4.3 The interaction of interaural time and level differences

Differences between the ear input signals are necessary in order for auditory events to appear laterally, away from the median plane. Specific types of differences arise as a consequence of diffraction, shadowing, and resonances introduced by the head and external ears. The effective components of these very different types of signal differences can be investigated in lateralization experiments using headphones. The last two sections described such experiments, and through these we can isolate two classes of attributes of interaural signal differences that can lead to lateral displacements of auditory events: interaural time differences and interaural level differences.

There are two important subclasses of interaural time differences. The auditory system can interpret time shifts in both the carrier and the envelope. Figure 2.85 shows the frequency ranges in which carrier time shifts, envelope time shifts, and level differences can have an effect. Carrier time shifts have an effect only below 1.6 kHz. Envelope time shifts have less of an effect as the frequency is decreased; the lowest frequency at which they have an effect depends on the shape of the envelope. Interaural sound pressure level differences are effective throughout the audible frequency range.

As a rule, evaluable interaural signal differences of the various kinds occur in combination in "natural" spatial hearing; that is, "natural" interaural signal differences include interaural attributes from the various classes and subclasses. We can then ask, What is the relative importance of the individual classes of interaural attributes, and how do they interact with each other?

Interaural time and level differences have the same effect on the position of the auditory event; both lead to its becoming displaced laterally. A possible way to compare the two parameters is to ask which time difference is equivalent to a particular level difference, and vice versa.

A frequently used technique for the measurement of this equivalence is the "trading" of time and level differences. This was first described by Klemm (1920) and Wittmann (1925). In a trading experiment the auditory event is displaced by means of a given time or level difference. Then one determines the opposing level or time difference that is needed to return the auditory event to the median plane.

The relationship determined in this way, measured in μs/dB, is called the "compensation factor" or "trading ratio." Röser (1965) surveyed a large number of results from the literature. Trading ratios measured up to that time ranged from approximately 2 to 200 μs/dB. Although considerable errors in measurement must be expected in trading experiments (see, e.g., Hershkowitz and Durlach 1969), these alone cannot account for this unusually wide range. Obviously the interactions between interaural time and level differences are too complicated to be describable by any one-number criterion.

The trading of impulse sounds (clicks) has been studied by David, Guttman, and van Bergeijk (1958, 1959), Deatherage and Hirsh (1959), Keidel, Wigand, and Keidel (1960), and Harris (1960). It was found that the trading ratio depends on loudness. When signals are stronger, a greater sound pressure level difference is necessary to compensate for a given interaural time difference. Figure 2.86 reproduces an often-quoted illustration that clearly shows this dependence. The trading curves are not straight lines, which would indicate a linear relationship;

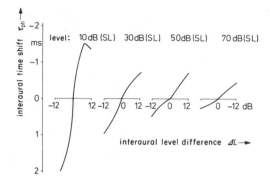

Figure 2.86
Trading curves of a typical subject for broadband clicks at various levels (after David, Guttman, and van Bergeijk 1959).

moreover, they become less and less steep with increasing loudness. David, Guttman, and van Bergeijk used two types of test signals: clicks shifted interaurally by a phase delay independent of frequency and noise uncorrelated between the two ears (produced by using two different noise generators). Only the envelopes had the same shape and could be shifted relative to one another. It is notable that almost the same trading curves resulted for both types of signals.

Harris pursued the problem of the loudness dependence of trading curves even further. He low-pass-filtered his impulse sounds. Under these conditions the loudness dependence of the trading curves first becomes significant when the signal includes components at frequencies above 1.6 kHz. If the spectrum is limited to frequencies below 1.6 kHz, the trading curves have only a moderate slope even at a low loudness level (figure 2.87). It is not wide of the mark to suggest that the observed loudness dependence is connected with the evaluation of interaural envelope displacements; this dependence affects only signals with frequency components for which there is no evaluation of time shifts of the fine structure.

From the results of trading experiments it may be concluded that the relative importance of interaural time and level differences depends on the type of sound signal. Interaural level differences have their greatest importance when the signal includes components above 1.6 kHz and the level is low.

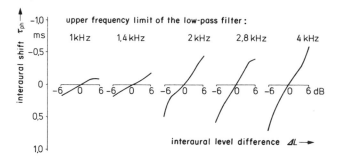

Figure 2.87
Trading curves of a typical subject for low-pass, band-limited clicks at a level of 20 dBSL (after Harris 1960).

Further analysis of such complicated interactions would be simpler if processes in the central nervous system were one and the same whether the auditory event is displaced laterally due to a time difference or due to a level difference. The relative importance of the different classes of attributes—and the behavior of the trading ratio—would then be determined only by the properties of peripheral components of the auditory system. In these peripheral components the information about the displacement of the auditory event would be translated from a time or level difference into the form in which it is represented in the central nervous system.

The literature includes two groups of hypotheses based on this simplified assumption. According to the first group, the central nervous system recognizes a displacement of the auditory event only through differences in arrival times of the nerve impulses from the two ears (e.g., Jeffress 1948, Kietz 1957, Deatherage and Hirsh 1959, Röser 1960, Sayers and Lynn 1968). In this group of hypotheses time differences between the ear input signals, and consequently between the nerve impulses, take on primary importance. The displacement of the auditory event in connection with level differences is explained by secondary effects. To mention two (see figure 2.88a):

1. The latency effect. A neuron fires only after a certain time lag, or latency time. This increases as the amplitude of the input signal becomes smaller. If the stimuli to the ears are signals of differing levels, the latency time at the more strongly stimulated ear is shorter. Consequently

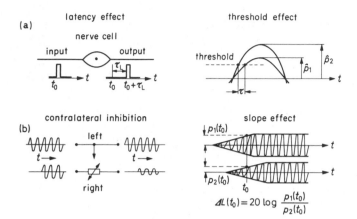

Figure 2.88
Transformation effects. a: Transformation of level differences into time differences.
b: Transformation of time differences into level differences.

the nerve impulses that ascend from that ear reach the central nervous
system sooner than those from the other ear.
2. The threshold effect. Two signals of the same shape but with different
amplitudes will exceed a given triggering level at different points in
time. In this case, too, the stronger signal releases the nerve impulse
earlier.

An extension of the "central" time difference hypotheses is the concept
that the central nervous system calculates a running average of the
interaural time difference, more or less by means of a running cross-
correlation (e.g., Licklider 1956, 1962, Sayers and Cherry 1957, Gruber
1967). A more detailed description of this concept is given in section
3.2.1.

According to the second group of hypotheses, differences in the number of impulses per unit time proceeding toward the central nervous
system from the two ears determine the displacement of the auditory
event (e.g., Boring 1926, Matzker 1958, van Bergeijk 1962, Elfner and
Tomsic 1968, Perrott 1969). If this were the case, then interaural sound
pressure level differences would be the primary attribute, since a stronger
ear input signal triggers more nerve impulses than a weak one. In order
for interaural time differences to be evaluated under these hypotheses
they must first be transformed into level differences. Two of the possible
effects that might do this are illustrated in figure 2.88b:

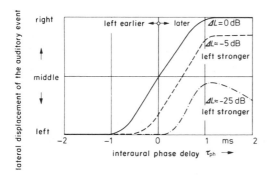

Figure 2.89
Schematic lateralization curves for frequency-independent interaural phase delay and simultaneous, opposite level differences. Valid for broadband signals.

1. Contralateral inhibition. Inhibitory impulses proceed from the ear receiving the first stimulus to the opposite ear, or to the nerve pathway from this ear, and so reduce the sensitivity at the opposite side.
2. Slope effect. On the onset slopes of the ear input signals, and on the rising slopes of the envelopes, a time difference leads to an interaural level difference for a short time.

For further details about both groups of hypotheses, reference to relevant literature is suggested, particularly to that in the field of physiology (e.g., Rosenzweig 1961, Schwartzkopff 1962a,b, 1968, Keidel 1966, Deatherage 1966).

Important objections may be raised against attributing exclusive validity to either of these two groups of simplifying hypotheses. For example, it may be stated in objection to the "central" time difference theories that an opposing time difference can no longer return the auditory event to the median plane in a trading experiment if the interaural level difference exceeds approximately 25 dB (Sayers and Cherry 1957, Guttman 1962). Figure 2.89 gives lateralization curves for this case. On the other hand, the central level difference theory cannot by itself fully explain the interpretation of envelope shifts. One needs in addition some mechanism that responds only to rising signal slopes. Differentiation of the envelopes, or a corresponding nerve process, could accomplish this (Franssen 1963).

Furthermore, the assumption that the central nervous system cannot distinguish interaural time differences from interaural level differences clearly does not hold. Rather, it seems quite clear that at least two types of information are encoded separately to a certain extent and conducted toward the center. One type has to do with interaural shifts in signal fine structure, and the other with sound pressure level differences or envelope shifts. This conclusion follows from the following observations.

Many investigators have pointed out that subjects in trading experiments do not have the same auditory event as in diotic presentations (reconfirmed systematically by Hafter and Carrier 1969). Particularly when interaural level differences are large (several dB), the auditory event appears broad or diffuse, or splits into two components. We noted this in section 2.4.2, but more details will be given here of the work of Whitworth and Jeffress (1961) that was cited in that section. They (and earlier Moushegian and Jeffress 1959) altered the classical trading technique by adjusting attributes so as to bring the auditory event not to the middle of the head but to a position at the side that was given by an acoustical pointer. Their subjects, who had normal hearing, were able to carry out the adjustment separately for the two parts of the auditory event. Figure 2.90 shows a typical result, which the authors themselves interpret as follows: "The . . . subjects . . . were able to perceive two separate, distinct sound images. One image . . . depended almost wholly upon the interaural time difference for its location. The other depended upon both the time difference and the intensity difference." The authors gave the name "time image" to the first component of the auditory event and the name "intensity image" to the other.

Hafter and Jeffress (1968) extended the investigation to 500 Hz pulsed sinusoids and to clicks with an energy maximum at 2.5 kHz. With both of these types of signals a time image and an intensity image were perceived separately. For clicks, the level dependence of the trading ratio was determined for both components of the auditory event. The trading ratio does not change much for the time image, but for the intensity image it clearly falls as the signal level rises (figure 2.91).

A comparison of these results with those shown in figures 2.86 and 2.87 gave rise to the following hypothesis (Blauert 1972b). For low-frequency signals that have no components over approximately 1.6 kHz, the time image determines the average displacement of the auditory event. The influence of interaural level differences is small in this case;

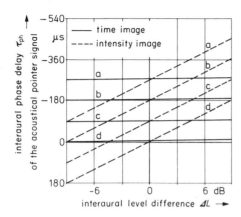

Figure 2.90
Lateral displacement of the two components of the auditory event that arise when a
500 Hz sinusoidal signal is presented binaurally (typical curves). Measured using an
acoustical pointer; loudness levels approximately 50 phon; interaural signal phase delays 270 μs (a), 180 μs (b), 90 μs (c), 0 μs (d)(after Whitworth and Jeffress 1961).

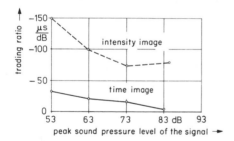

Figure 2.91
Trading ratio for the time image and intensity image in a trading experiment using
broadband clicks (after Hafter and Jeffress 1968; 3 subjects).

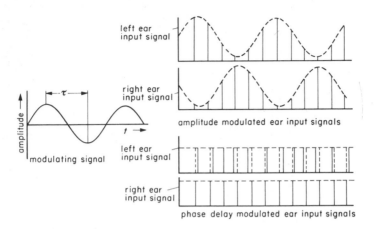

Figure 2.92
Schematic representation of ear input signals used in measuring the persistence of lateralization mechanisms.

the maximum trading ratio is approximately 40 μs/dB. For signals with components above 1.6 kHz, the intensity image may dominate even when there are also low-frequency components. In this case the displacement of the intensity image is determined by interaural envelope shifts and interaural level differences. Its trading ratio lies between 200 and 70 μs/dB. This falls distinctly with increasing loudness.

The significance of the time image and the intensity image in connection with the physiology of the inner ear will not be discussed further here; it is discussed briefly by Whitworth and Jeffress and by Hafter and Jeffress. Investigations by Jeffress and McFadden (1971) and McFadden, Jeffress, and Ermey (1971) are also of interest. These show that the relative importance of the time image and the intensity image can be different for different subjects.

A comparison of the dynamic properties of the auditory system in evaluating interaural time and level differences has shown less time persistence in the mechanism that establishes the intensity image than in the one that establishes the time image (Blauert 1970a). The concept of the experiments is illustrated in figure 2.92. An impulse train is presented to the subject's two ears; it is either amplitude-modulated interaurally or phase-delay-modulated interaurally. If the modulation frequency is low, the position of the auditory event oscillates inside the head. But if the modulation frequency exceeds a certain limit, the au-

ditory event no longer accurately traces the same path. When the interaural level difference is modulated, the shortest time for perception
of a complete cycle of the auditory event between the two sides is
approximately 162 ms; when the interaural phase delay is modulated,
a cycle requires at least 207 ms (80 Hz impulse train, approximately
60 phon, 40 subjects).

On the basis of what is known today about the evaluation of interaural
time and level differences in lateralization, the following summary
statements may be made:

1. The auditory system employs at least two evaluative mechanisms
that to a certain extent function independently of each other.
2. The first mechanism interprets interaural time shifts between the
fine structures of the ear input signals. Its influence on the displacement
of the auditory event is based only on signal components below 1.6
kHz.
3. The second mechanism interprets interaural sound pressure level
differences and also time shifts between the envelopes. There is some
indication that it may have a dominant influence on the displacement
of the auditory event if the signal has significant components above
1.6 kHz.
4. The second mechanism is time-variant; for example, it can be altered
by means of relearning processes (see section 2.4.2 and Held 1955).
To the best of my knowledge, time variance has not been demonstrated
separately for the first mechanism.
5. The relative importance of the two mechanisms can vary among
individuals.
6. The first mechanism appears to have more time persistence than
the second.

Further discussion requires another look at the interaural transfer
function, which describes the signal differences that occur in natural
hearing, in terms of frequency. Figures 2.36 and 2.38 show that the
average level difference and the average phase and group delays all
become greater as lateral displacement of the sound source increases.
They consequently have parallel effects in connection with the lateral
displacement of the auditory event.

For all sound sources the trend of the interaural sound pressure level
difference is to increase with frequency. As a first approximation it can

be said that the more that the signal energy lies in the higher frequency range, the greater is the average level difference.

Because envelope time shifts cannot without further assumptions be predicted by the interaural transfer function alone, a discussion of their relative importance in localization presents more difficulties. Nonetheless it may be noted that signals are crudely dissected spectrally in the inner ear, and that the envelope of each spectral component is then evaluated separately. The interaural envelope shifts of each spectral component can then be approximated by the average group delay in its frequency range. The way the results of evaluation in each individual spectral range contribute to the overall interpretation has not yet been investigated sufficiently. Research points to a higher weighting factor going to the envelope time shift of the frequency range in which energy density is highest (Flanagan et al. 1964).

The azimuth of the auditory event can depend on the type of signal while the direction of sound incidence remains constant. This fact is well known and can also be explained in terms of the foregoing discussion (see also figure 2.3). However, no one has sufficiently investigated whether the auditory system recognizes features of level difference and group delay and takes note of them in localization. Although it has been proven that dips or peaks in the group delay curve lead to changes in the position of the auditory event or to increases in localization blur, experiments relative to this problem have not used group delay curves characteristic of hearing in a free sound field (e.g., Licklider and Webster 1950, Schroeder 1961, Blauert, Hartmann, and Laws 1971).

Experiments using sinusoidal signals led to the following point of view, which was common in the early literature on spatial hearing. In the localization of broadband sounds, time differences and level differences work together in such a way that low-frequency components are localized on the basis of time differences of the fine structure, and high-frequency components on the basis of level differences. Figure 2.93 will help explain how this point of view came to be accepted. It shows the curves of lateralization blur for interaural time and level differences using sinusoidal signals, just as in figures 2.76 and 2.83, but it includes two additional curves, derived as follows. A loudspeaker was placed directly in front of a subject, and the smallest lateral displacement of the loudspeaker that led to a shift in the auditory event was measured. The interaural time and level differences of the ear input

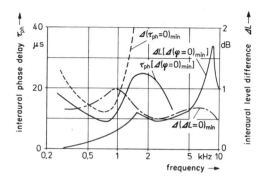

Figure 2.93
The interaural level differences $\Delta L[\Delta(\varphi = 0)_{min}]$ and phase delays $\tau_{ph}[\Delta(\varphi = 0)_{min}]$ corresponding to a just-noticeable lateral sound source displacement, compared with the curves of lateralization blur $\Delta(\Delta L = 0)_{min}$ and $\Delta(\tau_{ph} = 0)_{min}$. Valid for sinusoidal and narrow-band pulsed sinusoidal signals (after Mills 1960).

signals were approximately calculated for this displacement of the loud-speaker. The two solid lines are the result. It can be seen that, in the low-frequency range, the curve giving time differences for the just-noticeable loudspeaker displacement is close to the curve for lateralization blur connected with interaural time differences. Over a certain part of the high-frequency range, on the other hand, the curve giving the level differences for the just-noticeable loudspeaker displacement is very close to the curve of lateralization blur for interaural time differences. For sinusoidal signals, then, it is obviously a justifiable conclusion that low frequencies are lateralized or localized on the basis of interaural arrival-time differences, and higher frequencies on the basis of interaural level differences. But this conclusion, in this form, must not be generalized to all signals, for the following reasons:

1. It does not take interaural envelope shifts into account.
2. It gives equal weight to level differences and to fine-structure time differences. This relationship, however, is not proven with any generality.

To round out this section we offer some details about the role of interaural signal attributes in distance hearing. In section 2.2.2 it was pointed out that the interaural transfer function depends on the distance as well as on the direction of sound incidence. The dependence of interaural ear input signal attributes on the sound source distance has been called "acoustical parallax." Figures 2.27–2.29 show that this dependence is greatest with sound incidence from the side ($\varphi = 90°$ or 270°).

Proceeding from the physical effect of acoustical parallax, many authors have hypothesized that the auditory system, in forming the distance of the auditory event, makes use of monaural as well as interaural signal attributes (e.g., Thompson 1882, von Hornbostel 1923, Woodworth and Schlosberg 1954, Hirsh 1968). This is clearly the case. As an example, Feldmann (1972) gave a brief description of how two signals presented dichotically, with a pure time difference of 1 ms, lead to an auditory event somewhat outside the head. But if an additional interaural level difference is introduced such that the signal arriving later becomes the weaker one, the auditory event moves very close to the head or inside the head. Furthermore, anticipating an effect that will be discussed in more detail in section 3.1.1, the auditory event or parts of it appear very near the head or inside it when the sound source consists of two loudspeakers on each side, radiating signals identical except for a 180° phase shift. This effect occurs even if the loudspeaker distance is several meters. Hanson and Kock (1957) explained this effect in terms of the specific interaural signal differences that result from such an arrangement of the sound sources.

Given that acoustical parallax depends on the direction of sound incidence, one might think that in distance hearing localization and localization blur also depend on it. The available experimental results are, however, contradictory. Starch and Crawford (1909), for example, established that localization blur with respect to distance does not depend on the direction of sound incidence. Young (1931) noted that the distance of the auditory event depended on the direction of sound incidence if the sound source distance was held constant; however, he presented the sound by means of an arrangement like the one illustrated in figure 2.100 below (a so-called pseudophonic arrangement). Further experiments were carried out by Werner (1922), Cochran, Throop, and Simpson (1968), Gardner (1969a), and Holt and Thurlow (1969). The results of Werner, Gardner, and Holt and of Thurlow point to a dependence of distance localization blur on the direction of sound incidence, but these results do not agree with those of Cochran, Throop, and Simpson. Indeed, Werner found that localization blur with respect to distance is smaller when the sound incidence is from the front than when it is from the side. This result is the opposite of what would be expected as being due to acoustical parallax. Thus the complex of issues surrounding acoustical parallax and localization cannot be regarded as having yet been resolved.

2.5 Additional Parameters

Previous sections have dealt with spatial hearing under two restrictive conditions:

1. Discussion was limited to the relationship between attributes of the ear input signals and the direction and distance of auditory events. Other phenomena correlated with the position of the auditory event have not yet been investigated.
2. In all cases investigated to this point it has been required that the position of the subject's head not change relative to the position of the sound source. The subject's head was voluntarily held still or mechanically immobilized, or the sound signals were presented over headphones.

To this point, then, we have considered only those attributes of inputs to the subject that are available for evaluation in the auditory experiment illustrated in figure 2.11. In that experiment headphones were used to generate ear input signals like the ones that had previously been picked up at exactly the same points by probe microphones.

It is clear that both monaural and interaural attributes of the ear input signals contribute to forming the position of the auditory event. The essential monaural attributes of the ear input signals are time and level differences between the individual spectral components of each individual ear input signal; the essential interaural signal attributes are time and level differences between corresponding spectral components of the two ear input signals.

Experiments using two identical ear input signals have shown that monaural signal attributes serve primarily to define the front and rear sectors of the median plane, the angle of elevation, and the distance of the auditory event. Interaural signal attributes are correlated primarily with lateral displacements of the auditory event. It is a justifiable conclusion at this point, though not yet proven for every individual case, that monaural and interaural signal attributes contribute in specific combinations in forming the angles—both azimuth and elevation angles—and distances of auditory events.

In a free sound field, with the subject's head free to move and the surroundings lighted, a number of further attributes may be available. These contribute to evaluation by allowing additional inferences about the position of the sound source. This section will deal with these additional parameters of localization.

2.5.1 Motional theories

The external-ear transfer functions depend on the position of the sound source; that is, the linear distortions that sound signals undergo on their way to the eardrums depend on the direction and distance of the sound source relative to the subject's head. If the subject's head moves relative to the sound source while a sound signal is being presented, the monaural and interaural attributes of the signals at the eardrums will change in some particular way. Theories of spatial hearing that describe relationships between the position of the auditory event and the changes to the ear input signals during head movements are called motional or motoric theories.

Motional theories also describe changes to other attributes of auditory events during head movements, particularly attributes such as loudness and tone color from which the subject can obtain information about the position of the sound source. For example, marked voluntary searching and orienting movements of the head may be observed in persons who are deaf in one ear. These movements apparently serve primarily to facilitate the use of the (trainable) ability to discover the position of the sound source on the basis of changes in the loudness and tone color of the auditory event (Brunzlow 1925, 1939, Meyer zum Gottesberge 1940, Klensch 1949). Investigations have not yet been carried out to determine the extent to which head movements are correlated with the position of the auditory event for persons who are deaf in one ear.

Head movements in connection with spatial hearing may also be observed in subjects with normal hearing. Two classes of such movements can be distinguished:

1. A more or less unconscious, spontaneous (reflexive) movement of the head toward the position of the auditory event, and therefore toward

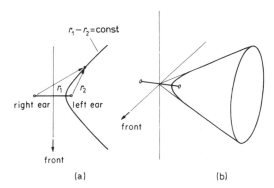

Figure 2.94
According to von Hornbostel and Wertheimer's model, the locus of all points at the
same distance from the left and right ears is a hyperbola in the horizontal plane (a)
and the shell of a cone at greater distances in three-dimensional space (b).

the most probable position of the sound source. The biological meaning
of such movements is obvious, but they require a more or less precisely
located auditory event before the movement begins. When the head
is moved, localization blur decreases, since the auditory event is brought
into the region of sharpest hearing.
2. Searching and orienting movements undertaken more or less consciously. Their goal is clearly to assemble more information in order
to establish a final position for an auditory event that is at first not
sharply located. Generally the location of the auditory event becomes
more definite during the head movement. In some cases the auditory
event changes its position in a specific way, for example from the front
to the rear or from the front to the front overhead. The following
sections deal primarily with this second class of head movements.

Motional theories first received attention as a supplement to the time-
difference theories of von Hornbostel and Wertheimer (1920). These
authors accepted two points separated by 21 cm as the simplest possible
model for sound collection with two ears (see section 2.2.2). In such a
model the differences between distances to the two ear points are the
same for all points on a particular hyperbola in the frontal plane (figure
2.94). The time difference at the two ears is the same for sound waves
that originate at any point on the hyperbola. For longer distances the
hyperbola may be approximated by its asymptotes; then, considering

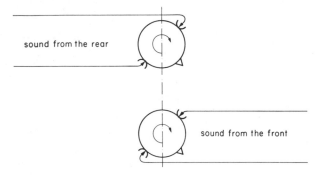

Figure 2.95
Changes in interaural ear input signal differences when the head is turned are opposite for sound waves arriving from the front and from the rear.

the model not only in a plane but in three dimensions, a conical shell describes the locus of all possible sound sources with the same time difference. If the interaural time difference is very small, the conical shell collapses toward the median plane. It is clear that an interaural time difference correlates only ambiguously to the direction of the sound source with this simple model (as it does with models that regard the head as an opaque sphere).

Van Soest (1929) seems to have been the first to point out that it is possible, despite this ambiguity, to determine the direction of sound incidence correctly by means of head movements. The principle that he recognized is illustrated in figure 2.95. Assuming, for example, that there is no interaural signal difference, sound will reach the two eardrums at the same time and at the same level. Then all directions in the median plane are possible as directions of sound incidence. Sound incidence can be from the front or the rear in the horizontal plane. If the subject then rotates his or her head to the right around a vertical axis, the left ear will come closer to the sound source if the source is at the front; the right will come closer if the sound source is at the rear. That is, for the same rotation of the head, the change in interaural time difference can be positive or negative depending on whether the sound waves arrive from the front or the rear. The same is true for the interaural level difference.

Van Soest assumed that the auditory system recognizes the polarity of the change in interaural time difference and makes use of this polarity in forming the position of the auditory event. It is easy to see, though, that the subject must recognize the direction of rotation of the head and in some cases the amplitude of head movement—not just the changes in the ear input signals—in order to obtain usable information. Information about head movement can be obtained through the organ of balance (vestibular organ), through the sense of vision, or, if necessary,through the position, tension, and posture receptors in the neck muscles. Motional theories, consequently, are heterosensory theories.

If we abandon von Hornbostel and Wertheimer's model and other models that assume a head symmetrical with respect to the axis of the ears, the situation immediately becomes more complicated. Taking into account the characteristic behavior of the external-ear transfer functions, it seems quite unlikely that ambiguities would occur between interaural signal differences and the direction of sound incidence in connection with broadband signals. But the case is different with narrow-band signals, for which it is still possible that the same interaural signal differences will occur in connection with sound incidence from different directions. Motional theories, then, are of importance to spatial hearing only when the effects of the head and the external ears have already been taken into consideration. The truth of this statement will be demonstrated in what follows.

Three groups of questions will now be addressed:

1. Do head movements occur at all in natural hearing with two ears? If so, how may these movements be described and anlayzed?
2. For particular head movements, which specific attributes of the ear input signals are available to the auditory system for interpretation?
3. What effect or effects do head movements have on the position of the auditory event?

The discussion will draw on work by Perekalin (1930), Young (1931), Wallach (1938/40), de Boer and Vermeulen (1939), de Boer and van Urk (1949), de Boer (1947), Klensch (1948, 1949), Koenig (1950), König and Sussman (1955), Burger (1958), Jongkees and van de Veer (1958), Fisher and Freedman (1968), Thurlow, Mangels, and Runge (1967), Thurlow and Runge (1967), and Thurlow and Mergener (1970).

The most thorough investigation of the first question was undertaken by Thurlow, Mangels, and Runge (1967), who observed more than 50 subjects with normal hearing attempting to determine the position of

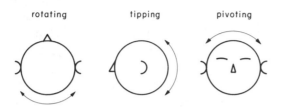

Figure 2.96
Classes of head movements (after Thurlow et al. 1967).

a sound source in an anechoic chamber. The subjects were blindfolded.
The sound source radiated narrow-band noise (500–700 Hz or 7.5–8
kHz). Ten sound source positions, well-distributed around the chamber,
were used. The subjects were permitted to move their heads freely
while addressing the task but were instructed to keep their torsos still.
Their head movements were recorded by a motion picture camera and
were subsequently interpreted. A classification in terms of rotating,
tipping, and pivoting movements was used in the interpretation (figure
2.96). The most important results of the interpretation are shown in
table 2.5.

As can be seen, the largest average amplitude is that of rotating
movements. The most frequent combination of classes of movements
involves rotating and tipping movements. As to the direction of the
movements, it may be stated that the first movement most subjects
undertook was such that they more nearly faced the direction of sound
incidence, though usually they did not carry this movement so far as
to face it squarely. More than 50 percent of the subjects moved their
heads back and forth, often more than once.

These experiments show that subjects, when permitted, actually do
initiate prolonged or repeated head movements in order to determine
the exact direction of the sound source. We now consider which specific
changes in the ear input signals occur during such head movements.
As regards rotating and pivoting movements, this question was investigated most thoroughly by Wallach (1938).

We have already demonstrated that a rotating movement (i.e., a
movement about the vertical axis) makes it possible to obtain information about whether the sound source is ahead of or behind the
subject; for a given direction of rotation of the head, the interaural

Table 2.5
Compilation of the results of Thurlow et al. (1967) on the head movements of 23 subjects asked to determine the direction of sound sources.

	Rotating	Tipping	Pivoting	Rotating, tipping, pivoting	Rotating, tipping	Rotating, pivoting	Tipping, pivoting
Average amplitudes and standard deviations							
500–1,000 Hz signals	42° ±20.4°	13.1° ±13.5°	10.2° ±9.6°				
7,500–8,000 Hz signals	29.2° ±18.6°	15.2° ±12.9°	11.6° ±8.3°				
Relative statistical frequencies with which subjects would exhibit specific combinations of movements							
500–1,000 Hz signals	48%	13%	3%	39%	70%	22%	4%
7,500–8,000 Hz signals	41%	15%	5%	36%	62%	19%	6%
Relative statistical frequencies with which subjects would exhibit specific classes of movements with amplitudes greater than 10°							
500–1,000 Hz signals	48%	1%	1%	10%	32%	3%	—
7,500–8,000 Hz signals	32%	3%	2%	17%	26%	7%	—

signal attributes change in a specific way. It is easy to see that the same principle, more generally, allows sound sources in the front hemisphere to be distinguished from those in the rear hemisphere. If, for example, it is true of a particular direction of sound incidence in the front hemisphere that the left ear comes closer to the direction of sound incidence during the head movement, then the same is true for all directions in the forward hemisphere. In addition to the rotating movement, a pivoting movement (i.e., a turning movement around the axis where the median and horizontal planes intersect) may be considered. Then, in a similar way, information may also be obtained about whether the sound source is in the upper or lower hemisphere.

The four sectors—forward and above, forward and below, behind and above, behind and below—may be distinguished by an evaluation of the direction in which interaural signal differences change during given rotating and pivoting head movements. Furthermore, if the degree of change of the interaural signals is evaluated as a function of head movement, then information can be obtained about the elevation angle of the sound source with respect to the horizontal plane and also about the corresponding angle with respect to the frontal plane.

To gain insight into this statement we consider two particular examples:

1. The sound source is in the horizontal plane, let us say at the front. The head is rotated until the sound source is exactly at the left side. During the course of the head rotation, the interaural signal differences increase from zero to their maximum value.
2. The sound source is exactly overhead. Once again the head rotates through 90° in the horizontal plane. The interaural signal differences remain zero throughout the rotation, since the sound source remains in the median plane.

It is immediately obvious that a continuum exists between these two limit cases (maximum change in the interaural signal differences on the one hand; no change on the other hand). In the final analysis the quantity that determines the interaural signal difference is the angle γ between the direction of sound incidence and the median plane. The geometric relationship of this angle to the azimuth angle φ and the elevation angle δ is

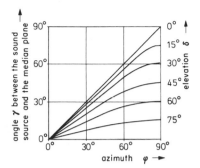

Figure 2.97
The angle γ between the direction of sound incidence and the median plane as a function of the azimuth φ and the elevation δ (after Wallach 1938).

$$\sin \gamma = \cos \delta \sin \varphi. \qquad (2.34)$$

Figure 2.97 shows γ as a function of δ and φ. The curves with the parameters $\delta = 0°$ and $\delta = 90°$ are immediately recognizable as representing the two limit cases mentioned above. The rate of increase of the curves as a function of δ is greater for large values of φ than for small ones.

A similar consideration of the amount of interaural signal change as a function of the amplitude of pivoting movements proceeds in a manner analogous to that for rotating movements. But the case of tipping movements—which are, as shown in table 2.5, not at all rare—is basically different. In this case the head turns around the axis of the ears. If the head is modeled as a simple sphere, the interaural signal differences remain constant. But with real heads, changes to interaural—and even more so, to monaural—signal attributes occur as functions of the direction of turning and the amplitude of the tipping movement. However, no investigations of this particular issue have yet been undertaken beyond those mentioned in section 2.2.3.

It may be concluded from the preceding theoretical considerations that interpretation of changes in the sound signals at the eardrums during head movement will always provide information about the position of the sound source. It will now be shown that this information is in fact used by the auditory system, perhaps in conjunction with other information, to form the position of the auditory event. Exper-

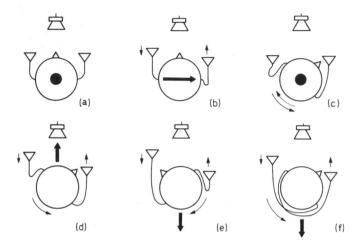

Figure 2.98
Schematic representation of the auditory experiments of Klensch (1948). The bold arrows and dots show the positions and directions of the auditory events. The light arrows indicate the movements of the funnels and the head (after Jongkees and van de Veer 1958).

iments demonstrating these relationships very vividly were undertaken by Klensch (1948) and were later confirmed by Jongkees and van de Veer (1958) (see figure 2.98).

Klensch inserted rubber tubes of equal length into the subject's two ears. A small metal funnel was attached to the end of each rubber tube. This eliminated the distortions characteristically introduced by the outer ear. In all cases the funnel opening faced the sound source. The following cases were investigated:

a. The head is not moved. The funnels are placed at an equal distance from the sound source. The auditory event appears in the middle of the head, as is usual with diotic headphone presentation.
b. The head is not moved, but the two funnels are moved back and forth in opposite directions, one toward the sound source when the other is moved away. The auditory event appears inside the head but moves on a path between the ears. This case corresponds to dichotic headphone presentation.
c. The funnels are placed at an equal distance from the sound source and are not moved. The head is rotated. This arrangement represents the general case in diotic headphone presentation. The ear input signals

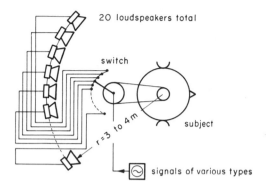

Figure 2.99
Schematic representation of the experimental apparatus of Wallach (1938, 1939, 1940). The subject's head movements led to the signal being switched among 20 loudspeakers.

do not change when the head is moved. The auditory event appears in the middle of the head.

d. The head is rotated. The funnels are moved in the same direction as the natural ears. The auditory event appears in front of the subject.

e. The head is rotated. The funnels are moved in a direction opposite to that of the natural ears. The auditory event appears behind the subject.

f. The head is rotated. Each hose leads from its funnel to the ear on the opposite side. The funnels are moved in the same direction as the head. The auditory event appears behind the subject.

It should be expressly noted that the auditory event did not appear in the middle of the head in cases d–f, though the sound was presented as if over headphones. Nothing, however, was said about the actual distance of the auditory events. From an article by de Boer and van Urk (1941) it may nonetheless be concluded that the auditory event appears in or near the head under these conditions.

The results of Klensch and Jongkees and of van de Veer agree fully with theoretical considerations, but they differ from natural hearing to the extent that the effect of the natural external ears is eliminated. Wallach (1938, 1939) carried out experiments incorporating this effect. His experimental apparatus is sketched in figure 2.99. Twenty loudspeakers were arrayed in an arc around the subject, whose head was connected to a rotary switch. The ratio between head movement and switch rotation was variable. The switch connected a signal (pulsed tones, music, speech, clicks) to one loudspeaker at a time, depending on the position of the head. Switching was almost transient-free.

In the first experiment the loudspeakers were arrayed in front of the subject and were connected to the switch in such a way that the signal was always radiated by the loudspeaker directly in front of the subject. The interaural signal differences therefore did not change as the head was rotated. For 10 of the 17 subjects, the auditory event appeared overhead, in agreement with theory. It sometimes first appeared at the front, then migrated upward as the head was rotated and stayed overhead. For 7 subjects the auditory event did not appear overhead or migrate overhead. These subjects heard it in front of them, behind them, diagonally above and in front, or had a diffusely located auditory event. They exhibited the same response when the experiment was repeated using a loudspeaker that was actually overhead.

The experiment was then altered so that the loudspeakers formed an arc in the subjects' frontal plane. The switch was also turned 90°, so that it was operated by a pivoting movement of the head. The auditory event appeared, with equal probability, in front of or behind all seven subjects in this experiment. According to theory, all positions on the axis where the median and horizontal planes intersect were possible.

In a further experiment, loudspeakers were placed at the front ($\varphi = 0°$, $\delta = 0°$), but the relationships that were simulated would occur if the head were rotated and the loudspeaker were behind. That is, the ratio between the rotation of the head and that of the switch was chosen to simulate rotation of the head with a loudspeaker behind the subject; the loudspeakers were switched in the same direction but through an angle twice as large as the head movement. The experiment succeeded with all 15 subjects. They reported that their auditory event at first appeared at the front, but that it immediately jumped to the rear when they moved their heads. Even when the head was once again held still, the auditory event remained at the rear; occasionally, after a while, it would once again jump to the front. A similar persistence of the auditory event is reported in a related context by Klensch (1948).

The experiment just described also succeeded in reverse; that is, it was possible to generate an auditory event at the front by means of loudspeakers at the rear, even though the experimental chamber was lighted. The auditory event, as described by the subjects, was at a position at which no sound source was visible.

Wallach undertook a number of further experiments in which he attempted to generate auditory events at specific angles of elevation. This effect was contrived by changing the ratio between head rotation and movement of the rotary switch. The switching between loudspeakers occurred more slowly than the head rotated. Elevation angles of $\delta = 78°$ and $\delta = 60°$ were generated in this way, precise to within a few degrees (4–7 subjects). A similarly altered experimental apparatus for tipping motions led to auditory events in directions diagonally away from the front. All of these results of Wallach's, and a number of additional ones, are fully in agreement with theory.

We have already established that motional theories are heterosensory; subjects must evaluate changes in the ear input signals at the same time as they evaluate the direction and amplitude of head movements in relation to the sound source. Wallach (1940) showed that the movements are still correctly registered under the following conditions:

1. The position, tension, and posture receptors of the neck muscles and cervical vertebrae do not furnish any information.
2. Only the vestibular organ furnishes information.
3. Only the sense of vision furnishes information.

These three experimental conditions were fulfilled in the following way. For the first the subject's head was immobilized with respect to the torso, and the entire body was rotated by means of a rotating chair. If, in addition, the eyes were blindfolded, the second condition was fulfilled. For the third condition the subject stayed in a fixed position but the entire visual space was rotated by means of an appropriate device (a movable curtain with vertical black and white stripes that surrounded the subject). Some of the experiments already described were then repeated, with the following results.

For passive movements with the eyes open (condition 1) results for all subjects were exactly the same as for active movements initiated by the subjects themselves. When the subjects were blindfolded (condition 2), discrepancies occurred for about 50 percent of the subjects, and the other half still reacted as the motional theories predict. In experiments using the rotating curtain the subjects had the impression that the curtain was standing still and they were rotating relative to it. Consequently, with a loudspeaker fixed in front of them, the auditory event appeared overhead, either immediately or after a short transitional period. A loudspeaker that circled the subjects at the same rate as the curtain but in the opposite direction led to the expected result with 20 subjects: The auditory event was in front when the loudspeaker was directly behind, and vice versa. It is definite, then, that the sense of vision plays an important role in registering head movements. Because information from the vestibular organs and from the receptors in the neck muscles is normally also available, head movements are registered with great certainty.

Given that the auditory system can evaluate information about the position of the sound source obtained by means of head movements, a question still remains: What is the position of motional theories in the context of other theories of spatial hearing? There is agreement in the literature that, in the case of normal spatial hearing, head movements improve the ability to determine the direction of sound incidence. With respect to localization, this means that the mutual discrepancies between the direction of sound incidence and the direction of the auditory event are smaller after head movements (Thurlow and Runge 1967, Thurlow and Mergener 1971). In particular, reversals of direction between the sound source and the auditory event are almost completely avoided (Perekalin 1930, Burger 1958, Fisher and Freedman 1968).

Head movements, especially consciously undertaken searching and orienting movements, can therefore lead to a change in the position of the auditory event if the signal lasts long enough. If information obtained by means of head movements is evaluated, it overrides information derived from monaural signal characteristics. This conclusion follows from Wallach's experiments; for example, it was possible in these experiments to generate an auditory event at the rear by means of loudspeakers at the front, even though the sound signals were broadband. This conclusion has been confirmed as follows (Blauert 1969): In the course of the auditory experiments using 1/3-octave noise described in section 2.3.1 (figures 2.45–2.48), sound was in some cases presented when the subjects' heads were not immobilized, and the subjects were expressly made aware that they could move their heads. The typical localization that is describable in terms of directional bands did not occur in this case. Without exception, the auditory event appeared in the direction of sound incidence. When the head was again immobilized and the signal was presented after 10 s, the direction of the auditory event corresponded in the great majority of cases to that of sound incidence. This behavior was significant even when another direction of the auditory event, corresponding to the directional bands, would be expected.

Thus head movements definitely make it possible to determine the direction of the sound source with great certainty. After head movements have been completed, the auditory event is almost always in the direction of sound incidence.

2.5.2 Bone-conduction, visual, vestibular, and tactile theories

The position of auditory events is primarily determined by the auditory system, which draws together the necessary information from the interaural and monaural attributes of the sound signals at the eardrums and from their changes during head movements. In section 1.2, however, it was noted that other of the subject's inputs may be involved in forming the position of an auditory event. Table 1.1 gave a systematic outline of the psychophysical theories of spatial hearing. The bone-conduction, visual, vestibular, and tactile theories listed in the outline remain to be discussed.

Bone-conduction theories   Sound signals can reach the inner ear not only over the eardrum–ossicle path, but also over the so-called bone-conduction path. Bone conduction occurs when oscillations of the skull are conducted directly to the inner ear through the temporal bone. For a description of the mechanisms that produce this effect, see von Békésy (1960) or Tonndorf (1966, 1972), which contain references to further literature. In considering the influence of bone conduction on the position of the auditory event, two cases may appropriately be distinguished:

1. Bone conduction resulting from air conduction. This is the normal way that bone conduction is produced in a sound field in air.
2. Bone conduction resulting from other causes, such as stimuli that set the body directly into vibration, or in underwater hearing.

In the first case a subject's threshold of hearing rises by as much as 40 dB if the auditory canals are plugged. It may then be concluded that the sound conducted through the bones of the skull is attenuated by at least 40 dB more than sound conducted through the external ear and middle ear. According to current psychophysical knowledge, it is improbable that components at the same ear 40 dB below the main signal have any influence on the auditory event. The hypothesis that bone conduction plays a role in normal spatial hearing (see, e.g., Wilson and Myers 1908, Hecht 1922a) consequently has, as a rule, received no support in recent years (Hecht 1922b, Carsten and Salinger 1922, Banister 1924, Kietz 1953, Blauert 1969a).

The situation is different when the component of the sound that reaches the inner ear by bone conduction is of a strength similar to that of the air-conducted sound. This can be true when the skull is stimulated by special transducers, when personal ear protectors are worn, or when the body is in a medium with a specific field impedance close to its own (such as water).

The lateralization of the auditory event for bone-conducted sound is used in audiometric practice. As an example, in Weber's test, a tuning fork is placed against the patient's forehead. Inferences about the type of hearing problem from which the patient is suffering can be drawn from the position of the auditory event (Langenbeck 1958, Plath 1969, Huizing 1970). Sone, Ebata, and Tradamoto (1968) investigated the effect of simultaneous presentation of bone-conducted signals and air-conducted headphone signals. The signals were identical except for a time shift. They established the possibility of generating auditory events outside as well as inside the head in this way. Plenge (personal correspondence) supplemented and confirmed these experiments. The work of Sone, Ebata, and Tradamoto includes a number of further auditory experiments in which bone-conducted stimuli are used. Veit (1971) investigated whether bone conduction would be useful in generating precisely located auditory events in aids for the blind, but he came to the conclusion that it was not as suitable as other means. From audiometry it is known that the interaural attenuation of bone-conducted sound (stimulus at the mastoid process of the temporal bone) is at least 10–20 dB. This may be attributed to the fact that the inner ear is embedded in pneumatic parts of the skull, that is, in highly porous bone that contains air. This structure, which humans have in common with several mammals—notably the whale, an underwater mammal— shields the inner ear from sound conducted through the body (see Meyer zum Gottesberge 1968, Blauert and Hartmann 1971).

Water is a medium of approximately the same acoustic field impedance as the skull. In underwater hearing, then, the conditions for stimulation by means of sound transmitted through the body are good. In
fact, it has been shown that the threshold for hearing under water is
determined by stimulation of bone conduction by the skull; when the
head, with the exception of the entrances to the auditory canals, is
covered with a hood, the threshold of hearing rises (Nordmark, Phelps,
and Whightman 1971). Investigations have also shown that, if head
movements are used, it is possible to determine the direction of sound
incidence under water to an accuracy of about 20° (Feinstein 1966;
Norman et al. 1971, which contains references to the literature; Goeters
1972). However, sound transmitted over the "normal" eardrum–ossicle
path also seems to contribute information; when the entrances to the
auditory canals are covered, the ability to identify the direction of sound
incidence is reduced. This phenomenon has not yet been subjected to
precise investigation. It should be noted that interaural time differences
are greatly decreased under water, since the speed of sound is five times
as great as it is in air. Acoustically one might say that the head shrinks
to the size of a golf ball (Bauer and Torick 1966). Auditory events
appear closer to the median plane than they do with the same direction
of sound incidence in air; they often appear at the surface of the head
or inside it.

Visual theories   The assumption underlying visual theories may be
stated as follows: What the subject sees during sound presentation, and
where the subject sees it, are factors determining the position of the
auditory event. A number of observations confirm such a relationship.
For example, it is a matter of daily experience that a person watching
television hears an announcer's voice at the position where the announcer appears on the screen. Only with the eyes closed is the auditory
event clearly at the side of the screen, in the direction of the loudspeaker.
Stratton (1887), using eyeglasses that turned the visual field upside
down, established that the auditory event is also inverted as long as it
lies within the visual field. Klemm (1918) reported an experiment in
which he arrayed two microphones at the right and left in front of a
subject and presented the signals from the microphones to the opposite
ears over headphones. A sound-generating hammer device was placed
in front of each microphone, and the two devices produced sounds in

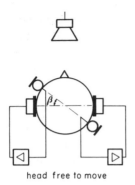

head free to move

Figure 2.100
Pseudophonic experimental arrangement.

alternation. With the subject's eyes closed, the hammer blows were heard on the sides opposite the devices. But if the subject watched the hammer devices attentively, the hammer blows were heard on the same sides as the devices. If, after a few minutes, the subject closed his or her eyes, this relationship was maintained for a while but then, gradually, the positions of the auditory events reversed themselves with respect to the visual events and returned to the positions that would be expected on the basis of the ear input signals. Held (1955) equipped subjects with what he called a "pseudophonic" apparatus, after a similar device created by Thompson (1879) (figure 2.100). Two microphones were affixed to the head, spaced the same distance apart as the ears but on an axis that stood at an angle to the axis of the ears. With the subject's eyes closed, the auditory event, as expected, appeared displaced with respect to the direction of sound incidence. The angle by which the auditory event was displaced was the same as that between the axis of the microphones and that of the ears. With open eyes, on the other hand, the subject noticed no discrepancy between the position of the sound source and that of the auditory event.

Jeffress and Taylor (1961) seem to have succeeded in bringing an auditory event from the inside of the head to the outside with at least a few of their subjects by turning on a lamp in front of the subjects. Sound presentation was over headphones. Gardner (1968b) describes a phenomenon that he calls the "proximity–image effect." In experiments having to do with distance hearing, the auditory event usually

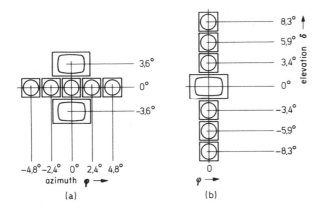

Figure 2.101
The experimental apparatus of Blauert (1970b) used in measuring localization blur with a simultaneous optical stimulus. a: Test series 1 (horizontal plane). b: Test series 2 (median plane).

appeared at the position of the nearest of a number of loudspeakers arrayed one behind the other ahead of the subject, as long as the subject's eyes were open.

Klemm (1909) used the evident tendency of visual and auditory events to merge spatially as the basis for the formulation of a rule of "spatial complication." According to this rule, there is a general tendency for perceptions of different senses to merge spatially when stimuli are presented simultaneously to the different senses. He supported this formulation with an observation that the positions of both the visual and the auditory events moved toward each other when light and sound stimuli were presented simultaneously.

There are exceptions to the rule of spatial complication. Ewert (1930) discovered one using an experimental apparatus like Stratton's but with a lens system instead of prismatic eyeglasses to distort visual space. He found that his subjects could learn to form a direction of the auditory event corresponding to the direction of the sound source, despite the distorted visual field. Blauert (1970b) measured the localization blur of speech from the front with and without a simultaneous television image of the person speaking. The experimental apparatus is shown in figure 2.101. The loudspeakers, 7 m in front of the subject, were switched on in random order. A 5 s sequence of logatomes (speech fragments) was presented over each loudspeaker. The subjects were required to say whether their auditory event was above or below, to the left or right of the forward axis. When the television picture was turned on, they were instructed to concentrate on it. Localization blur of the direction of the auditory event in both the horizontal and median planes proved not to depend on whether the visual image of the person speaking was shown (20 subjects, 35 phon).

Thus optical inputs are evaluated along with other inputs in forming the auditory event. Whether acoustical or optical inputs dominate when the two contradict each other depends on, among other factors, the task that is being emphasized. This is similar to the situation in which monaural signal attributes are evaluated, when the subject can suppress certain information about the position of the sound source at will and focus on other information.

Visual theories of spatial hearing, taken in a narrow, carefully defined sense, must be distinguished from the visual theories according to which the movements of the subject's own body are registered. These latter theories play a role in the context of the motional theories discussed in section 2.5.1 (Wallach 1940). Visual theories must also be distinguished from the audiovisual reflex, an involuntary turning of the eyeballs to face the direction of the sound source (Paulsen and Ewertsen 1966), since this reflex must be preceded by at least a coarse awareness of the direction of the sound source. Shifts in the auditory event do occur, though, as the eyes are moved (Goldstein and Rosenthal-Veit 1926, Ryan and Schehr 1941, and, even earlier, Pierce 1901). A point of view expressed in this context by Güttich (1937) and Meyer zum Gottesberge (1940) may be at least partly valid, namely, that eye movements are indispensible if the most accurate agreement between the direction of the sound source and the directions of the auditory and visual events is to be achieved.

Vestibular theories   In vestibular theories it is assumed that the vestibular organ participates in spatial hearing. This means that one must investigate physical parameters correlated to the position of the auditory event that are processed by the vestibular organ, not just those that stimulate the cochlea.

The concept of the "vestibular organ" or "organ of balance" embraces those parts of the inner ear that are innervated by the pars vestibularis

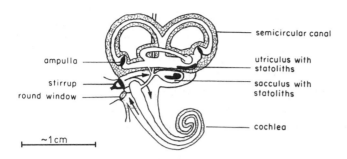

semicircular canal

ampulla

utriculus with statoliths

stirrup

sacculus with statoliths

round window

cochlea

~1cm

Figure 2.102
Simplified diagram of the inner ear showing the cochlea and vestibular organ (after de Burlet 1934).

of the nervus statoacustici (figure 2.102). These are the three semicircular canals, the utriculus, and the sacculus. The sensitive parts of the semicircular canals are the ampullar organs, and those of the utriculus and sacculus are the statolithic organs. For more details and further references see, for example, Bischof (1966) or Groen (1972).

We first offer a few notes about the input to the vestibular organ. Its adequate stimuli are mechanical forces: for the semicircular canals, angular accelerations and the resulting forces in the ampullar organs; for the statolithic organs, gravity, inertia, and centrifugal forces, from whatever direction they may be applied. There are a number of nonphysiological stimuli that are also possible, including the technique of caloric stimulation of the semicircular canals, which is widely used in otological practice. One way of applying this technique is to pour cold or warm liquid into the auditory canal. A temperature gradient results in the semicircular canals, and this leads to movement of the endolymph. A question that has often been debated, and is relevant here, is whether sound in the inner ear can stimulate the vestibular organ. Because of the mechanical character of sound and the particular anatomical position of the vestibular organ, this question does not appear at all inappropriate.

The output of the vestibular organ is the perception of the position and orientation of the head, as well as alterations of this perception, that is, percepts in terms of spatial coordinates. When the semicircular canal system, for example, is stimulated, subjects perceive themselves as turning with respect to their surroundings. Stronger stimuli to the semicircular canals also elicit involuntary rhythmic movements of the eyeballs, called nystagmus. Dizziness can also occur. When the head is not moving, the statolithic organs furnish the perception of the vertical (gravity). When the head is moving, they furnish, more generally, the perception of the head's position and of linear changes in its position.

In discussing the possible participation of the vestibular organ in forming the position of the auditory event, three cases may be crudely distinguished according to the type of stimulus:

1. Stimulation of the vestibular organ by means of normal head movements.
2. Nonphysiological stimulation, such as by means of strong accelerations or decelerations or by caloric means.
3. Stimulation by means of sound.

Section 2.5 may be recalled in connection with the first case. There it was confirmed that in forming the position of the auditory event, the auditory system evaluates alterations in the ear input signals during head movements. One way that head movements are registered is by means of the vestibular organ. In this sense the vestibular organ has an indirect effect on the forming of the position of the auditory event.

A number of publications discuss the second point. Münsterberg and Pierce (1894), Holt (1909), Frey (1912), Allers and Bénésy (1922), Clark and Graybiel (1949), Arnoult (1950), and Jongkees and van de Veer (1958) investigated directional hearing after suddenly stopping rotational movements effected using a rotating chair or a similar device. The subject experienced what might be called postrotational dizziness for a short time after the rotation was stopped. During this time the direction of the auditory event often shifted with respect to that of the sound source, usually in the opposite direction from the original rotation. Sometimes, though, it shifted in the same direction, or it oscillated. The same was true of visual events. After caloric stimulation (Rauch 1922, Güttich 1937, Jongkees and van de Veer 1958), changes in directional hearing were also observed—for example, increases in localization blur. The changes in spatial hearing that occur following strong rotational stimuli or caloric stimuli are clearly both due to the importance of the vestibular organ to the subject's sense of spatial orientation. Consequently they confirm the indirect influence of the vestibular organ on spatial hearing.

In the overall context of our subject it is a question of particular interest whether the vestibular organ has a direct as well as an indirect role in spatial hearing, that is, whether it not only registers body movements but also evaluates attributes of sound signals and so participates directly in the hearing process (the third point above). In the older literature (e.g., Preyer 1887, Arnheim 1887, Münsterberg 1889), but also more recently (e.g., Kraus 1953), the point of view has been expressed purely speculatively from time to time that forming the position of the auditory event might be partly a function of the vestibular organ. This hypothesis can be regarded by now as having been disproven. One fact pointing away from this hypothesis is that patients with totally nonfunctional vestibular organs but with normal or nearly normal hearing have no significant deficiencies in spatial hearing when compared with normal persons (Güttich 1937, 1939, 1940, Diamant 1946, Jongkees and van de Veer 1958).

On the other hand, it has been shown in a number of studies that very strong sound stimuli can elicit responses from the vestibular organ under experimental conditions. Tullio (1929), after exposing the semicircular canals of animals, was able to produce currents and turbulences of the lymph using sound as a stimulus. He observed nystagmus under these conditions. The same has been reported by von Békésy (1935), Retjö (1938), Trincker and Partsch (1957), and Jongkees (1953). Meurman and Meurman (1954) confirmed disturbances to spatial hearing in subjects whose semicircular canals had been surgically opened; these disturbances might possibly be related to sonic stimulation of the semicircular canals. Parker, von Gierke, and Reschke (1968), Reschke, Parker, and von Gierke (1970), and Parker and von Gierke (1971) have proven that responses in the semicircular canal system can be elicited by strong, low-frequency sound stimuli even when the inner ear has not been surgically modified. These articles contain further references to the literature. Bischoff (1966) lists several authors who also believe this to be true of the statolithic system.

Despite these findings, there are no confirmed results showing that the vestibular organ processes sound stimuli in the unmodified inner ear. All hypotheses of this type must be regarded as speculative.

Tactile theories   Tactile theories are doubtless the least substantial of all the theories mentioned up to this point. Tactile theories take into consideration not only sound at the eardrum but also sound presented to touch and vibration receptors as determining the position of the auditory event. Tactile regions that have been mentioned are those of the pinnae and of the hairs of the nape of the neck.

By locally anesthetizing the entire external ear, Güttich (1937) showed that tactile stimuli in the region of the pinna probably play a very small role. Perekalin (1930) and Blauert (1969a) covered the entire nape of the neck, or the entire head except the external ears, with felt and also had negative results. On the other hand, it is well known that sound leads to tactile perceptions under conditions of high intensity and low frequency. The spatial location of the tactile events is, however, not at the position of the auditory event but within the body. A special case occurs, to be sure, when the sound source is within the reach of the subject and can be felt with the hands. In this case, just as in that of visual theories, the rule of spatial complication may be applicable.

3 Spatial Hearing with Multiple Sound Sources and in Enclosed Spaces

Chapter 2 surveyed the functioning of spatial hearing when there is only one sound source and when sound waves can propagate freely in space. The topics examined there will now be generalized in two ways: to sound fields originating frcm multiple sound sources and to sound fields that cannot propagate freely (as in enclosed spaces in the presence of obstacles or reflecting surfaces).

According to the Huygens-Fresnel principle, any disturbed sound field can be conceived of as an undisturbed field generated by multiple elementary sound sources—in the limit, by an infinite number of such elementary sources. Spatial hearing in a disturbed sound field may thus be considered one example of the more general problem of spatial hearing of sound generated by multiple sources. This generalization is especially easy to understand in the case of reflections from planar surfaces that are large in comparison with the wavelength of the propagating sound. Here the sound field may be represented very simply as a superposition of the sound field of the original sound sources and that of (virtual) mirror-image sound sources (see figure 1.15).

When there are multiple sound sources, just as when there is only one, attributes of the sound signals at the eardrums are the subject's most important input. The communications channel from the sound source to the eardrum behaves linearly, in the sense of systems theory, in the range of levels of interest (L less than approximately 80–90 dB). Consequently the ear input signals can be described by a superposition of components originating with each individual sound source. In carrying out calculations, the transfer functions given in section 2.2.3, measured using one sound source, are still applicable. When there are n sound sources, $2n$ sound paths must be taken into consideration (figure 3.1).

The signals radiated from multiple sound sources may have identical time functions or may differ more or less from one another. The normalized cross-correlation function (Lee 1960, Fischer 1969) can be used as a formal mathematical index for the similarity of the waveforms of

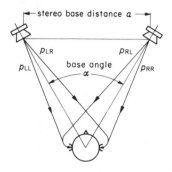

Figure 3.1
In calculating the ear input signals for n sound sources, $2n$ air paths must be taken into consideration. The example shows two loudspeakers in the standard stereophonic arrangement.

signals to each other. In its form for two alternating, unbiased signals, this function may be expressed as*

$$\Phi_{xy}(\tau) = \lim_{T \to \infty} \frac{\dfrac{1}{2T} \displaystyle\int_{-T}^{+T} x(t)y(t+\tau)\,\mathrm{d}t}{\dfrac{1}{2T}\sqrt{\displaystyle\int_{-T}^{+T} x^2(t)\,\mathrm{d}t \int_{-T}^{+T} y^2(t)\,\mathrm{d}t}} = \frac{\overline{x(t)y\,(t+\tau)}}{x_{\mathrm{rms}} \cdot y_{\mathrm{rms}}}. \tag{3.1}$$

Two signals whose normalized cross-correlation function has the absolute value 1 for any value of τ, that is, two functions for which

$$\max |\Phi_{xy}(\tau)| = 1, \tag{3.2}$$

will be called "coherent." This is somewhat different from the use of the word in other areas of science.† As defined here, two signals are coherent if they are identical, or if they differ only in one or more of the following ways:

1. Different amplitudes but the same waveform; that is, a level difference ΔL that is independent of frequency.

---

*This is the form for power signals, that is, for signals with finite power. For energy signals, that is, for signals with finite energy, the limit and the division by $1/(2T)$ are omitted, and the expression is integrated from $-\infty$ to $+\infty$.
†See Cremer (1976) for a more recent discussion of the use of the terms "coherence" and "correlation."

2. A pure delay of one with respect to the other; that is, a difference in phase delay τ_{ph} that is independent of frequency.
3. Inversion of one with respect to the other; that is, a phase difference of 180° or π radians. Note that the envelope of a signal is the same whether or not it is inverted; we therefore regard signals as coherent in this case.

Signals that differ in other ways are partially coherent or incoherent (section 3.2).

Superposition may be used to describe sound transmission only up to the eardrum when we are examining spatial hearing with multiple sound sources. The psychophysical relationships between attributes of the ear input signals and the positions of auditory events are, however, as a rule not describable in terms of linear systems. In particular, the auditory event or events that appear when there is more than one sound source are not superpositions of the individual events that would appear in connection with each individual sound source. When there are multiple sound sources, additional laws and rules apply to the auditory event; the phenomena on which these laws and rules are based do not occur when there is only one sound source.

3.1 Two Sound Sources Radiating Coherent Signals

The subject of this section is spatial hearing in the sound fields of two sound sources radiating coherent signals. These sound sources could be two loudspeakers driven by coherent electrical signals. In considering the auditory events that appear under these conditions, three important cases must be distinguished:

1. One auditory event appears at a position that depends on the positions of the two sound sources and the signals radiated by them.
2. One auditory event appears, but its position is determined by the position of and the signals radiated by only one of the two sound sources. The other sound source has no role in determining the position of the auditory event.
3. Two auditory events appear. The position of one depends more or less exclusively on the position of one sound source and on the signals it radiates; the position of the other depends on the other sound source and its signals.

The first case occurs when the levels and times of arrival of the two radiated signals differ only slightly. In establishing the position of the auditory event, the auditory system interprets the resulting two ear input signals approximately as if they arose at a single "phantom" sound source. The term "summing localization," as defined by Warncke (1941), is used in this case. The summing-localization effect provides the basis for the stereophonic sound transmission process with reproduction via loudspeakers (room-related stereophony). One special case of summing localization occurs when the loudspeaker signals are 180° out of phase.

If the signals differ by more than about 1 ms at the position of the listener, then the position of the auditory event is determined in most cases only by the position of and the signals radiated by the sound source whose signal arrives first. The signal components that arrive at the eardrum first are taken into consideration, and the later ones are suppressed in the interpretation process. This effect, especially important in architectural acoustics and electroacoustic sound reproduction technology, is called "the law of the first wavefront" (Cremer 1948). In the Anglo-American literature, summing localization and the law of the first wavefront are frequently subsumed under the term "precedence effect" (Wallach et al. 1949).

If the delay between the two signals exceeds a certain upper limit, which depends heavily on the experimental conditions, two auditory events appear one after the other. One is connected with each sound source. The second auditory event is called the echo of the first one.

Von Békésy (1971) described an effect contrary to the law of the first wavefront that he observed to occur when the delay between the two signals is approximately 70 ms. Such an effect would imply that the components of the ear input signals that arrive first are not used for evaluation, and only the later ones determine the position of the auditory event. This effect will be called "inhibition of the primary sound." It remains a largely unexplored subject at this time.

3.1.1 Summing localization

Figure 3.1 shows a sound source array normally used in reproducing stereophonic signals. Two loudspeakers are positioned in front of the subject, symmetrically with respect to the median plane. The angle α between the loudspeakers from the subject's position is usually about

60°. If both loudspeakers are driven with identical signals, the subject perceives a single auditory event in the median plane, as a rule at the front and, if the signal level is appropriate, at the distance of the loudspeakers. A delay or weakening of one of the two loudspeaker signals leads the auditory event to migrate from the middle toward the loudspeaker that is radiating the earlier or stronger signal.

It is possible, then, to place the direction of the auditory event within a specific range of azimuths at will by choosing the delay and level difference between the two loudspeaker signals generated by this array. Blumlein (1931) was the first to recognize the relevance of this possibility to electroacoustic communications technology. (Head-related or binaural stereophonic transmission, that is, with headphone reproduction, was introduced even earlier; for the early history of stereophony see Eichhorst (1959).) In 1933 a musical concert was transmitted stereophonically from Philadelphia to Washington; a two-loudspeaker array, among others, was used in reproduction (Fletcher 1934). Steinberg and Snow (1934) reported similar experiments in sound reproduction.

Beginning with de Boer (1940a,b), a number of authors have investigated the independent influence of time and level differences between the loudspeaker signals on the direction of the auditory event (e.g., Jordan 1954, Leakey 1959, Brittain and Leakey 1956, Hanson 1959, Franssen 1959, 1960, 1963, Wendt 1960a, 1963, 1964, Mertens 1960, 1965, Bauer 1960, 1961a, Harvey and Schroeder 1961, Ortmeyer 1966a,b; but see also Warncke 1941, Snow 1953, Sandel et al. 1955, Clark et al. 1957, Katzvey and Schröder 1958, Olson 1959, Kasynski and Ortmeyer 1961, Makita 1962).

Figures 3.2–3.4 show measured results for the relationship of a pure level difference or pure time difference between different types of loudspeaker signals and the direction of the auditory event. Figure 3.2 shows de Boer's classic curves (dashed lines). These are nearly linear for azimuth angles of approximately $\varphi < \pm 20°$ and for both level and time differences between the loudspeaker signals. The results of Wendt (1963) are also included. Especially for time differences, Wendt's curves are less linear and less steep; in some parts of his investigation, however, Wendt immobilized the subjects' heads. In other experiments in which the subjects were free to move their heads, Wendt obtained curves that largely agreed with de Boer's. Leakey (1957) also confirms that curves of summing localization are less steep when the head is immobilized

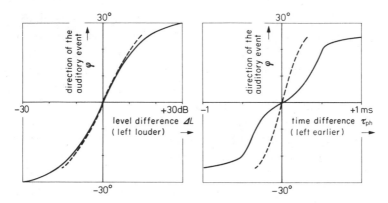

Figure 3.2
The direction of auditory events when the loudspeakers are arranged as in figure 3.1.
Left: Loudspeaker signal levels different from each other. Right: Loudspeaker signals
shifted in time relative to one another (after Wendt 1963). Dashed curves: Speech,
head free to move. Solid curves: Impulses, head immobilized, 10 subjects, $\alpha = 60°$,
anechoic chamber.

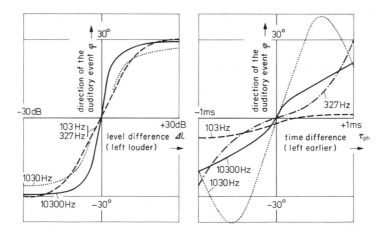

Figure 3.3
The direction of auditory events when the loudspeakers are arranged as in figure 3.1.
Left: Loudspeaker signal levels different from each other. Right: Loudspeaker signals
shifted in time relative to one another. 1/3-octave pulsed sinusoids similar to Gaus-
sian tone bursts, head immobilized, 10 subjects, $\alpha = 60°$, anechoic chamber (after
Wendt 1963).

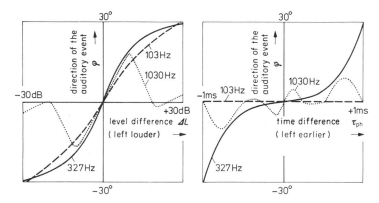

Figure 3.4
The direction of auditory events when the loudspeakers are arranged as in figure 3.1.
Left: Loudspeaker signal levels different from each other. Right: Loudspeaker signals
shifted in time relative to one another. Sinusoidal signals, head immobilized, 10 subjects, anechoic chamber, $\alpha = 60°$ (after Wendt 1963).

than when it is free to move. This is consistent with the observation
that the auditory event moves to some degree as the head is turned,
and in the same direction as the turning. Wendt's results apply to a
point source and an anechoic chamber. If a directional radiator is used
and the surroundings are not anechoic, results differ (Ortmeyer 1966a).

Figure 3.3 shows measurements made by Wendt using a 1/3-octave
pulses similar to a Gaussian tone burst. When a level difference is
introduced, the curve is approximately the same as for broadband
impulse sounds; however, the slope at the center depends on frequency.
Curves for 1/3-octave noise are similar. When a time difference is
introduced, the curves depend heavily on the center frequency of the
pulsed signals. Auditory events may in some cases appear outside the
range of angles bounded by the loudspeakers. Figure 3.4 shows
summing-localization curves for sustained sinusoids; it can be seen that
these curves are strongly dependent on frequency. Wendt could not
obtain useful results for frequencies above 1,030 Hz, apparently because
the directions reported by the subjects were too divergent.

Table 3.1 gives results that are useful in establishing a value for the
blur of summing localization. For each constellation of sound signals,
50 percent of the directions of auditory events appeared within the
given range of azimuth angles. A wide range indicates that the directions

Table 3.1
Data on summing-localization blur; shown are limits of intervals around the average angle $\bar{\varphi}$ in which 50 percent of the auditory event occurred for 10 or more subjects (calculated from results of Wendt 1963).

	Brief broadband impulses	Pulsed (Gaussian) signals				Sinusoidal signals		
		103 Hz	327 Hz	1,030 Hz	10.3 kHz	103 Hz	327 Hz	1,030 Hz
Loudspeaker signals with level differences of:								
0 dB	±1.3°	±2.5°	±2°	±2°	±8°	±3.5°	±3.5°	±5.5°
6 dB	±1.5°	±4°	±4°	±4.5°	±6°	—	—	—
12 dB	±3°	—	—	—	—	±5°	±5°	±10°
30 dB	±3.5°	±2.5°	±2.5°	±3.5°	±2°	±5.5°	±5.5°	±6°
Loudspeaker signals with pure time differences of:								
0 ms	±1.3°	±2.5°	±2°	±2°	±7.5°	±4.5°	±4.5°	±5.5°
0.3 ms	—	±3.5°	±6.5°	±6°	±5.5°	—	—	—
0.5 ms	±4.5°	—	—	—	—	±4°	±4.5°	±11°
1 ms	±6°	±6°	±7.5°	±5.5°	±4.5°	±7.5°	±8°	±11.5°

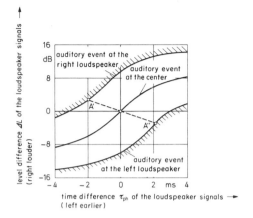

Figure 3.5
The direction of auditory events when the loudspeakers are arranged as in figure 3.1 and there are simultaneous time and level differences of the loudspeaker signals (after Franssen 1963).

of the auditory events as reported by the subject were highly divergent. There are two possible explanations for the divergence: Either the direction of the auditory event changes from one presentation to the next, or the auditory events are located imprecisely, that is, are smeared in space. It can be seen that, as a rule, the reported range of angles increases with increasing lateral displacement of the auditory event. Only with pulsed signals do exceptions to this rule sometimes occur.

Measured results examined to this point have to do with summing localization when there are only level differences or only time differences between the loudspeaker signals. If simultaneous level and time differences cooperate with each other (in other words, if the earlier signal is stronger), the lateral displacement of the auditory event is greater than it would be if only a time or a level difference were present. When level and time differences conflict, the displacement is smaller, or it is zero. These relationships can clearly be shown in a sort of nomogram (figure 3.5). Each point in the region between the two limit curves represents a combination of time and level differences between the loudspeaker signals and the azimuth angle of the auditory event in the range between the two loudspeakers. The line $A'-A''$ is a characteristic working line for a specific stereophonic transmission process. The curves in figure 3.5 apply to broadband signals. These curves have not yet

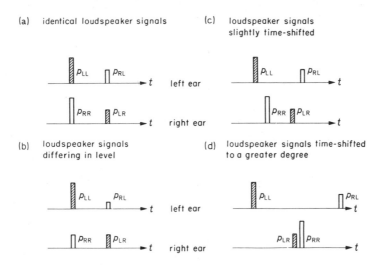

Figure 3.6
Ear input signals for brief impulses when the loudspeakers are arranged as in figure 3.1.

been sufficiently verified by measurement to be useful other than for qualitative study.

In order to understand how the phenomenon of summing localization comes about, it is necessary to analyze the ear input signals. Only an approximate analysis has been carried out, and only for certain specific types of signals. It is appropriate first to consider the ear input signals in the case where the loudspeakers radiate very short impulse sounds. Figure 3.6 shows the ear input signals corresponding to three cases: those of loudspeaker signals that are identical, that differ in level, and that differ in time. The impulses are indicated by rectangles. The nomenclature for the signal components is the one indicated in figure 3.1.

When the loudspeaker signals are identical, the ear input signals are as shown in figure 3.6a. Each signal consists of a component that originates at the loudspeaker on the near side and a second, delayed and attenuated component that originates at the loudspeaker on the far side. Both ear input signals are the same. The auditory event appears in the median plane. Part b illustrates the situation in which the levels of the two loudspeaker signals are different. The magnitude of the left loudspeaker signal is chosen to be twice that of the right signal. The positions of the components of the ear input signals in time are not different from those shown in part a, though their magnitudes differ. At the right ear the magnitude of the first component is smaller, and at the left ear the magnitude of the second component is smaller as compared with part a. Not only is the first signal component stronger, but also the total energy is greater at the left ear as compared with the right one. The auditory event appears to the left of the median plane.

Parts c and d illustrate cases in which the left loudspeaker radiates its signal earlier than the right loudspeaker. The time difference is smaller than the interaural delay in part c, and greater in part d. The position in time of the components of the ear input signals is no longer as it was in case a, though their magnitude is the same. The earliest signal component is still found at the left ear and originates at the left loudspeaker. When the time difference is small, the earlier component at the right ear originates at the right loudspeaker; when the time difference is greater, it originates at the left loudspeaker. In both cases the auditory event is displaced to the left of the median plane—more so in case d than in case c.

The influence of the individual signal components on the direction of the auditory event might also be investigated. Synthetically generated groups of impulses might, for example, be presented over headphones. The individual signal components would then be variable at will. Investigations of this type have been carried out by von Békésy (1930a), Wallach, Newman, and Rosenzweig (1949), Guttman, van Bergeijk, and David (1960), David and Hanson (1962), Harris, Flanagan, and Watson (1963), Sayers and Toole (1964), Toole and Sayers (1965a,b), and Guttman (1965). Some of the results from these works will now be discussed briefly as they relate specifically to summing localization.

A study of figure 3.6 might lead to the hypothesis that the direction of the auditory event is determined only by the signal components that arrive first at the two ears. The problem would then be the same as that of directional hearing with one sound source, since the direction of the auditory event could be determined from the time and level differences between whichever signal components arrived first. The actual case is more complicated, since the second components of the signal can also participate in determining the position of the auditory event. This can be shown using an auditory experiment described by Wallach, Newman, and Rosenzweig (1949), in which the signal sequence shown in figure 3.7a was presented to the subject. The first impulses

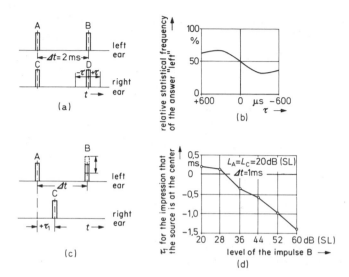

Figure 3.7
Lateralization experiments investigating summing localization with impulse-type signals. a: Signal combinations with two ear signal components each. b: Relative statistical frequency of the answer "left" as a function of the position in time of the impulse D in signal combination a (after Wallach, Newman, and Rosenzweig 1949). c: Signal combinations with an impulse pair at the left and a single impulse at the right. d: The time shift of the impulse C relative to the impulse A necessary to create the impression that a sound source is at the center, as a function of the level of the impulse B in signal combination c (after Guttman, van Bergeijk, and David 1960).

reached both ears at the same time, but the second component was either delayed or advanced at the right ear in comparison with the left ear. The auditory event was displaced from the median plane. The relative number of "left" judgments is shown in part b. The average time interval between the first and second groups of impulses was 2 ms.

A number of experiments that lead to some significant conclusions have been carried out using a combination of three impulses; one impulse was presented to one ear, and two were presented to the other (figure 3.7c). One task presented to subjects was to adjust the timing of the C impulse, τ_1, so that the auditory event appeared in the median plane. Guttman et al. (1960) varied the level of the B impulse and determined that the τ_1 necessary to position the auditory event in the median plane varied as shown in part d. Thus the level as well as the timing of the second ear input signal is of importance in summing localization.

Harris et al. (1963) used the same experimental procedure, except that they held the levels of A, B, and C constant and equal. They varied Δt instead of the level. Within the range of interest with regard to summing localization—that is, for values of Δt under approximately 1 ms—the subjects found two positions at which the auditory event appeared in the median plane: $\tau_1 = 0$ and $\tau_1 = \Delta t$. The authors expressly note that only one auditory event was perceived. This was, however, not sharply located in space but had two "centers of gravity," either of which could be brought into the median plane.

The experiments of Toole and Sayers (1965a,b) led to further observations of this type. In these experiments, too, one impulse was presented to one ear and a pair of impulses was presented to the other. The subjects' task, however, was not to adjust τ_1 to bring the auditory event into the median plane. Rather, they were asked to evaluate the lateral displacement of the auditory event as τ_1 was continuously changed by the person conducting the experiment. When this was the task, the subjects could, after some practice, clearly distinguish different components of the auditory event, following different paths in space as τ_1 was varied. Two components were particularly easy to distinguish: a "low-pitched" component whose path was determined by the positions of the A and B impulses relative to the C impulses, and a "high-pitched" component whose lateral displacement was determined only by the relative position of the A and C impulses.

We shall omit the details, but it can be established that the first signal components to arrive at the ears, as well as the later ones, play a role in summing localization with impulse-shaped signals. However, the direction of the auditory event can be determined only approximately from figure 3.2. A more precise analysis shows that the auditory events possess a complicated spatial structure.

The discussion so far has been limited to cases in which the sound source radiates only very brief, broadband impulses. Only in these cases can the ear input signals also be approximated as series of very brief impulses. The next case to be considered, the summing localization of sinusoidal signals, will go to the other extreme. The ear input signals corresponding to this case have been calculated approximately by Leakey (1959), Wendt (1963, 1965), and others. Here we shall only outline the quantitative analytical approach employed and discuss four examples that can be understood without the mathematical details. As shown in figure 3.1, the sound pressure generated at the left ear by the left loud-speaker is called $p_{LL}(t)$. The two loudspeaker signals differ by a frequency-independent phase delay $\tau_{ph}*$ and by a frequency-independent real amplitude factor q. The sound pressure generated at the right ear by the right loudspeaker is then

$$p_{RR}(t) = q p_{LL}(t - \tau_{ph}*). \tag{3.3}$$

When $\tau_{ph}*$ is positive, $p_{RR}(t)$ arrives later at the ear facing the source than does $p_{LL}(t)$, according to the equation written in this form. The sound pressure components at the ear facing away from the source may be derived as

$$p_{LR}(t) = |A(f)| p_{LL}[t - \tau_{ph}(f)], \tag{3.4}$$

$$p_{RL}(t) = q |A(f)| p_{LL}[t - \tau_{ph}* - \tau_{ph}(f)]. \tag{3.5}$$

In these equations $|A(f)|$ and $\tau_{ph}(f)$ are the magnitude and phase delay of the interaural transfer function for the angle of sound incidence of the loudspeakers, that is, for $\varphi = \alpha/2$.

With $\tau_{ph}* = b*/2\pi f$ and $\tau_{ph}(f) = b/2\pi f$, and using complex notation, we find

$$\underline{p}_{LL} = \hat{p}, \tag{3.6}$$

$$\underline{p}_{RR} = \hat{p} q e^{-jb*}; \tag{3.7}$$

Consequently the total ear input signals can be represented as

$$\underline{p}_{left} = \underline{p}_{LL} + \underline{p}_{RL} = \hat{p}[1 + q|A(f)|e^{-j(b*+b)}], \tag{3.8}$$

$$\underline{p}_{right} = \underline{p}_{RR} + \underline{p}_{LR} = \hat{p}[q e^{-jb*} + |A(f)|e^{-jb}]. \tag{3.9}$$

The solutions to these equations are, of course, sinusoids since we are dealing with a linear system.

Since $|A(f)|$ is almost exactly unity at low frequencies, a surprising result follows: A difference in the levels of the loudspeaker signals at low frequencies leads only to a time difference between the ear input signals, and conversely, a time difference between the loudspeaker signals leads only to a level difference between the ear input signals. The two phasor diagrams at the left in figure 3.8 clarify this situation. In part a the right loudspeaker signal is taken as having twice the amplitude

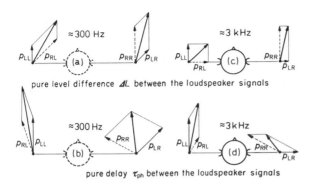

pure level difference ΔL between the loudspeaker signals

pure delay τ_{ph} between the loudspeaker signals

Figure 3.8
Phasor diagrams of the ear input signals for summing localization with sinusoids.
a, b: Level or time difference between the loudspeaker signals, low signal frequency,
no interaural attenuation. c, d: Level or time difference between the loudspeaker signals, medium signal frequency, interaural attenuation taken into consideration.

of the left loudspeaker signal. Interaural attentuation is 0, since $|A(f)|$
$= 1$. It can be seen that the resulting phasor differs only with respect
to phase. In part b the amplitudes of the loudspeaker signals are equal,
but the right signal is radiated earlier. The resulting phasors have the
same phase but different amplitudes. Note that in this special case the
ear input signal on the side of the lagging loudspeaker may even be
the stronger one!

The two phasor diagrams at the right in figure 3.8 are examples of
relationships at higher frequencies, at which interaural attenuation must
be taken into consideration. It can be seen that level differences and
time differences between the loudspeaker signals both lead to combinations of level and phase changes in the ear input signals. Evaluation
of equations 3.8 and 3.9 using measured values of $|A(f)|$ and $\tau_{ph}(f)$
shows that for sinusoids, a relationship between loudspeaker signals
and ear input signals, useful for stereophonics, exists only below about
800 Hz. Most characteristics of the summing-localization curves in
figure 3.4 can be explained in this way.

Since this author knows of no analysis of summing localization gen-
eralizable to all signals, only speculation can be presented here. It can
be stated with some certainty that the ear input signals are dissected
spectrally in the inner ears into components of approximately constant
relative bandwidth. Interaural differences are apparently evaluated sep-

arately for the different spectral components. As was shown in section 2.4.3, interaural differences in the fine structure of signals are most important for low-frequency components, and interaural differences between the envelopes are most important for high-frequency components. In this context the summing-localization curves for pulsed signals of constant relative bandwidth (figure 3.3) are seen to be similar to those for sinusoids if the center frequency is low, and similar to those for impulses if the center frequency is high.

Calculation of interaural differences between low-frequency spectral components is similar to that for sinusoids. The methods of Leakey (1959) and Mertens (1960, 1965) should be mentioned in connection with the calculation of interaural differences at higher frequencies. Leakey gives approximations for interaural envelope shifts, and Mertens calculates the interaural time differences between energy peaks for Gaussian tone bursts.

After the interaural signal characteristics of interest have been determined for all important spectral components, it is still necessary to determine the dominant direction of the auditory event. The rules that apply in this situation are still largely unknown, and there is some indication that interaural signal attributes in the middle frequency range (0.5–2 kHz) dominate the average direction of the auditory event for signals whose energy is constant with frequency (Flanagan, David, and Watson 1962, 1964, Toole and Sayers 1965a). However, it should be recalled at this point that the constellation of auditory events may be quite complicated in summing-localization situations. It is by no means certain that a single, precisely located auditory event will occur. Careful evaluation by trained listeners reveals multiple or split auditory events in the majority of cases.

Summing localization, of course, is not limited to the arrangement of sound sources shown in figure 3.1. An auditory event whose position depends on several sound sources at once can appear in connection with two or more sound sources placed anywhere, as long as their time and level differences at the position of the subject do not exceed certain limits. The cases examined up to this point can be taken as examples of how lateral directions are established via the process of summing localization. We now offer two additional examples of summing localization relative to directional hearing in the median plane.

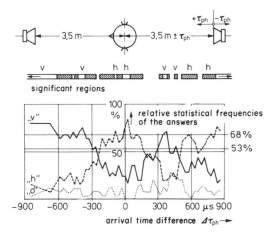

Figure 3.9
On summing localization in the median plane. Top: The experimental arrangement;
the loudspeakers radiate identical signals. Bottom: Relative statistical frequencies of
the answers "front" (*v*), "back" (*h*), and "overhead" (*o*); 25 subjects. Signals: 1.7 s
white-noise pulses (after Blauert 1971, scales defined as in figure 2.45b). Similar
curves are obtained using music and speech as signals.

The top part of figure 3.9 shows an experimental arrangement in
which a subject is positioned in an anechoic chamber exactly halfway
between two loudspeakers, one at the front ($\varphi = 0°$, $\delta = 0°$) and the
other at the rear ($\varphi = 180°$, $\delta = 0°$). The subject's head is immobilized.
Both loudspeakers are driven with identical broadband signals. The
distance of the rear loudspeaker may be varied by ±30 cm. At the
position of the subject a delay difference of ±880 μs may be generated
in this way between the signals that arrive from the front and rear
loudspeakers. The level difference that is unintentionally generated at
the same time is under 0.5 dB and can be ignored in this case. The
auditory events appear in the median plane, since the signals that arrive
at both ears are largely identical. If the rear loudspeaker is moved and
the subject is asked to report the direction of the auditory event, then,
using the scale of judgments from figure 2.45, the result is the distribution
of answers shown as a function of delay in figure 3.9. The ranges in
which one of the three possible answers is more probable than the
other two together are shown at the top of the graph. It should be
emphasized that subjects were asked to identify only the direction of

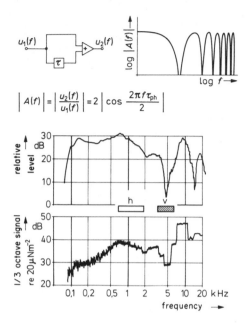

$$\left| A(f) \right| = \left| \frac{u_2(f)}{u_1(f)} \right| = 2 \left| \cos \frac{2\pi f \tau_{ph}}{2} \right|$$

Figure 3.10
Top: Magnitude of the transfer function (in terms of level) for a system with one reflection. Bottom: Transfer function of the experimental apparatus and 1/3-octave level diagram of the test signal at the position of the subject for $\tau_{ph} = -111\ \mu s$. Also indicated are two important directional bands. In 60 percent of the cases the auditory event appeared behind the subject.

whichever component of the auditory event was dominant. Changes in the extent and distance of the auditory event were not examined.

The results shown in figure 3.9 can be explained as follows. The electroacoustic system used in the experiment includes a delay element, due to different air paths from the speakers to the subjects, as shown schematically at the top of figure 3.10. The transfer function of this system is characteristic of a comb filter. The amplitude of the transfer function in log-log coordinates is also shown at the top of the figure. The positions of the maxima and minima are a function of τ_{ph}, as set by the distance of the rear loudspeaker. In section 2.3.1 it was shown that the direction of auditory events in the median plane is formed on the basis of the spectrum of the ear input signals. It may therefore be assumed that the transfer function of the electroacoustic system used in this experiment is responsible for the results shown in figure 3.9;

the positions of the maxima and minima of the amplitude of the transfer function as a function of τ_{ph} would be of special significance. In figure 3.10 this assumption is confirmed for one specific case (for further examples see Blauert 1971. Somerville et al. 1966 report related effects).

Another example of summing localization in directional hearing in the median plane uses the standard stereophonic loudspeaker arrangement of figure 3.1. In auditory experiments using this arrangement the auditory event frequently appears at a certain angle of elevation δ rather than in the horizontal plane. If the subject moves toward the loudspeakers in the plane of symmetry of the array, the auditory event becomes elevated by a greater angle; when the subject is exactly midway between the loudspeakers, the auditory event appears directly overhead (δ = 90°). In the literature this is called the "elevation effect."

Early explanations of the elevation effect were based on motional theories (section 2.5.1). For example, de Boer (1946, 1947) and Wendt (1963) showed that when the head is turned through an angle α with respect to a two-loudspeaker array, the changes in the interaural level and time differences between the ear input signals are similar to those that occur when a single sound source is elevated through an angle δ = α/2. The relationship

$$\left(\frac{d\tau_{ph}}{d\gamma}\right)_{\gamma=0} = -\text{const} \cdot \cos\frac{\alpha}{2} = -\text{const} \cdot \cos\delta, \tag{3.10}$$

for example, approximates the changes in interaural time difference when the head is rotated out of the plane of symmetry by an angle γ.

An elevation effect also occurs when subjects do not turn their heads, and the effect must then be explained in terms of the spectrum of the ear input signals. Damaske (1969/70) investigated this case in detail. He also used a two-loudspeaker array symmetrical about the subject's median plane. The base angle could be varied between 0° and 360°. The loudspeakers, in other words, could be moved in an arc around the subject in the horizontal plane, one on the left side and one on the right. The subjects were expressly instructed to keep their heads still. The results are shown in figure 3.11. The solid line shows the measured directions of the auditory event; the dashed line represents a prediction based on the spectra of the ear input signals and their relationship to the directional bands.

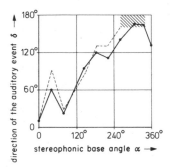

Figure 3.11
The direction of the auditory event's "center of gravity" as a function of the stereo-phonic base angle α of an arrangement such as that shown in figure 3.1 (after Da-maske 1969/70). Test signals: Noise, 0.65–4.5 kHz. Solid line: Average values for ten subjects. Dashed line: Prediction according to the energy distribution in the directional bands.

Finally, we examine the case in which two loudspeakers in the standard stereophonic arrangement radiate broadband signals that are identical but 180° out of phase. Several particularly striking effects are then observed (see, e.g., Sandel et al. 1955, Schodder 1956b, Lauridsen and Schlegel 1956, Hanson and Kock 1957, Jeffress 1957, Leakey 1957, Lochner and Burger 1958, Mertens 1965, Scherer 1966, Keibs 1966, Gardner 1969b, Plenge 1971b, 1972). The auditory event splits up into at least two components of different tone colors. A "low-pitched" com-ponent is located more or less diffusely near or inside the back of the subject's head. If the head is moved slightly from side to side, the place where this component is strongest moves in an arc around the back of the head in the same direction as the head is moved. The perception of this component of the auditory event is linked with an unpleasant feeling of pressure. A "high-pitched" component appears at the usual position between the loudspeakers and is often the less noticeable of the two. If the head is moved more than a small amount, other peculiar effects occur, but these will not be described here. The effects that have been described occur when the signals include components below ap-proximately 2 kHz. If the signals are high-pass-filtered, the subject is not aware whether the wires to one of the loudspeakers have been reversed.

A closer look at the sound field generated by loudspeakers 180° out of phase in a standard stereophonic arrangement reveals the following properties:

1. If the head is immobilized exactly in the median plane, the ear input signals are 180° out of phase at all frequencies. Consequently $\tau_{gr}(f) = d\pi/d2\pi f = 0$, and $\tau_{ph}(f) = \pi/2\pi f$ decreases as the frequency increases (see figure 2.66).*
2. Sound pressure in the plane of symmetry between the loudspeakers is zero at all frequencies, representing an interference minimum. By means of small, sideward movements of the head, the subject can, at will, place the entrance to the left or right ear canal into the plane of symmetry of the loudspeakers.

The auditory effects that occur in connection with this experimental situation can be explained at least partly in terms of the foregoing attributes of the sound field. In connection with point 1, the auditory system evaluates interaural envelope shifts of components at frequencies above approximately 1.6 kHz; but in this case the envelopes of both ear input signals are identical. Time differences in the fine structure of the signal are evaluated for frequency components below 1.6 kHz, and in this case these time differences increase as the frequency is lowered. These facts explain why the auditory events connected with high-pass-filtered signals are the same whether the ear input signals are in or out of phase, and also why the dull-sounding components of the auditory event appear to be spatially diffuse.

In connection with point 2, by moving the head slightly the subject can place one ear in the plane of symmetry and make the signal at that ear largely disappear. A signal is still present at the other ear. This is similar to the situation in which a sound source is placed near the other ear. Small head movements can reverse the situation with respect to the two ears. According to Hanson and Kock (1957), this fact may explain why the auditory event appears inside or close to the head. When the head is immobilized, in fact, the auditory event appears not close to the head but diffusely behind the subject.

---

*The same is true for other frequency-independent phase shifts between the loudspeaker signals, including, for example, the Hilbert transform, which has a 90° phase shift. However, the signals are not coherent in the sense of equation 3.2 if the phase shift is other than 0° or 180°.

Further characteristics of the ear input signals when the loudspeaker signals are 180° out of phase, including cancellation of the lower frequencies or dips and peaks in the spectrum due to interference, have not yet been investigated systematically with respect to their effect on the position of the auditory event.

3.1.2 The law of the first wavefront

The following discussion, once again, assumes two loudspeakers in the standard stereophonic arrangement of figure 3.1. It is further assumed that both loudspeakers radiate nonperiodic, coherent signals. As long as both signals are radiated simultaneously and at the same level, the auditory event appears exactly in front. If one of the signals is delayed, with the delay increasing continuously from $\tau_{ph} = 0$, the direction of the auditory event migrates toward whichever loudspeaker radiates the earlier signal. This phenomenon was discussed in the last section. When the delay time is 630 μs $< \tau_{ph} < 1$ ms, the auditory event will have reached the position of the loudspeaker radiating the earlier signal. If the delay time is increased beyond 1 ms, it can be established that the direction of the auditory event remains nearly constant. The position is then determined primarily by the components of the ear input signals originating with the loudspeaker that radiates its signal first. Cremer (1948) called this effect the "law of the first wavefront." It is of great importance to phenomena pertinent to hearing in enclosed spaces.

Several common terms from room acoustics will be useful here: The "primary sound" S_0 is the signal radiated first, and the "reflection" S_T is the delayed signal. The term reflection is used because the delayed signal corresponds to one that would appear if the primary signal were reflected from a surface.

The law of the first wavefront has been known for many years. According to Gardner (1968c), the first published account of the phenomenon was given by Henry (1849). The law is applicable to sound-source arrangements other than the standard stereophonic arrangement, and it seems to be applicable to all directions of sound incidence. Only for directions in the median plane are there observations inconsistent with this law (Somerville et al. 1966, Blauert 1971, Wagener 1971, Kuhl and Plantz 1972). Wagener's work is especially valuable. It includes thorough topographic data for auditory events occurring in connection with a primary sound from the front when the reflections are from various directions in the upper hemisphere and at various levels and delay times.

The transition to summing localization defines the lower boundary of the range of delay times to which the law of the first wavefront is applicable. This boundary may be regarded as the delay time at which the direction of the auditory event undergoes a just-noticeable change. For the standard stereophonic loudspeaker arrangement and with signals of equal level this boundary lies between 630 μs and 1 ms. There is also an upper boundary for delay times to which the law is applicable, but the threshold at the upper boundary is more difficult to define. As the delay time is increased, a considerable number of changes occur in the auditory event, of which the change in direction is only one. The change audible at any particular delay time depends strongly on the type of signal, the level, and the direction of sound incidence.

In order to arrive at a definition of a threshold, one might ask whether the auditory event exhibits any particular attribute that allows an inference that a reflection is present in addition to the primary sound. For example, a test might be conducted by switching the reflection off and on and listening for audible differences. Such a threshold of perception for reflections, based on the criterion of a change in the auditory event without regard to the specific type of change, was defined by Seraphim (1961), who gave it the name "absolute threshold of perceptibility" (absolute Wahrnehmbarkeitsschwelle: aWs); it is more widely known as the "masked threshold."* However, when the level of the reflection is equal to that of the primary sound, the reflection exceeds this absolute perceptual threshold regardless of the delay time. For example, if $\tau_{ph} \geq 1$ ms, the reflection is noticeable in that the auditory event is louder and has a greater spatial extent than when the reflection is not present. If the reflection is to be "absolutely" inaudible, its level must be decreased with respect to that of the primary sound. The masked threshold, consequently, can be defined as the level difference between the primary sound and the reflection at which the reflection becomes "absolutely" audible. For the case in which a single

---

*Masking is defined as a process whereby the threshold of audibility of one sound event is raised by another sound event (the masker). When the event being masked and the masker do not occur at the same time, the situation is called forward or backward masking (resp. premasking or postmasking) depending on whether the masker occurs before or after the event being masked.

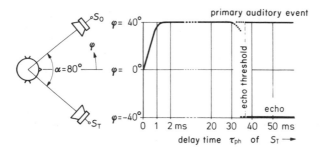

Figure 3.12
Paths of the directions of the auditory events as a function of the delay of the reflection; illustrated schematically for speech of average speed and a level of the primary sound equal to that of the reflection (approximately 50 dB).

reflection is present, this threshold has been measured with reference to the type of signal, the direction of sound incidence, and the delay time by Burgtorf (1961), Burgtorf and Oehlschlegel (1964), and Schubert (1966), as well as Seraphim (1961). In the context of interest to us here, involving the directon of the auditory events and the attributes of the reflection, the masked threshold is of secondary importance. We shall state here only that this threshold exhibits the lowest values of any threshold of perceptibility for attributes of reflections.

In seeking a more appropriate definition for a threshold, we might once again increase the delay beyond 1 ms. The signal will be taken to be speech at average speed, with the primary sound and reflection at the same level. The reflection is already audible when $\tau_{ph} = 1$ ms, since the auditory event is louder and has a greater extent in space than when the primary sound is presented alone. As the delay time is increased, further changes in the auditory event are noticeable. The tone color of the auditory event changes, and its spatial extent increases. Moreover, the "center of gravity" of the auditory event may sometimes shift somewhat toward the direction of incidence of the reflection. When a certain delay time is exceeded, the auditory event finally separates into two events in different directions. The direction of the first event is determined by the primary sound and generally agrees with the direction of incidence of the primary sound. The second auditory event generally appears in the direction of incidence of the reflection. We call the second auditory event the "echo" of the first one and the shortest delay time at which the second auditory event becomes audible the

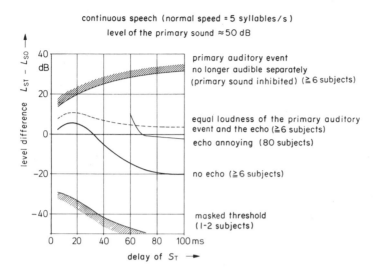

Figure 3.13
A comparison of various thresholds for reflections; standard stereophonic loudspeaker arrangement, base angle $\alpha = 80°$ (data of Haas 1951, Meyer and Schodder 1952, Burgtorf 1961, Seraphim 1961).

threshold of perceptibility of the echo, or the "echo threshold." Figure 3.12 illustrates this definition of the echo threshold.

The echo threshold represents a sensible way of indicating the upper limit of validity for the law of the first wavefront. This threshold has been measured under differing experimental conditions by Haas (1951), Meyer and Schodder (1952), Lochner and Burger (1958), Kietz (1959), Burgtorf (1961), Thurlow and Marten (1962), Boerger (1965a,b), and Damaske (1971a), among others.

Related definitions might be based on the criterion "primary auditory event and echo equally loud" (see, e.g., Haas 1951, Meyer and Schodder 1952, Snow 1954, Lochner and Burger 1958, David 1959, Franssen 1959, 1960, 1963, David and Hanson 1962) or the criterion "echo annoying" (see, e.g., Bolt and Doak 1950, Haas 1951, Muncey, Nickson, and Dubout 1953). Compare also the "threshold of indistinction" defined by Petzold (1927), Stumpp (1936), and others.

Figure 3.13 shows the different thresholds as measured using the standard stereophonic loudspeaker arrangement, with $\alpha = 80°$, speech presented at a rate of approximately 5 syllables per second, and the

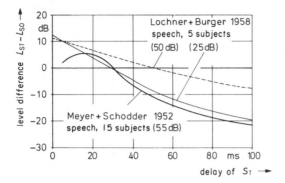

Figure 3.14
Echo thresholds for continuous speech of average speed ($\approx$ 5 syllables/s); standard
stereophonic loudspeaker arrangement, base angle $\alpha = 80°$.

level of the primary sound approximately 50 dB at the position of the
subject. The lowest threshold values (i.e., the lowest levels of reflection)
are for the masked threshold. The level that corresponds to the echo
threshold is considerably higher than that for the masked threshold. If
the delay time is less than approximately 32 ms, the level of the reflection
can even be as much as 5 dB higher than that of the primary sound
without the echo becoming audible. The curve of equal loudness for
the primary auditory event and the echo is, again, at a higher level
than the echo threshold, though their shapes are similar. At a delay
time of 15 ms, the reflection must be more than 10 dB stronger than
the primary sound to lead to an equally loud auditory event. The echo
is perceived as annoying at threshold values that intersect the curve of
equal loudness at a delay time of approximately 65 ms and increase
sharply as the delay time is decreased. At delay times less than 50 ms,
echoes are no longer perceived as annoying even if the reflection is
considerably stronger than the primary sound. This is known as the
"Haas effect," due to its description by Haas (1951). The level above
which the primary auditory event disappears is shown in the uppermost
curve. This curve will be discussed further in section 3.1.3.

In measuring the echo threshold, it is important that the threshold
criterion be thoroughly discussed and settled with the subjects. Figure
3.14 gives results of several measurements of the echo threshold. Meyer
and Schodder (1952) used the criterion "echo barely inaudible," Lochner

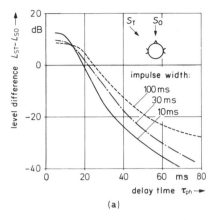 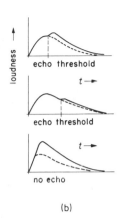

(a)   (b)

Figure 3.15
a: Echo thresholds for noise pulses of various durations (Damaske 1971a; level of the primary sound not given, direction of incidence of S_0 from the front, S_T from left front or right front, 1 subject). b: Sketches illustrating a hypothesis of Damaske (1971a) that the echo is audible whenever the curvature of the time function of total loudness exceeds a certain positive threshold value.

and Burger the criterion "echo clearly audible." This is apparently one of the reasons why Meyer and Schodder's curve, measured using the same level of the primary sound, is lower than that of Lochner and Burger. The criteria used also explain the marked discrepancies between the curves at short delay times. Meyer and Schodder's subjects regarded the echo as audible even when it could not be heard as a separate auditory event; what was recognizable was a change in direction of the primary auditory event. In other words, the criterion changed when summing localization came into play. Lochner and Burger's curves, on the other hand, represent the echo threshold more accurately as we define it in this book. They also show that the echo threshold depends on the level of the primary sound.

Damaske (1971) investigated the echo threshold for noise pulses as a function of pulse width (figure 3.15a). However, he did not use the standard stereophonic arrangement but, rather, incidence from the front for the primary sound and from the side, near the front, for the reflection. Meyer and Schodder's threshold criteria were used. At delay times below approximately 15 ms, increasing impulse width leads to a decrease in the threshold value; at delay times over 15 ms they lead to an increase. At τ_{ph} greater than 15 ms, dependence of the echo threshold

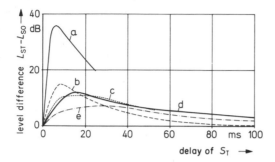

Figure 3.16
Curves of equal loudness of the primary auditory event and the echo for various
types of signals. Curve a: High-pass filtered clicks (400 Hz, 60 dB, several subjects;
after David and Hanson 1962). Curve b: Speech (50 dB, 5 subjects; after Lochner and
Burger 1958). Curve c: Speech (50 dB, 15 subjects; after Hass 1951). Curve d: Speech
(55 dB, 20 subjects; after Meyer and Schodder 1952). Curve e: Pulsed sinusoids (50
dB, 100 ms, 5 subjects; after Lochner and Burger 1958).

on the level of the primary sound (Lochner and Burger) and on the
impulse width (Damaske) is similar, if the loudness of the auditory
event is used as a parameter in both cases.

Damaske (1971) hypothesized that loudness as a function of time
can serve as a basis for criteria for pinpointing when an echo becomes
perceptible. Figure 3.15b shows several time functions of loudness calculated according to an analog model constructed by Zwicker (1968).
The solid lines represent the primary sound and reflection together;
the dashed curve represents the case in which the reflection is not
present. Damaske's hypothesis is that an echo always appears when
the curvature of the loudness function exceeds a certain positive threshold value.

Figure 3.13 made it clear that the curve of equal loudness between
the primary auditory event and the echo is similar to the echo-threshold
curve; the former, however, is at a higher level. Figure 3.16 shows
several curves of equal loudness corresponding to different types of
signals. It may be hypothesized that the relationships shown in this
figure apply also to the echo threshold. For example, the maximum of
the curve is higher and occurs at a lower delay time as the signals
become more impulse-like. In fact, this relationship is similar to the
one derived from the measurements of Damaske (1971), and it, too,
can be explained in terms of the loudness time functions.

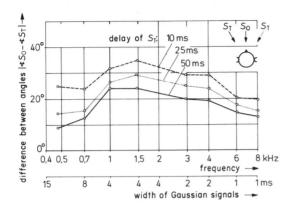

Figure 3.17
Echo thresholds corresponding to different angles between the primary sound and the reflection as a function of frequency for critical-band-wide Gaussian tone bursts (4 subjects, level of the primary sound equal to that of the reflection, 75 dB peak level at 1 kHz, and equally loud at other frequencies; after Boerger 1965a,b).

The echo threshold depends not only on the type of signals presented, but also on the delay time of the reflection and on the level of the primary sound. These relationships can be seen in the curves already discussed. The directions of sound incidence are also important parameters. Their importance becomes clear when it is considered that the primary sound and the reflection undergo linear distortions on their way to the eardrums—distortions that depend on the direction of sound incidence. Boerger (1965a,b) measured the dependence of the echo threshold on the direction of sound incidence. A fixed loudspeaker at the front radiated Gaussian tone bursts one critical band wide. A second loudspeaker could be moved continuously through a range of angles in the horizontal plane. This second loudspeaker radiated the reflection, with delay times set at $\tau_{ph} = 10$, 25, and 50 ms. Figure 3.17 shows the minimum azimuth at which an echo became audible. Measurements were also taken with the primary sound incident from $\varphi = 25°$; the resulting curves were different.

The law of the first wavefront—that is, the fact that the reflection is not taken into consideration in forming the direction of the auditory event—points to the existence of inhibitory processes in hearing. Clearly components of the ear input signals that originate with the reflection are not fully evaluated; in one way or another, their evaluation is totally or partially suppressed. The term "masking" may also be used in this context, in those cases where the reflection becomes absolutely inaudible. Conclusions about details of inhibitory processes can be gained by means of auditory experiments using dichotic presentation over headphones. Several relevant works will now be discussed.

One interesting special case occurs when the primary sound is presented only to one ear, and the reflection only to the other. This condition can be easily arranged using dichotic headphone presentation; and in a particular range of delay times, the law of the first wavefront holds true. Just as with symmetrical sound presentation in a free sound field, the lower boundary of the range of validity lies between 630 μs and 1 ms. The processes that occur below this range were discussed in section 2.4.1. The upper boundary, again, is established by the echo threshold. Measured results of the echo threshold under these conditions are assembled in table 3.2.

The smallest echo thresholds are for single clicks. Under some conditions these thresholds are less than 2 ms. The threshold depends on the level; as the signal level is raised, the delay time at which an echo appears becomes shorter. For ongoing signals the delay time representing the echo threshold is longer than for single impulses. For speech it is approximately 20 ms. The steeper the slopes of the signals, the shorter the delay time at which the auditory event dissociates into a primary auditory event and an echo. This statement agrees with the observation that narrow-band noise of constant relative bandwidth produces an echo at a shorter delay time the higher the center frequency (figure 3.18). If the level of the reflection is raised with respect to that of the primary sound, the echo appears at a shorter delay time (figure 3.19); if the level of the reflection is lowered, it appears at a longer delay time (Blodgett, Wilbanks, and Jeffress 1956; Babkoff and Sutton 1966).

The validity of the law of the first wavefront even when the primary sound is presented to one ear and the reflection to the other indicates that contralateral inhibitory processes are at work. Reception of a signal by one ear leads to an inhibition of signal reception at the other ear. It may be assumed that these contralateral inhibitions also play an important role when sound is presented in a free sound field. Evidence confirming this assumption includes the fact that the delay time corresponding to the echo threshold is greater for ongoing signals than for single impulses and that this relationship holds true for the primary

Table 3.2
Survey of measurements of the upper limit of the range of validity of the law of the first wavefront with dichotic headphone presentation (primary sound on the left, reflection on the right, or vice versa: level of the primary sound equal to that of the reflection).

Reference	Signal	Approximate level (dBSL)	Type of threshold	Value of threshold (ms)
Klemm (1920)	Clicks	—	Echo threshold	c. 2
Rosenzweig and Rosenblith (1950)	Clicks	—	Echo threshold	2
Cherry and Taylor (1954)	Speech of average speed	—	Echo threshold	20
Blodgett, et al. (1956)	Narrow-band noise around 425 Hz	—	Equal-loudness threshold	7.6
	Broadband noise 0.1–4.8 kHz	—		9.4
Guttman (1926)	Clicks	36	Echo threshold	3
		16		4.6
Babkoff and Sutton (1966)	Clicks	50	Echo threshold	2.6
		20		3.6
Schubert and Wernick (1969)	Sinusoids 0.25, 0.5, and 2 kHz, with triangular envelope	40	Echo threshold (envelope shifted but fine structure of signal not shifted)	
	duration 20 ms			5–7
	duration 50 ms			7–12
	duration 100 ms			up to 100 ms
	Noise, high- or low-pass-filtered (cutoff at 1 kHz), with triangular envelope	40	Echo threshold (envelope shifted but fine structure of signal not shifted)	
	duration 20 ms			5.5 (HP), 6 (LP)
	duration 50 ms			8 (HP), 12 (LP)
	duration 100 ms			16 (HP), 22 (LP)

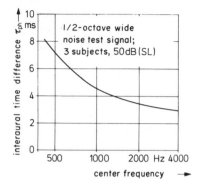

Figure 3.18
Dependence of the echo threshold of interaural delay on the center frequency of narrow-band noise (after Kirikae et al. 1970).

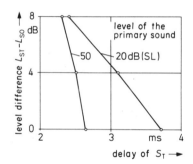

Figure 3.19
Dependence of the echo threshold of interaural delay on the interaural level difference for broadband clicks (after Babkoff and Sutton 1966).

sound being presented to one ear and the reflection to the other, just as it does in the free sound field case. Furthermore, the dependence on the level of the reflection is similar in both cases; also in both cases the rule holds true that high-frequency signal components lead to shorter delay times than do low-frequency components. On the other hand, the influence of the level of the primary sound cannot yet be compared well, since the data are insufficient. In binaurally separate presentations of primary sound and echo, the delay time necessary for an echo to appear becomes shorter as the level rises. Such a relationship is characteristic of contralateral inhibition, as Hall (1965) confirmed by means of physiological investigations. In a free sound field the same relationship is observed at very short delay times, but the opposite relationship is observed at longer delay times (figure 3.14). Data relative to longer delay times with binaurally separate presentation are not available.

When only the reflection is presented to one ear, only contralateral inhibition can explain the law of the first wavefront. In a free sound field, on the other hand, ipsilateral inhibition must also be assumed to play a part (see, e.g., David 1959, Guttman, van Bergeijk, and David 1960, Harris, Flanagan, and Watson 1963, Guttman 1965, Toole and Sayers 1965b). An experiment by Harris et al. (1963) was especially effective in casting light on this subject (figure 3.20). An impulse pair was presented to one of the subject's ears, using headphones. The time interval between the impulses was fixed at a value Δt. A single impulse was presented to the other ear, and its time of occurrence could be adjusted by the subjects. The task was to use this adjustment to make the auditory event appear in the center of the head. If multiple auditory events occurred, each was to be adjusted individually to appear in the center. The probability density for auditory events to appear in the middle is shown at the right side of the figure as a function of the position of the single impulse. The spacing Δt of the impulse pair is varied as a parameter. When $\Delta t = 1$ ms or 4 ms, it can be seen clearly that an auditory event appears in the center whenever the single impulse occurs simultaneously with one of the impulses of the pair. But when $\Delta t = 2$ ms, the auditory event corresponding to the second impulse of the pair disappears. Evidently the first impulse of the pair masks the second when their spacing is 2 ms. When the spacing is 1 ms, this effect does not yet occur; when the spacing is 4 ms, the effect no

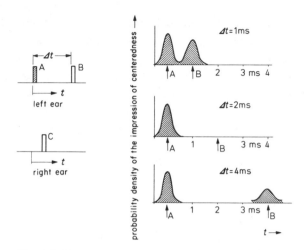

Figure 3.20
Probability density for the impression of centeredness as a function of the time of occurrence of a single impulse at one ear relative to that of a pair of impulses at the
other ear. The parameter varied between top and bottom is the interval between the
two impulses of the pair.

longer occurs. It follows that ipsilateral forward inhibition may be of
importance relative to the law of the first wavefront.

Ebata, Sone, and Nimura (1968a) carried out a series of experiments
dealing with the dependence of the echo threshold on signal duration.
Impulse pairs, as shown in figure 3.21a, were presented to the subjects,
and the echo threshold was determined. Under the experimental conditions indicated in the figure, the echo threshold was 10 ms. In a
second experiment pulsed sinusoidal signals were presented. The primary auditory event was determined by the rising slopes of the envelopes, and the secondary auditory event by the falling slopes of the
envelopes. The echo threshold was between 175 and 215 ms (figure
3.21b). Similar results were obtained using noise pulses. The fact that
the echo threshold increases so markedly beyond its value in case a is
obviously due to the presence of the carrier signal, filling up the time
interval between the rising and falling slopes. The rise in the delay time
corresponding to the echo threshold can also be achieved in case a by
inserting additional impulse pairs between the original first and second
pairs. In a free sound field these would correspond to additional reflections (see section 3.3).

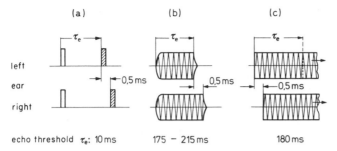

Figure 3.21
Echo thresholds for dichotically presented impulse pairs and pulsed sinusoids. a: The impulse pair shown in outline leads to the primary auditory event; the shaded impulse pair leads to the echo. b: The rising slopes of both pulsed sinusoids lead to the primary auditory event, and the falling slopes lead to the echo (rise and fall time, 0.75 ms). c: The rising slopes lead to the primary auditory event. The echo threshold is reached when the auditory event begins to migrate toward the center of the head (after Ebata, Sone, and Nimura 1968a; level of the primary sound 45 dBSL for the impulses, 60 dBSL for the pulsed sinusoids).

Another way to study the inhibitory effect of the primary sound with respect to the reflection is illustrated in figure 3.21c. Pulsed sinusoidal signals of long duration with steep rising slopes were presented. At first the rising slopes led to an auditory event to the left of the median plane. After 180 ms, however, this auditory event began to migrate toward the center of the head. The influence of the rising slopes has clearly begun to decrease. The time interval of 180 ms, moreover, agrees very well with results of Blauert (1968a, 1970a) and Plath, Blauert, and Klepper (1970). Using Gaussian tone bursts, noise pulses, amplitude-modulated noise, or impulse trains, these authors alternately stimulated first one ear and then the other. They asked subjects to determine the shortest switching interval at which perception of complete oscillation of the auditory event between left and right was still possible.

3.1.3 Inhibition of the primary sound

When a primary sound and a reflection are presented at the same level, summing localization occurs when the delay of the reflection is short. With increasing delay, the law of the first wavefront comes into play. Once the echo threshold has been passed, a primary auditory event and an echo appear. Finally, when the delay time is very long, more than several seconds, the echo is perceived as completely independent of the primary auditory event.

Von Békésy (1971) suggested that under some experimental conditions it may also be possible for the echo to dominate or to appear alone, and for the primary auditory event to be only weakly audible or inaudible. In other words, under some conditions the reflection may cause partial inhibition or even masking of the primary sound.

Backward masking has been discussed repeatedly in the literature (see, e.g., Pickett 1959, Raab 1961, Burgtorf 1963, Robinson and Pollack 1971; for a survey see Elliott 1962). All of these experiments involved the threshold at which the primary sound becomes "absolutely" audible, that is, the masked threshold. The results show that, for a delay time of 20 ms, the level of the reflection must be at least 40 dB higher than that of the primary sound for backward masking to occur, even under conditions favorable to masking. When the reflection and the primary sound are equally strong, backward masking never occurs.

Another threshold may be considered besides the masked threshold: a threshold analogous to the echo threshold, at which the primary auditory event becomes audible or inaudible as a separate auditory event. This threshold is represented by the uppermost curve in figure 3.13. Depending on the delay time, the reflection must be approximately 15–30 dB stronger in order to inhibit a separate primary auditory event. Further clues about inhibition of the primary auditory event are given by Rosenzweig and Rosenblith (1950), who found that the echo is often louder than the primary auditory event when the primary sound and reflection are equally strong. Chistovich and Ivanova (1959) found backward inhibition effects even at delay times of 500 ms if the subject was asked to regard the primary auditory event as separate. However, the reflection had to be stronger than the primary sound.

An experiment reported by von Békésy (1971) deserves particular attention here. The levels of the primary sound and the reflection were the same at the position of the listener, but the primary auditory event was markedly inhibited when the reflection was delayed by 70 ms. Since the results, to the degree that they may be generalized, are clearly relevant in the fields of architectural acoustics and sound reproduction, the basic experiment will be described here (figure 3.22).

Subjects sat before a ring of loudspeakers (A), with an additional loudspeaker (B) at the center of the ring. The loudspeakers in the ring were switched on and off simultaneously, and the loudspeaker at the center was switched on and off separately from them. The primary

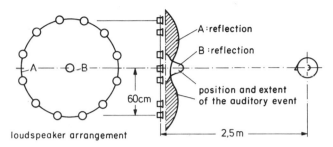

Figure 3.22
A loudspeaker arrangement used in investigating inhibition of the primary sound. The primary sound is presented over either A or B, and the reflection over B or A (delay of the reflection 70 ms, 35 ms pulsed sinusoids of approximately 1 kHz or pulsed noise at 90 dB) (after von Békésy 1971).

sound was presented over the ring and the reflection over the central loudspeaker, or vice versa. The signals were 35 ms pulsed sinusoids or 35 ms noise pulses. (In order to make it easier to distinguish the primary sound from the reflection, their carrier frequencies were made somewhat different—1 kHz and 1.5 kHz—or one carrier was a sine wave while the other was a square wave with the same fundamental frequency.) The inhibition of the primary auditory event was maximal at the chosen delay time of 70 ms. The figure shows the positions and extents of the auditory events as described by three trained subjects. If the reflection was radiated by the central loudspeaker, the auditory event was of small extent and at the center; if the reflection was radiated by the ring of loudspeakers, the auditory event was spread out over the entire ring.

In further experiments as well, von Békésy (1971) arrived at similar results in which the echo predominates over the primary sound. In these experiments the directions of incidence of the primary sound and the reflection differed by 90° or 180°. The question of inhibition of the primary sound as described by von Békésy needs further investigation before the effect can be accepted as established.*

*The present author, in a later investigation, failed to reproduce von Békésy's results (Blauert and Tütteman 1978/80).

3.2 Two Sound Sources with Partially Coherent or Incoherent Signals

The last section dealt with the relationships between sound events and auditory events observed when two spatially separate sound sources radiate signals that are fully coherent with each other. If the degree of coherence k is defined as the maximum absolute value of the normalized cross-correlation function of two signals $x(t)$ and $y(t)$, or

$$k = \max_{\tau} |\Phi_{xy}(\tau)|, \tag{3.11}$$

then only the case in which $k = 1$ has been considered up to this point. Here the discussion moves on to partially coherent and incoherent signals, that is, to cases in which $0 \leq k < 1$. When $k = 0$, the signals are incoherent; when $0 < k < 1$, they are partially coherent.

The following two techniques, among others, may be used either separately or together to generate partially coherent or incoherent signals:

1. The distortion technique. By means of linear or nonlinear systems, one or more distorted signals are derived from an original signal. The derived signals are partially coherent or incoherent with the original signal or with one another.
2. The superposition technique. One or more signals that are coherent with the original signal and with each other are derived from an original signal. Additional signals that differ from one another are superimposed on these; the additional signals are incoherent with respect to each other and the original signal. The resulting signals are, then, partially coherent or incoherent with the original signal.

The usual methods for measuring correlation can be used in measuring degrees of coherence (on this subject see, e.g., Lange 1962, Kuttruff 1963).

Figure 3.23 will serve as an aid in our discussion of the ear input signals generated when two sound sources present partially or totally incoherent signals. The figure shows the differing transmission paths from the two sound sources to the eardrums. All of the symbols represent functions of frequency, that is, Fourier transforms. S_R and S_L are the signals at the position of each sound sources when it alone radiates sound. When the sources are loudspeakers, these signals are the input

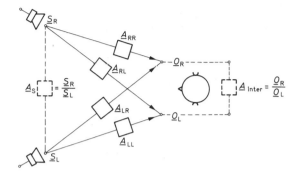

Figure 3.23
Block diagram showing how ear input signals are calculated when there are two sound sources radiating partially coherent or incoherent signals; S and Q are Fourier transforms of the signals; A the transfer functions (linear, time-invariant systems).

voltages as modified by the transfer functions of the loudspeakers. A total of four transmission paths between the sound sources and the ears must be considered. These paths may be regarded as linear, time-invariant systems and are designated by the transfer functions A_{RR}, A_{RL}, A_{LL}, and A_{LR}. The ear input signals Q_L and Q_R may be calculated as follows from the signals S_L and S_R at the sound sources:

$$Q_R = S_R A_{RR} + S_L A_{LR}, \tag{3.12}$$

$$Q_L = S_R A_{RL} + S_L A_{LL}. \tag{3.13}$$

It follows that the ratio of the two ear input signals is described by

$$\frac{Q_R}{Q_L} = \frac{\dfrac{S_R}{S_L} A_{RR} + A_{LR}}{\dfrac{S_R}{S_L} A_{RL} + A_{LL}} = \frac{A_{RR}}{A_{RL}} + \frac{\dfrac{A_{RR}}{A_{RL}}\left(\dfrac{A_{LR}}{A_{RR}} - \dfrac{A_{LL}}{A_{RL}}\right)}{\dfrac{S_R}{S_L} + \dfrac{A_{LL}}{A_{RL}}}. \tag{3.14}$$

This can be simplified to

$$\frac{Q_R}{Q_L} = A_1 + \frac{A_2}{\dfrac{S_R}{S_L} + A_3}. \tag{3.15}$$

Equation 3.15 makes it clear that the ear input signals can be transformed into each other by a linear, time-invariant system, as long as the ratio of the signals at the sound sources can be described by a linear, time-invariant transfer function. In other words, as long as $S_R/S_L = A_R$, then $Q_R/Q_L = A_{inter}$. Without further mathematical proof we can, as a rule, make the following additional statements. If S_R and S_L are related by a system that is linear and time-variant, nonlinear and time-invariant, or nonlinear and time-variant, then Q_R and Q_L are related in the same way. If the relationship between S_R and S_L cannot be described analytically, then neither can that between Q_R and Q_L. When the signals at the sound sources are random, then so are the ear input signals.

It is possible to make the following qualitative statements about the relationship between the degree of coherence of the signals at the sound sources and that of the ear input signals. The degree of coherence of the signals at the sound sources is, as a rule, different from that of the ear input signals. Incoherent signals at the sound sources lead to ear input signals that are partially coherent (one exception is sound presented over headphones). Completely coherent signals at the sound sources also lead to partially coherent ear input signals (exceptions are diotic headphone presentation or presentation by means of two loudspeakers symmetrical with respect to the median plane). As a rule, the range of variation of the degree of coherence of the ear input signals is smaller than that of the signals at the sound sources, though there are exceptions to this rule as well (e.g., the TRADIS process of Damaske and Mellert 1969/70; see section 3.3).

Section 3.2.1 will discuss the results of auditory experiments with two sound sources and signals of differing degrees of coherence. In explaining some of the relationships observed under these conditions, it is helpful to use a model that regards the auditory system as deriving a running cross-correlation function of the ear input signals. In this model spatial characteristics of the auditory event are determined according to characteristics of this cross-correlation function. This so-called correlation model of hearing is based on the ideas of Jeffress (1948), Licklider (1956), and Sayers and Cherry (1957). It, too, will be discussed in some detail in section 3.2.1. Section 3.2.2 deals with phenomena that come under the headings "binaural signal detection" or "binaural unmasking" in the literature. These phenomena have to do with the ability to detect signals in the presence of other, interfering signals. Interaural differences occur between the components of the ear

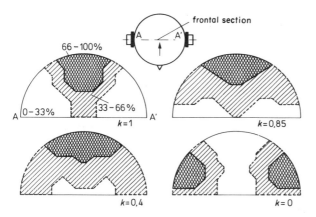

Figure 3.24
Position of the auditory events projected onto a frontal section of the upper half of
the head for broadband noise of various degrees of interaural coherence presented
over headphones. The differently shaded areas indicate regions of different salience of
the auditory events (after Chernyak and Dubrovsky 1968).

input signals corresponding to the signals to be detected; other interaural
differences occur between components corresponding to the interfering
signals. Both types of differences affect the ability to detect the desired
signals.

3.2.1   The influence of the degree of coherence

The sound events to be discussed in this section are presented to the
subject by means of two sound sources and have a degree of coherence
$k < 1$. The phenomena that occur under these conditions will be introduced through description of a simple auditory experiment. Two
broadband noise signals are presented; the degree of coherence of the
signals can be varied between zero and unity. Subjects are asked to
describe the position and extent of what they hear. Figure 3.24 illustrates
the results of such an experiment. The subjects were given a piece of
paper on which a semicircular area with a radius of 10 cm had been
outlined. This area was intended to represent a frontal section of the
upper half of the head. The task was to sketch a projection of the
position of the auditory events onto this plane. The figure shows the
parts of the plane in which auditory events appeared with a given
relative statistical frequency over several repetitions of the experiment.

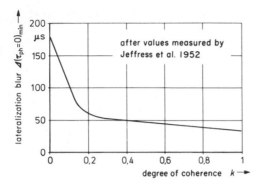

Figure 3.25
Lateralization blur $\Delta(\tau_{ph} = 0)_{min}$ as a function of the degree of coherence of the ear input signals. Low-pass filtered noise, $f_g = 2$ kHz, level approximately 90 dB, 7 subjects. The measured value for $k = 0$ corresponds to complete uncertainty in connection with the experimental arrangement in use.

The results indicate the following principles. When the ear input signals are fully coherent, a single auditory event of relatively limited extent appears. Its "center of gravity" is in the median plane. As the degree of coherence decreases, the position of the center of the auditory event at first remains largely unchanged, but the area over which components of the auditory event are found becomes greater. When $k = 0.4$, components of the auditory event occur over practically the entire upper half-plane. As the degree of coherence sinks even further, two spatially separated auditory events finally appear, one at each ear, correlated with the ear input signal at that ear.

In this experiment partially coherent ear input signals clearly lead to auditory events over a greater area than do coherent signals. However, it is not apparent whether the auditory event is sharply located—though it appears over a wider range of areas—or whether it loses spatial definition as the range increases, becoming more diffusely located. Zerlin (1959) and Jeffress, Blodgett, and Deatherage (1962) suggest an answer to this question; they report measurements of lateralization blur $\Delta(\tau_{ph} = 0)_{min}$ as a function of the degree of coherence. Figure 3.25 shows the result. Lateralization blur increases slowly as the degree of coherence is reduced. Below $k \approx 0.2$ (which is also the value below which two auditory events appear), the curve begins to rise rapidly, reaching a final value of approximately 190 ms. This limit value cor-

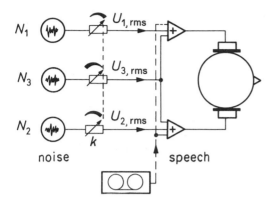

Figure 3.26
Experimental arrangement used in generating noise signals with a variable degree of coherence (superposition technique). Also shown is a way of superposing interaurally identical speech signals.

responds to total uncertainty with the apparatus used in this experiment; in other words, no additional lateral displacement is observed when the interaural time difference is over 190 ms. The increase in lateralization blur as the degree of coherence is lessened is to be interpreted as an increase in diffuseness of the spatial location of the auditory event.

As a postscript to the description of these two auditory experiments, it should be indicated how ear input signals with variable degrees of coherence were generated. The superposition method was used. A block diagram of the experimental apparatus is shown in figure 3.26. Three noise generators N_1, N_2, and N_3 generate three broadband noise signals that are incoherent with each other. The rms values of these signals are U_1, U_2, and U_3. Sum signals are fed to the two headphones by way of attenuation elements and adders. The signal at one ear is derived from $U_1 + U_3$, and that at the other ear from $U_2 + U_3$. In all cases $U_1 = U_2$. The degree of coherence of the ear input signals can thus be calculated as

$$k = \frac{U_3^2}{U_3^2 + U_2^2} \quad \text{with} \quad U_1 = U_2. \tag{3.16}$$

For the derivation of this formula see Jeffress and Robinson (1962).

In 1948 Licklider carried out a pioneering experiment using a similar apparatus. In addition to the three noise generators he used a source

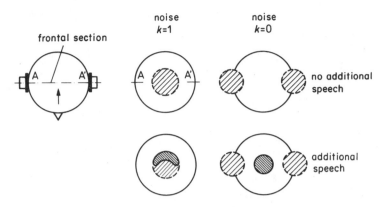

Figure 3.27
The position of auditory events, projected on the frontal plane, when broadband noise
with $k = 0$ and $k = 1$ is presented along with interaurally identical speech signals
(after Licklider 1948).

of speech signals, which he incorporated into the circuit shown in figure
3.26, among other ways. Some of Licklider's most important results
are given in figure 3.27. The positions of the auditory events are shown
as before, projected onto the frontal plane. The upper two diagrams
correspond to the cases $k = 1$ and $k = 0$ in figure 3.24. When the ear
input signals are coherent and no level or time difference exists between
them, a single auditory event appears in the median plane. The auditory
event does not appear at the top of the head, as it did with Chernyak
and Dubrovsky (figure 3.24). Instead it appears in the middle of the
head. This difference seems to be connected with the differing experimental technique and possibly also with the signals used; it will be
ignored here. When the ear input signals are incoherent, two auditory
events appear, one at each ear.

The two lower diagrams in figure 3.27 show the situation that results
when identical speech signals are presented to each ear in addition to
the coherent or incoherent noise signals. These speech signals lead to
an auditory event of speech. When the noise signals are coherent, this
appears at the approximate position of the auditory event of noise and
largely fuses with it spatially. When the noise signals are incoherent, a
total of three auditory events appears: the two auditory events of noise,
and a separate one of speech in the middle of the head. This last case
is of particular interest. It can be generalized further: If more signals
are fed to the headphones besides the noise signals and the speech

signal, then, under favorable conditions, other simultaneous auditory events appear, each of which is connected with one of the additional signals.* By "favorable conditions" we mean that the additional signals are presented in such a way that they lead to auditory events that are sufficiently separate from each other spatially. Under other conditions localization shifts of one auditory event toward another may occur, as may a fusing of auditory events. "Sufficient" spatial separation can be achieved by introducing interaural time or level differences into the additional signals.

The following rules can be derived from the experimental results reviewed to this point. The auditory system is capable of identifying coherent components of partially coherent ear input signals and of forming a separate auditory event with respect to each of these components. If incoherent components are also present, then the auditory events are less sharply located than if this is not the case. If the ear input signals contain no coherent components, or only very minor ones, a separate auditory event is formed from each ear input signal just as if each ear input signal were presented monotically.

The same rules apply to sound presented in a free sound field. It must be taken into consideration, though, that the signals radiated by the sound sources are not identical with the ear input signals, which are generated in accordance with the linear transformations indicated symbolically in figure 3.23.

Figure 3.28 shows a few results obtained by Damaske (1967/68) using sound from two sources. The sources were placed slightly above the horizontal plane ($\delta = 18°$) and radiated incoherent broadband noise signals. The azimuth of each loudspeaker could be varied. The diagrams indicate ranges of solid angles within which components of auditory events were found. Different shading, once again, represents different relative statistical frequency. At the lower left in the figure the equal-area projection of the upper hemisphere used in the diagrams is shown. The upper row gives two examples of cases in which largely separate auditory events appear—cases in which the auditory system recognizes two components in the ear input signals that are each totally or largely

---

*A more precise analysis in terms of cognitive theory would show that the several auditory events are never perceived simultaneously but are perceived in a rapid sequence, one after the other. It is unnecessary, however, to take this fact into account in the present context.

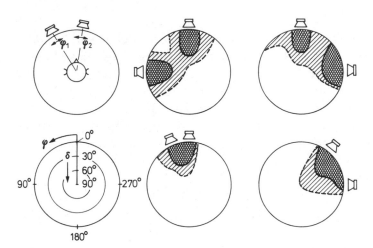

Figure 3.28
Directions of auditory events when two incoherent noise signals are presented from
various directions in the horizontal plane. The ranges of solid angles in which the auditory events appear are indicated in an equal-area projection of the upper hemisphere (after Damaske 1967/68; level at the position of the subject 75 dB,
loudspeaker 2.6 m from the position of the subject, two experienced subjects).

coherent interaurally. The second row shows two examples in which
the loudspeakers are placed closer to one another. The solid angles of
the auditory events fuse into a single range. What appears is apparently
only a single, extended, diffusely located auditory event.

Plenge (1972) reported an experiment in which the degree of coherence
of sound signals from two loudspeakers in the standard stereophonic
arrangement was varied. The experimental apparatus and some typical
results are shown in figure 3.29. Two incoherent noise signals were
combined so that they added at one loudspeaker's inputs and subtracted
at the other's inputs. The ratio between the two noise signals could be
varied. The degree of coherence of the loudspeaker input signals can
be represented by

$$k = \left| \frac{U_2{}^2 - U_1{}^2}{U_2{}^2 + U_1{}^2} \right| . \tag{3.17}$$

Then $k(U_1 = 0) = 1$, $k(U_2 = U_1) = 0$, and $k(U_2 = 0) = 1$. If the
ratio U_2/U_1 is varied from large positive values toward zero while the
overall level is held constant, the degree of coherence decreases at first,
passes through a minimum when $U_2/U_1 = 1$, and then rises again. The

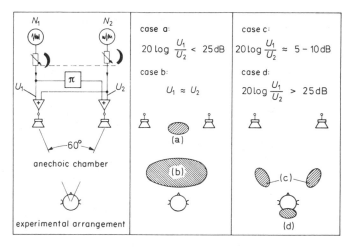

Figure 3.29
The position of the auditory events for one specific subject when broadband noise
was presented as shown in the diagrams (after Plenge 1972). Results using other subjects differ considerably from the ones shown here in cases b and c.

reported positions of the auditory events are completely in agreement
with the rules stated up to this point, taking into account that the degree
of coherence of the ear input signals is not identical with that of the
loudspeaker signals. When $U_2/U_1 = 0$, the ear input signals are 180°
out of phase. This case was discussed in more detail in section 3.1.1.

In the experiments described to this point the degree of coherence
of the sound signals was varied by means of the superposition technique.
We now offer examples of the distortion technique, in which two partially
coherent signals are derived from a single original signal by means of
linear or nonlinear distortion processes.

An example of the generation of two incompletely coherent sound
signals by means of linear distortion is the reflection of sound from a
surface with a frequency-dependent coefficient of reflection. This example is of considerable practical importance. The reflection as it arrives
at the position of the listener is not fully coherent with the primary
sound. This state of affairs can lead to masked thresholds, echo thresholds, and thresholds of annoyance different from those that occur when
the reflection is fully coherent (Haas 1951, Meyer and Schodder 1952,
Babkoff and Sutton 1966). Since the degree of coherence between the
primary sound and the reflection is usually still quite high even when

the reflection is frequency-dependent, no effects occur here that are basically different from the ones that occur when the reflection is frequency-independent.

Some interesting practical applications of the distortion technique have arisen in investigations of the problem that a one-channel (monophonic) signal reproduced over a single loudspeaker usually leads to a sharply defined auditory event. The spatial complexity of the original sounds is lost in such reproduction; it is therefore sometimes desirable to generate a certain spatial distribution of auditory events by means of a suitable process (figure 3.30). Such processes are called "pseudo-stereophonic." In all of them two partially coherent signals are derived from one original signal and are then reproduced over two loudspeakers.

Technique a is based on a suggestion of Janovsky (1948). The signal is divided by means of a low-pass and a high-pass filter, both with gentle cutoff slopes so that the high-frequency components are reproduced mostly by one loudspeaker and the low-frequency components mostly by the other. In technique b two complementary comb filters replace the low-pass and high-pass filters (Lauridsen 1954). The spectral components at both loudspeakers are balanced in this case, but noticeable distortions of tone color still occur. Technique c, described by Schroeder (1961), partly circumvents this problem by using different group delay distortions of the signals to the two loudspeakers. Banks of all-pass filters are used to generate these distortions. Amplitude distortions, which are the the primary factor leading to distortions of tone color, do not occur. Technique d is largely similar in its effect to technique c. Partial coherence of the loudspeaker signals is achieved by means of a reverberation chamber (Schroeder 1958, Lochner and Keet 1960). The microphones are at different positions inside the reverberation chamber. A reverberation plate or spring may be used instead of the reverberation chamber. Technique e has been described by Lauridsen (1954), Schodder (1956b), and Lauridsen and Schlegel (1956). One part of the loudspeaker signal is derived by delaying the original signal, attenuating it, and recombining it in phase at one loudspeaker and out of phase at the other.

The techniques just described are particularly effective if the original signal changes over time. Normal music and speech always fulfill this condition, so that the position and extent of the resulting auditory events also change with time. In technique f changes in the original

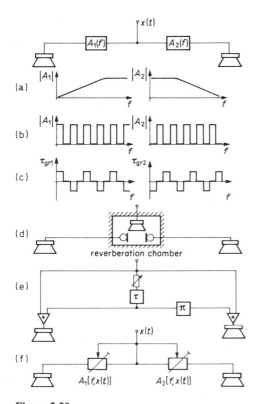

Figure 3.30
"Pseudostereophonic" processes. a: A highpass and a lowpass filter (Janovsky 1948). b: Two complementary comb filters (Lauridsen 1954). c: Two all-pass filter banks (Schroeder 1961). d: Reverberation chamber (Schroeder 1958, Lochner and de Keet 1960). e: Lauridsen effect (Lauridsen 1954, Schodder 1956b). f: Two time-variant, controllable filters controlled by the signal (Enkl 1958).

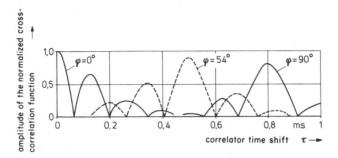

Figure 3.31
The magnitude of the normalized cross-correlation function of the ear input signals of a dummy head for bandpass-filtered noise (0.18–6.3 kHz) radiated by a source in the horizontal plane. The parameter varied between the three curves is the azimuth φ (after Damaske 1969/70).

signal are also used to determine a control variable that continually changes the characteristics of the two filters A_1 and A_2 (see, e.g., the process suggested by Enkl 1958).

In "true" stereophony, that is, when the collection, transmisison, and reproduction of sound are both over two separate channels, the partial or total incoherence of the loudspeaker signals involves both superposition and distortion processes. Consequently true stereophony, within the technical limits of this technique, makes it possible to a certain extent to reproduce an image of the spatial distribution of auditory events. This is not the case with pseudostereophonic processes. With these processes the spatial distribution of the auditory events as reproduced is independent of the distribution where the sound was picked up.

In the context of this section it should be noted again that, even in the case of only one sound source, the ear input signals are only coherent if the source is in the median plane. If the source is displaced laterally, the degree of coherence can fall below 0.5. Measurements of the degree of coherence of the ear input signals when there is only one sound source have been carried out by Rimski-Korsakov (1962) and Damaske (1969/70), both of whom used dummy heads. Some of Damaske's results are shown in figure 3.31. The decrease in the degree of coherence of the ear input signals with lateral displacement of the sound source is consistent with the simultaneous increase in localization blur (figure 2.2).

It is difficult to resist the hypothesis that correlation processes occur in the evaluation of signals by the auditory system, considering its behavior in connection with partially and totally incoherent signals— particularly its ability to identify interaurally coherent components within largely incoherent ear input signals.

The possibility that the auditory system makes use of correlation processes in signal interpretation was first considered by Licklider (1951), though in another context. He suggested that the system carries out a running (short-term) autocorrelation of the ear input signals and uses this to help establish the pitch of perceived tones. This hypothesis was developed further in later papers (Licklider 1956, 1959, 1962). An introduction to this complex of problems may also be found in Nord-mark (1970) or Duifhuis (1972); a critical assessment is given by Whit-field (1970).

In 1956 Licklider hypothesized that correlation processes also par-ticipate in the formation of the position of the auditory event—spe-cifically that a cross-correlation analysis of the two ear input signals takes place. Cherry and Sayers (1956) came to the same conclusion by another route. On the basis of this hypothesis, a functional model of the auditory system was sketched out that was capable of explaining a number of the phenomena of spatial hearing (Licklider 1956, 1959, 1962, Sayers and Cherry 1957, David, Guttman, and van Bergeijk 1959, Danilenko 1969). Some of the principles and applications of this model will be explained here.

The nonnormalized interaural cross-correlation function can be ex-pressed in the form

$$\Psi_{x,y}(\tau) = \lim_{T \to \infty} \frac{1}{2T} \int_{-T}^{+T} x(t)y(t + \tau)\,\mathrm{d}t. \tag{3.18}$$

Let $x(t)$ and $y(t)$ be physiological signals derived respectively from the two ear input signals. Since

$$\Psi_{x,y}(\tau) = \Psi_{y,x}(-\tau), \tag{3.19}$$

then

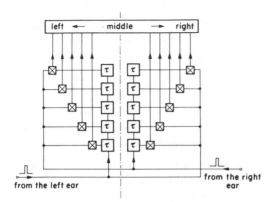

Figure 3.32
Block diagram of the coincidence model for the evaluation of interaural time differences between ear input signals (after Jeffress 1948). The nerve impulses from each of the two ears are only transmitted farther if they arrive simultaneously at one of the multipliers.

$$\Psi_{x,y}(\tau) = \lim_{T \to \infty} \frac{1}{2T} \int_{-T}^{+T} y(t)x(t - \tau)\, dt. \tag{3.20}$$

This form of the equation is more suitable than the first one, in that positive values of τ represent a delay in the signal, not an advance (which is a physiological impossibility).

We must now ask whether there exist physiological processes that correspond to these formulas. An answer is usually sought in connection with the so-called coincidence model of the evaluation of interaural time differences. This model was proposed first by Jeffress (1948) and later, in a similar form, by Matzker (1958), Röser (1960), and Franssen (1960, 1963), among others. Its principle is illustrated in figure 3.32. A nerve impulse arriving from one of the two ears is transmitted along a delay line on the same side as the ear and, once delayed, is led to a series of (binary) multiplier cells of the sort called "and-gates" in digital electronics. The nerve impulse is led directly to the multiplier cells on the far side, without being delayed. Each multiplier cell releases an impulse at its output when two impulses appear simultaneously at its input. Since one of the two input impulses originates at each ear, only one multiplier cell corresponds to any given time difference between the impulses from the two ears. The model may thus be viewed as carrying out a time–space transformation by associating specific inter-aural time differences with particular multiplier cells. One advantage of this model is that it appears to be physiologically realizable. The delays might be realized by means of latency intervals, and the multiplier cells by means of synaptic connections. However, the actual existence of such an evaluative mechanism has not yet been proven. It should also be noted that this model cannot without further assumptions explain the evaluation of monotically presented signals.

The coincidence model includes all elements necessary to calculate the product $y(t)x(t - \tau)$. The steps of the delay lines in the model must be sufficiently fine, and all of the elements shown must exist in large numbers, operating in parallel. The cross-correlation function can then be constructed simply by integrating the output impulses of all of the multiplier cells that correspond to a specific delay time. Integration cannot, however, encompass time extending indefinitely into the past; rather, a running integration must be carried out, more or less like that accomplished by an RC circuit. A mathematical representation leads to a short-term correlation according to

$$\Psi_{xy}(t, \tau) = \int_{-\infty}^{t} y(\vartheta)x(\vartheta - \tau)G(t - \vartheta)\,d\vartheta, \qquad (3.21)$$

$$\Psi_{yx}(t, \tau) = \int_{-\infty}^{t} x(\vartheta)y(\vartheta - \tau)G(t - \vartheta)\,d\vartheta. \qquad (3.22)$$

The first operation is carried out if $x(t)$ is the earlier signal, and the second if $y(t)$ is earlier. Note that $\Psi_{xy}(t, \tau) = \Psi_{yx}(t - \tau, -\tau) \neq \Psi_{yx}(t, -\tau)$. $G(t - \vartheta)$ is a weighting function that gives less and less significance to the values of the product $y(\vartheta)x(t - \vartheta)$ or $x(\vartheta)y(t - \vartheta)$ the farther they lie in the past. This function also sets all future values of these products equal to zero (figure 3.33). The function

$$G(s) = \begin{cases} e^{-s/\tau_{RC}} & \text{for } s \geq 0 \\ 0 & \text{for } s < 0 \end{cases} \qquad (3.23)$$

is commonly used; the constant τ_{RC} is certainly smaller than a few milliseconds (Licklider 1951, Atal, Schroeder, and Kuttruff 1962, Gruber 1967).

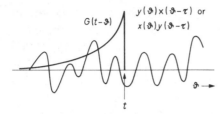

Figure 3.33
Illustration of how the short-term cross-correlation function is derived.

Any possible short-term cross-correlation by the auditory system according to the preceding rules must also be subject to the following restrictive assumptions:

1. The maximum interaural time difference for which cross-correlation can be evaluated must be taken to be limited. Under normal (free sound field) conditions, in any case, the maximum time difference is approximately 0.6 ms.
2. The delays generated within the auditory system are likely to vary over time; there might be a random variation whose extent increases as the delay time increases. Consequently a random variable will be superimposed on the delayed signals. The maxima and minima of the cross-correlation function, then, become broader, and their amplitudes decrease, as τ becomes larger. This is the case even when the ear input signals are completely coherent.

Some of the fundamental principles of a signal-processing model using interaural cross-correlation are assembled in figure 3.34, as they apply to the problem of forming spatial characteristics of auditory events. Principles discussed to this point are incorporated in the diagram, though it describes only such operations as do not seem improbable in the light of current physiological knowledge. First, the ear input signals are spectrally dissected into ranges of approximately equal relative bandwidth.* The signals at the outputs of the filters, $x_1(t)$, $x_2(t)$, . . . , $x_m(t)$ and $y_1(t)$, $y_2(t)$, . . . , $y_m(t)$, are rectified and low-pass-filtered. Above approximately 1.6 kHz this means that the envelope of the signals is

---

*Information about the probable transfer function of these bandpass filters, which represent the spectral sensitivity of the peripheral ear, can be found in the literature (e.g., Duifhuis 1972).

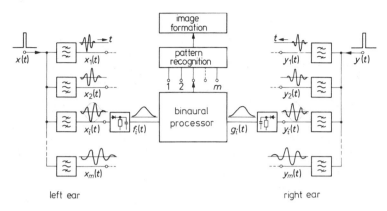

Figure 3.34
Principles of a functional model of the auditory system that determines spatial attributes of auditory events on the basis of interaural cross-correlation functions.

derived, that is, the signals are amplitude-demodulated. The output signals of the demodulating elements are then subjected to short-term cross-correlation (equations 3.21 and 3.22) in each frequency range. The figure shows the cross-correlation process for one pair of signal components, $f_i(t)$ and $g_i(t)$. The short-term cross-correlation functions corresponding to all components may then be assumed to be fed into a "pattern-recognizing" processor, which decides which of a predetermined array of patterns best matches the one at the input. The pattern recognizer passes on information representing its decision, and this information is used in forming one or more spatially defined auditory events.

The basic idea behind this and all other correlation models of hearing is that the information necessary to form the position and extent of auditory events can be derived in an especially simple way by cross-correlation of the two ear input signals. For example, the presence of interaurally coherent components of the ear input signals can be indicated by maxima of the cross-correlation functions. Conclusions about the degree of coherence can be drawn from the height and width of the maxima; conclusions about the average interaural time differences, from the position of the maxima along the τ axis. And from the interaural time differences, in turn, conclusions can be drawn about the lateral displacements of sound sources. Interaural level differences, however, cannot be determined by means of the cross-correlation function alone.

At least three different attempts have been made, up to 1972, to extend the model to include them, though with limited success so far:

1. An ear input signal at a higher level triggers more sensory cells than one at a lower level. Therefore, when there is an interaural level difference, more nerve impulses proceed from one ear than from the other. An attempt has been made to show that, in the coincidence model of Jeffress (1948), the probability of coincidences on the side with more impulses is greater than on the other side (see, e.g., David, Guttman, and van Bergeijk 1959). The statistical considerations underlying this assertion are, however, erroneous, at least for the model as it stands.
2. The assumption has been made that the auditory system translates level differences into time differences. Possible mechanisms were discussed in section 2.4.3 (see figure 2.88a). In that section it was also noted, however, that the auditory system evaluates time and level differences separately under some conditions; the correlation model cannot explain this fact at present.
3. Sayers and Cherry (1957) used the relationship between the areas under the two partial short-term correlation functions to derive a function relating only to the specific case of a decision whether the auditory event is to the left or the right of the median plane. For this limited case, it is possible to use the levels of the ear input signals as weighting functions for the areas, thus taking the level difference between the ear input signals into consideration.

In summary, it can be said that a model using an interaural cross-correlation analysis of the ear input signals can filter out components of the ear input signals that are interaurally coherent or partially coherent. It can, furthermore, provide information about the lateralization and lateralization blur of auditory events due to interaural time differences. The model as proposed does not provide any information beyond this; for example, it does not provide information about angles of elevation or about distances. One phenomenon of spatial hearing that is well explained by cross-correlation is the decrease in lateralization blur as signal duration is increased up to approximately 250 ms (Tobias and Zerlin 1951, Houtgast and Plomp 1968; see figure 2.77). Also deserving of mention are the results of lateralization experiments in which pulsed signals of slightly differing center frequencies were presented to the two ears (see, e.g., Ebata, Sone, and Nimura 1968a,

Perrott, Briggs, and Perrott 1970). A single auditory event appears only until the relative difference $\Delta f/f$ between the center frequencies reaches a certain value. This value increases as the signal duration is decreased. Thurlow and Elfner (1959) observed that a single auditory event appears in connection with two sinusoidal signals that differ greatly in frequency if the ratio of the two frequencies is an integer. This phenomenon may also be interpreted in terms of cross-correlation.

Absolute thresholds of perception for changes in the degree of interaural correlation of the ear input signals were measured by Pollack and Trittipoe (1959) and Pollack (1971). (The degree of correlation is the value of the normalized cross-correlation function at $\tau = 0$.) It became evident in the course of their experiments that a change in the spatial extent of the auditory event was the most important criterion used by the subjects. If the degree of interaural correlation is varied periodically, it becomes evident that the auditory event expands, becoming more diffusely located, and contracts, becoming more precisely located, with the same period. This effect goes by the somewhat imprecise name "binaural correlation beats" in the literature. It was investigated thoroughly as a function of various parameters by Gruber (1967), who varied the degree of correlation of the ear input signals by driving both headphones with a noise signal that originated with the same generator. Both headphone signals were amplitude-modulated by square-wave signals of the same frequency, and the modulation indices were 100 percent. By altering the switching times of one square wave relative to those of the other, any desired degree of correlation could be obtained.

3.2.2   Binaural signal detection

The following situation is often observed in daily life. Several people are engaged in lively conversation in the same room. A listener is nonetheless able to focus attention on one speaker amidst the din of voices, even without turning toward the speaker. But if the listener plugs one ear, the speaker becomes much more difficult to understand. This interesting psychoacoustic phenomenon is called the "cocktail party effect," after Cherry (1953). It arises from the fact that a desired signal S with a certain direction of incidence is less effectively masked by an undesired noise N from a different direction when subjects listen binaurally (with two functioning ears) than when they listen monaurally (e.g., with one ear plugged).

A quantitative treatment of this subject proceeds from the concept of the masked threshold of audibility of the signal S. This is the level of the signal at which it is just audible in the presence of the noise N. The masked threshold in dB for monotic presentation is generally used as a reference quantity, from which the masked threshold in dB under the binaural conditions being studied is subtracted. The difference between the two masked thresholds is called the binaural masking level difference (BMLD). In experiments using speech as a signal, the masked thresholds are replaced by the levels corresponding to a given degree of intelligibility. The difference between these levels is called the binaural intelligibility level difference (BILD).

A large amount of work has been done on the behavior of the BMLD or BILD under various conditions. Pioneers included Hirsh (1948), Licklider (1948), Hirsh and Webster (1949), Kock (1950), Hawkins and Stevens (1950), and Jeffress, Blodgett, and Deatherage (1952). Green and Henning (1969) surveyed and discussed the literature then available. The problems of binaural signal detection are only indirectly relevant to spatial hearing, since they are concerned primarily with the auditory detectability of signals and not necessarily with the spatial attributes of auditory events. One link between these two areas is that the way the two ears work together is a subject of interest in connection with both spatial hearing and binaural signal detection. Another link is that a BMLD or BILD greater than zero occurs, as a rule, when signals and noise, presented at different times, lead to auditory events in separate positions. This point will be discussed in more detail at the end of this section.

We shall only offer a brief summary of the problem of binaural signal detection. The type of sound presentation will be indicated, as in most of the literature, by the following symbols:

S for the (desired) signal
N for (interfering) noise, with the indices:
m   for monotic presentation
0   for diotic presentation with the interaural phase term 0
φ, π for dichotic presentation with the interaural phase term φ or π
τ for dichotic presentation with the interaural time difference τ
u   for dichotic presentation with interaurally uncorrelated signals.

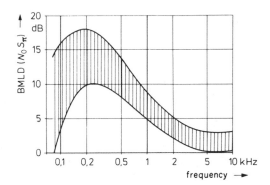

Figure 3.35
Dependence of the BMLD of a sinusoidal signal on frequency for N_0S_π. The interfering signal was broadband noise at various levels.

The expression $N_\pi S_m$, then, represents dichotic presentation with the noise out of phase and the signal presented monotically. $N_m S_m$ represents monotic presentation of the signal and noise to the same ear.

Hirsh has evolved the following hierarchy for the BMLD that occurs with combinations of signals and noises that are easily generated using headphones:

$N_m S_m$: BMLD = 0 dB (reference condition)*
$N_\pi S_\pi$: BMLD = 0 ?
$N_0 S_0$: BMLD = 0–1.5 dB ?
$N_\pi S_m$: BMLD = 0 ?
$N_0 S_m$: BMLD = 6–9 dB
$N_\pi S_0$: BMLD = 9–12 dB
$N_0 S_\pi$: BMLD = 12–15 dB.

The BMLD depends on the frequency of the signal. Figure 3.35 shows the dependence of the N_0S_π BMLD on the frequency of a sinusoidal signal when the interfering signal is broadband noise. The shaded area represents the data of six authors (Hirsh 1948, Webster 1951, Hirsh

*Sometimes diotic presentation of signal and noise, that is, N_0S_0 presentation, is used as a reference. The BMLDs are hardly affected by this.

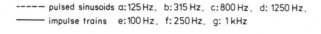

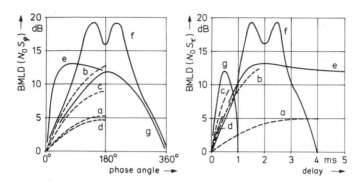

Figure 3.36
The BMLD for N_0S_φ and N_0S_τ as a function of the interaural phase difference or time difference of the signal. The desired signals were pulsed sinusoids or 100 μs impulse trains; the interfering noise was broadband noise at a level of 60–70 dB (data from Schenkel 1964, Flanagan and Watson 1966; 4 subjects and 1 subject, respectively).

and Burgeat 1958, Durlach 1963, Schenkel 1964, Rabiner, Laurence, and Durlach 1966). The BMLD reaches a maximum between 200 and 300 Hz, falling off with increasing signal frequency beyond this point. Above approximately 3 kHz it settles to a constant value of approximately 3 dB.

The wide range of measured values at low frequencies is apparently due to the differing signal levels used; it should be noted in this context that the threshold of audibility increases at lower frequencies, as shown in figure 2.54. The dependence of the BMLD on level will be discussed in more detail later in this section. The decrease in the BMLD at higher frequencies is often explained by saying that the interaural phase delay is the determining variable for the BMLD. As Schenkel (1966) correctly notes, the BMLD would have to approach zero asymptotically at higher frequencies if this were the case, since

$$\lim_{f \to \infty} \tau_{\mathrm{ph,max}} = \lim_{f \to \infty} 2/f = 0. \tag{3.24}$$

Figure 3.36 shows the BMLD as a function of interaural phase and time differences for N_0S_φ and N_0S_τ for pulsed signals and impulse trains. The maximum BMLD occurred with an interaural time difference of

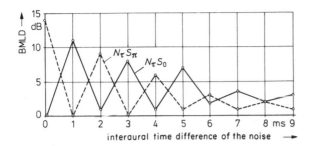

Figure 3.37
The BMLD of a 500 Hz sinusoidal signal as a function of the interaural delay of band-limited noise (0.1–1 kHz, level 50 dB; after Langford and Jeffress 1964).

1.5–2 ms. The information that the interaural time difference is 1.5–2 ms is repeatedly presented to the auditory system at the greatest possible rate by sinusoidal signals or impulse trains whose fundamental frequency is 250–333 Hz. This fact apparently explains the position of the maximum in figure 3.35.

Langford and Jeffress (1964) carried out an experiment showing the dependence of the BMLD on the interaural time difference. They investigated the BMLD of a 500 Hz sinusoidal signal with $N_r S_0$ and $N_r S_\pi$ as a function of the interaural time difference of the interfering signal. Figure 3.37 shows results for the case in which the interfering noise is band-limited white noise with a center frequency of approximately 500 Hz. The BMLD reaches a maximum whenever the interaural phase relationship of the signal is opposite that of the noise. However, the height of the maxima decreases as the interaural delay of the noise increases. When τ_{ph} is more than 9 ms, the noise signals at the ears must be regarded as largely independent of one another; in other words, the delayed component at one ear is no longer recognized as being related to the component presented earlier at the other ear. This behavior may well reflect the ringing times of the ear's peripheral filters.

We have already noted that the BMLD depends on level. Dolan (1968) and Schenkel (1964, 1966), for example, give curves like those shown in figure 3.38. These curves show the BMLD as the difference between the masked thresholds between $N_0 S_0$ and $N_0 S_\pi$. The masked threshold for $N_0 S_0$ shows a linear increase as the level of the masking noise rises; for $N_0 S_\pi$ the increase is nonlinear. These different increases in the masked thresholds lead to the level dependence of the BMLD.

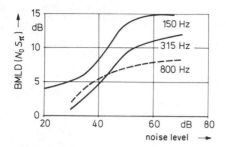

Figure 3.38
The BMLD of sinusoidal signals as a function of the sound pressure level of broad-band noise (after Schenkel 1964, Dolan 1968; 4–5 subjects).

McFadden (1968), like many other authors, explained the specific dependence of the BMLD on the noise level in terms of this noise's being superimposed on internal (physiological) noise generated inside the auditory system. McFadden cited an interesting clue reported by Diercks and Jeffress (1962), who noted that the BMLD at medium and high noise levels is approximately 0 dB for $N_0 S_0$ and 9 dB for $N_0 S_m$. On the other hand, when the level of the noise is lower, and also at the threshold of hearing with no noise present, the desired signal is easier to recognize with $N_0 S_0$ than with $N_0 S_m$. Two considerations will help explain this situation:

1. A test signal presented without interfering noise is perceived at a level approximately 2.5 dB lower when presented diotically than when presented monotically (see, e.g., Pollack 1948). In other words, the threshold of audibility is lower when the signal is presented to both ears than when it is presented to only one ear.
2. The internal physiological noise signals of the two ears are only slightly correlated with each other. The internal noise can be separated into two components: the fully uncorrelated "fundamental" noise of the ears and a smaller component that apparently stems from circulatory and muscle sounds and has a slight positive correlation (see, e.g., Shaw and Piercy 1962).

The only slightly correlated, internal noise of the ears dominates over the fully correlated external interfering noise when the level of the external noise is very low. The BLMD decreases along with the interaural

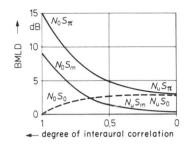

Figure 3.39
Dependence of the BMLD on the degree of interaural correlation of the interfering noise; conceptual illustration.

correlation of the total noise; finally, at the threshold of audibility, this phenomenon leads to the 2.5 dB lower level for N_0S_0 than for N_0S_m.

Robinson and Jeffress (1963), Dolan and Robinson (1967), and Wilbanks and Whitmore (1968), among others, have examined in more detail the dependence of the BMLD on the interaural correlation of the interfering noise. Figure 3.39 shows the N_0S_m BMLD as a function of the degree of correlation; that is, it shows the BMLD along the continuum between N_0S_m and N_uS_m. The BMLD between N_0S_π and N_uS_π is higher and approaches a value of 2.5–3 dB asymptotically. The same asymptotic value applies to the curve from N_0S_0 to N_uS_0. The degree of correlation was controlled in these experiments by superposing the outputs of three independent noise generators so as to generate the necessary signals.

We have so far examined the dependence of the BMLD on the signal frequency, the interaural phase or time difference, the level, and the interaural correlation. Other relationships examined in the literature include that with the duration of the desired signal (Jeffress et al. 1956, Green 1966, Schenkel 1967a); that with interfering noises of differing bandwidth (Jeffress, Blodgett, and Deatherage 1952, Schenkel 1964, Sondhi and Guttman 1966, Whightman 1969a,b, Hafter and Carrier 1970); and that with interaural level differences (Schenkel 1966, Dolan and Robinson 1967). An area in which little work has yet been done is the study of the BMLD in connection with desired signals and interfering noises that are not presented simultaneously. Works that can be mentioned are those of Deatherage and Evans (1969), Dolan and Trahiotis (1970), and Gruber and Boerger (1971). These authors found

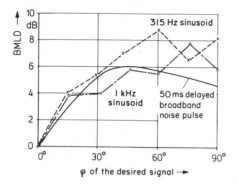

Figure 3.40
The BMLD in a free sound field as a function of the azimuth φ of the desired signal.
The interfering noise—a noise of 1 critical bandwidth (level 60 dB) or a broadband
noise pulse (level 75 dB)—arrives from the front (after Suchowerskyj 1969, Burgtorf
and Oehlschlägel 1964; 5 subjects and 1 subject, respectively).

that a BMLD may also be observed in connection with both forward
and backward masking.

All of the foregoing investigations of the BMLD were carried out
using headphones. Sound presented in a free sound field has been used
by Ebata, Sone, and Nimura (1968b) and Suchowerskyi (1969). All
works concerned with the masked threshold of reflections are relevant
in this context. Besides those listed in section 3.1.2, the work of Burgtorf
(1963), Burgtorf and Wagener (1967/68), and Damaske (1969/70)
should be mentioned. The appropriate reference threshold is that for
the case in which the signal and the noise arrive from the same direction.
If the two directions of sound incidence differ, the threshold generally
becomes smaller than under reference conditions; the BMLD is then
positive. Figure 3.40 shows examples in which sound incidence is from
directions in the horizontal plane. Note that the measured results can
depend strongly on level (Ebata, Sone, and Nimura 1968b). A masking
level difference can, by the way, exist even when the sources of both
the signal and the noise are in the median plane (Burgtorf and Oehlschlägel 1964).

The phenomena of binaural signal detection in a free sound field,
like those of spatial hearing, may be ascribed to the linear distortions
imposed by the head and external ears on sound signals on the way to
the eardrums. This has been proven explicitly for some particular cases

(Suchowerskyj 1969, Damaske 1969/70). Ebata, Sone, and Nimura (1968b) hypothesized that the BMLD is especially large if the subject knows the direction of incidence of the desired signal; however, Suchowerskyj (1969) could not confirm this hypothesis.

We now turn to the BILD, the binaural intelligibility level difference. The intelligibility of speech can be measured by presenting to subjects meaningless one-syllable words, called logatomes. The percentage of syllables understood correctly is called the "degree of syllabic intelligibility." The "syllabic intelligibility level" is defined as the sound pressure level of speech, measured broadband, in connection with which a given degree of syllabic intelligibility (usually 50 percent) is attained. Instead of logatomes, words with meanings (e.g., two-syllable words or spondees) or short sentences may be used. Their intelligibility is called, respectively, "word intelligibility" and "sentence intelligibility." The test material should be balanced phonemically so as to be representative of normal conversational speech.

The fundamental work on the BILD is that of Licklider (1948), who presented speech and broadband noise over headphones. The noise level was 80–90 dB. The following BILDs were typically obtained: $N_u S_0$ and $N_u S_\pi$, approximately 0.5–1 dB; $N_0 S_\pi$ and $N_\pi S_0$, approximately 3–3.5 dB. The hierarchy of BILDs corresponds to that of the BMLDs, though the BILDs are generally much smaller than the corresponding BMLDs (see Feldmann 1963). Later investigations have confirmed this observation. It is worth noting that an interfering noise at one ear cannot mask speech at the other; in other words, there is no contralateral masking.

Flanagan and Watson (1966), Carhart, Tillman, and Johnson (1966), and Carhart, Tillman, and Greetis (1969a,b), among others, investigated the masking of speech by other speech or by square-wave-modulated noise. The masking effect of modulated noise was very nearly the same as that of meaningful speech when the envelope repetition frequency of the noise, f_m, was 4 Hz, the envelope duty cycle was 50 percent, and the modulation depth m was about 60 percent. When logatomes were substituted for meaningful speech, their level had to be about 3 dB higher to produce the same masking effect. If the valleys of the envelope curves of the square-wave-modulated noise are lengthened, its masking effect is reduced. The term "window effect" is used in this context (see also Kaiser and David 1960).

The dependence of the BILD for N_0S_τ on interaural time differences of the desired signal has been investigated by Levitt and Rabiner (1967a), who determined that the BILD is practically constant, approximately 3 dB, for time differences from 0.5 to 10 ms and falls toward zero when the time difference decreases from 0.5 ms to zero. The corresponding BMLD with time differences in the range 0.5–10 ms is approximately 12 dB. For purposes of comparison we should mention the values these authors measured for N_0S_π: BILD = 6 dB, BMLD = 13 dB. Levitt and Rabiner asked—as had Schubert and Schultz (1962) and Flanagan and Watson (1966)—which frequency components of speech are most important in determining the BMLD and BILD. Schubert and Schultz, like Flanagan and Watson, hold the lower frequency range (250–500 Hz) particularly responsible, but Levitt and Rabiner confirm this assertion only for the BMLD. They argue that higher-frequency components also make a contribution to the BILD. In a later work (Levitt and Rabiner 1967b) the authors give a method for calculating the BILD when the BMLD is known. They assume that the BILD is based on the same frequency-dependent release from the masking effect of the interfering noise as is the BMLD.

Carhart, Tillman, and Johnson (1968) and Carhart, Tillman, and Greetis (1969b) determined the intelligibility level difference when several noises were presented simultaneously from different directions. The increase of the degree of intelligibility of speech as compared to monotic presentation is markedly better in this case than with only one interfering noise. Under favorable conditions the BILDs attain values up to 9 dB. Using various interfering signals, Carhart, Tillman, and Greetis (1969b) obtained the following values for $N_\pi S_0$:

Interfering noise	BILD
White noise, 75 dB	7.2 dB
Modulated white noise, $f_m = 4$ Hz, $m = 62\%$	5.5 dB
1 speaking voice	4.3 dB
1 speaking voice + white noise	5.7 dB
1 speaking voice + modulated white noise	5.2 dB
2 speaking voices	9.0 dB
2 speaking voices + white noise	6.4 dB
2 speaking voices + modulated white noise	6.6 dB

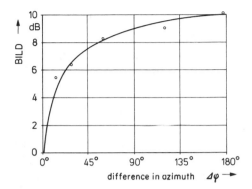

Figure 3.41
The BILD for one speaking voice against broadband noise as a function of the difference in azimuth between the speaking voice and the source of the interfering noise (10–15 subjects, level of the speaking voice 60 dB, relative word intelligibility 60 percent, head free to move; after Wendt 1959).

Pollack and Pickett (1958) presented up to seven speaking voices to one ear, and up to seven others to the other ear, all simultaneously. The desired signal, another speaking voice, was presented diotically. Under these conditions, $N_{1,m}N_{2,m}S_0$, the BILD with one interfering speaking voice at each side was 12 dB; with seven voices at each side it was 5.5 dB.

The BILD for sound presentation in a free sound field has been measured by Wendt (1959), Thomson and Webster (1963), and Tonning (1971). Figure 3.41 gives, as an example, the BILD, measured at 60 percent word intelligibility, for one desired speaking voice and one broadband interfering noise source in the horizontal plane. The subjects were allowed to turn their heads freely. In another case the interfering sound was radiated coherently by six loudspeakers placed at 60° angles in the horizontal plane; here the BILD was approximately 3 dB.

For binaural signal detection, just as for spatial hearing, models have been devised to describe how the auditory system evaluates the ear input signals. All of these proceed from the assumption that the signal is dissected spectrally as it arrives in the inner ear—for example, into components one critical band wide. Furthermore, binaural processing is postulated only between components whose center frequency is the same. The models differ only with respect to the assumptions they make about the mechanism by which corresponding components of the two ear input signals are processed.

The oldest model is that of Jeffress et al. (1956), based on previous work of Jeffress (1948) and Webster (1951), among others. It is usually called the "vector model." The assumption underlying the model is that the spectral components of the desired signal and interfering noise can be regarded as sinusoidal over short time intervals. If the interaural phase difference of the signal and the noise is the same at both ears, there is also no interaural phase difference between the two components that result from the signal and the noise. But if the interaural phase differences of the signal and the noise are not the same, the resulting components also differ interaurally. The ultimate, evaluated characteristics are the interaural time differences between the elicited nerve impulses from each ear. Jeffress makes use of his coincidence model, published in 1948, as an explanation of an evaluative mechanism for these time differences. This mechanism was described in detail in section 3.2.1. The advantage of the vector model lies in its clarity and the fact that it takes physiological considerations into account. Disadvantages are the impossibility of making quantitative statements about it, and the indefiniteness of a number of its aspects (see, e.g., Schenckel 1967b). A related model that allows quantitative statements and takes interaural level differences into consideration was put forward by Hafter (1971). The models of Jeffress et al. and of Hafter have been called "lateralization models" because they are based on the same interaural attributes that determine the lateral displacement of auditory events. Further literature on this subject is cited in Jeffress (1972).

Another model, called the "equalization and cancellation model" (EC model), based on an idea of Kock (1950), was developed further by Durlach (1963) and has been constantly refined since then (see Durlach 1972). The basic idea is that the auditory system attempts to eliminate the interfering noise by transforming one ear input signal with respect to the other. The interfering noises of both ear input signals are transformed in such a way that they become equal (equalization), and then one ear input signal is subtracted from the other (cancellation). The details of the transformation of the ear input signals depend on the interaural level and time differences between the desired signal and interfering noise that compose the ear input signals. The range of application of the model is basically determined by a catalog of transformations that are regarded as achievable by the auditory system. A disadvantage of the EC model is that it does not relate directly to

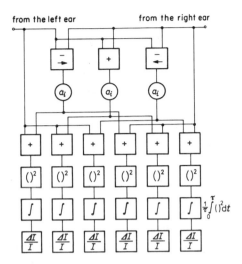

Figure 3.42
Accumulation scheme of Schenkel (1967b) as an example of a model of interaural evaluation in binaural signal detection.

physiological considerations, but rather regards the central nervous system as a sort of general-purpose computer (Green and Henning 1969).

Schenkel (1967b) describes an "accumulation model" that requires no internal time delays but instead "linearly superimposes upon the input signal a term characteristic of the phase shift, time delay, or level difference between the two ears, and so strengthens (accumulates) the desired input signal." Figure 3.42 illustrates this concept. If it is assumed that the signal and the noise are at the same level but are 180° out of phase interaurally ($N_0 S_\pi$ or $N_\pi S_0$), one of the adders in the third row will have an output signal whose desired signal component is three times as great as its interfering noise component. Further interpretation is by means of a running calculation of the rms value and by threshold detectors. Schenkel's model is applicable to interaural phase, delay, and level differences of both the desired signal and interfering noise. Even when the noises are only partially correlated, measured curves correspond well to theoretical values derived using this model. The accumulation model alone does not explain the BMLD of impulses, or forward and backward masking. This difficulty has been only partially solved by expansions of the model.

The last model that we shall mention is the "correlation model" of Osman (1971). This is a purely mathematical model based on statistical decision theory according to which the auditory apparatus, as a receiving system, chooses the more probable of two possible hypotheses: signal alone, or signal and superimposed noise. The decision is based on the variable

$$D = A \int_0^T x_L^2(t)\, dt + B \int_0^T x_R^2(t)\, dt + C \int_0^T x_L(t) x_R(t)\, dt, \qquad (3.25)$$

that is, on a weighted sum of the energy in the left ear input signal, the energy in the right ear input signal, and the degree of interaural correlation. The coefficients A, B, and C must be chosen according to the result desired. The model is applicable to BMLDs for various combinations of interaural time and phase differences of the signal and the noise, as well as for various degrees of interaural correlation of signal and noise. In order for this model to fit the measured data well, an internal noise in the auditory system must be assumed; the same is true of all of the other models we have mentioned. The idea that the auditory system operates as a correlation receiver is not new (see, in addition to the works listed in section 3.2.1, Lehnhart 1961, Lange 1962).

In closing this section we return once more to the relationship between binaural signal detection and spatial hearing. In the study of binaural signal detection, in connection with the BMLD, masked thresholds have been considered. Which specific attributes of the auditory event are used as perceptual clues has not been taken into consideration. In the context of spatial hearing, however, it is a significant question whether the subject might detect the presence of the desired signal on the basis of spatial attributes of the auditory event. In this case the phenomena of binaural signal detection could be attributed to spatial hearing. Evidence supporting this hypothesis includes the fact that a positive BMLD occurs, as a rule, if signal and noise, presented separately, lead to auditory events at different positions. The effect described by Curthoys (1969) lends further support: the direction of an auditory event connected with a desired sound event can be affected by an interfering sound event (see also Butler and Naunton 1964). However, some investigators of the relationship between spatial hearing and binaural signal detection argue that the underlying phenomena may not be fully identical. A few relevant experimental results will be mentioned here.

Egan and Benson (1966) determined that for N_0S_m subjects were able to detect the signal when it was at a far lower level than was necessary for them to state correctly the side from which it was presented. McFadden (1969), Jeffress and McFadden (1970, 1971), and others have investigated BMLDs and lateralization thresholds in connection with various interaural level differences of the signal and the noise for N_0S_m, N_0S_0, and N_0S_π. They demonstrated that lateralization thresholds and BMLDs depend in different ways on interaural time and level differences. However, Hafter et al. (1969) found that BMLDs and lateralization thresholds behave largely analogously. An interesting work in this context is that of Taylor and Clarke (1970), who compared the measured BMLD for N_mS_τ as a function of interaural signal delay with the hypothetical BMLDs that would be expected in connection with a simple lateralization or correlation model. Both hypotheses lead only to a partial agreement with the measured curve.

It is possible that lateralization thresholds are not the most suitable index for spatial changes in the auditory event near the masked threshold. In parallel with the attributes of auditory events by which coherent reflections are detected (section 3.1.2), it might be hypothesized that changes in the spatial extent of the auditory event are noticeable at lower signal levels than are lateral displacements or changes in direction.

3.3   More than Two Sound Sources and Diffuse Sound Fields

This section will generalize the results of the preceding sections to spatial hearing in sound fields that are generated by more than two sources. One particularly important example is that of sound fields in enclosed spaces; the reflected sound can then be thought of as being generated by mirror-image sound sources.

Summing localization is observed when two sound sources radiate coherent signals or signal components whose time and level differences at the position of the listener are below certain limit values; in other words, one auditory event appears, and its position depends on the signals from both sound sources. When there are more than two sound sources, regardless of where they are placed, summing localization can

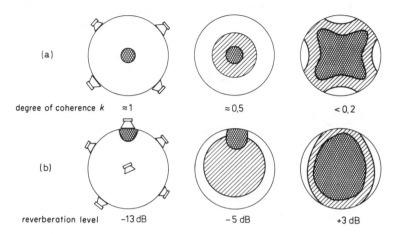

Figure 3.43
a: Directions of auditory events for 4 bandpass-filtered noise signals whose degree of coherence with each other is variable (after Damaske 1967/68; level at the position of the listener 75 dB, two experienced subjects). b: Directions of auditory events when a direct sound (level 70 dB) and five mutually incoherent reflections (reverberation, delayed by 80 ms) are presented. The signal was music at a fast tempo. More than 20 subjects (after Wagener 1971). An explanation of the graphic representation is given in figure 3.28.

also occur. In establishing the position of the auditory event, the auditory system takes into consideration (subject to certain other conditions) coherent components of the ear input signals that arrive within up to a couple of milliseconds after the first component. Consequently all signal components that constitute a significant part of the ear input signals within this time interval contribute to summing localization.

Summing localization with more than two sound sources has not yet been investigated systematically; only specific examples can be given here. For example, four loudspeakers arranged in a circle around a subject and radiating coherent signals lead to an auditory event directly above the subject (figure 3.43a, left).

Figure 3.44 shows a loudspeaker arrangement with which the present author attempted some years ago to generate an auditory event that would circle around a subject's head in the horizontal plane. Six loudspeakers were driven with signals whose carriers were identical but whose sinusoidal envelopes were phase-shifted by 60° between loudspeakers. The angles indicated numerically in front of the loudspeakers in the figure represent the phase angles of the respective envelopes,

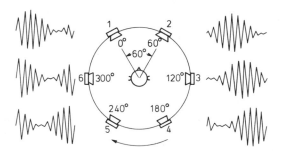

Figure 3.44
An arrangement for generating moving auditory events. The loudspeakers are driven
with amplitude-modulated or phase-delay-modulated signals. The modulating signal is
sinusoidal and phase-shifted by 60° between one loudspeaker and the next.

referred to that at loudspeaker 1. At the moment when the envelope
at one loudspeaker reaches its maximum — that is, when its signal is at
its maximum level — the signal at the opposite loudspeaker reaches its
minimum level. The maximum level rotates at the frequency of the
envelope; an acoustical "rotary field," so to speak, is generated. However, the auditory event does not appear, as intended, in the horizontal
plane; rather, it follows an elliptical path at an angle of elevation of
approximately 60°, approximately parallel to the horizontal plane. This
path does not change significantly even if, in addition to the amplitude
modulation described above, a simultaneous delay modulation with a
maximum phase delay of ± 500 μs is performed. (In other words, the
strongest part of each signal is advanced by 1 ms in comparison with
the weakest part. Because of equipment limitations at the time, this
part of the experiment could only be carried out using an impulse train
as the carrier signal; see also figure 2.92.) The auditory event appears
in the horizontal plane and moves along a circular path passing through
the positions of the loudspeakers only when the phase-delay modulation
of the signals is increased to more than approximately ± 3 ms. Then
the position of the auditory event is determined only by the three signals
radiated earliest; only these three take part in summing localization.

Several additional effects may be placed under the heading of summing
localization with more than two sound sources. Among these are effects
that occur in connection with sound presented by means of one or
more loudspeakers arranged so that they cannot be regarded as approximations of point sources. Examples are one-, two-, and three-

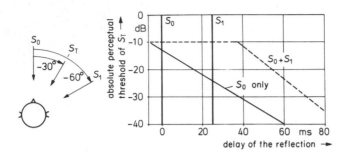

Figure 3.45
The masked threshold of a test reflection with and without an additional reflection
between the primary sound and the test reflection (speech, level S_0 = level S_1 = 70
dB, 1 subject; after Seraphim 1961, 1963).

dimensional arrays of loudspeakers. Such loudspeaker arrays must be
considered to be constituted, in the limit case, of an infinite number
of elementary radiators whose signals are superposed at the subject's
ears, leading to a unified auditory event. An auditory event generated
in this way is distinguished in some cases by its relatively diffuse locatedness (see in this context Kuhl and Zosel 1956, Aschoff 1958,
Ortmeyer 1966a,b).

The law of the first wavefront, like summing localization, can be
generalized to a primary sound with more than one reflection. A basic
rule is that a particular reflection (the test reflection) is less likely to be
audible if additional reflections are present between the primary sound
and this reflection. This rule is applicable to the masked threshold, the
echo threshold, the threshold of equal loudness of the primary sound
and the echo, and the threshold of annoyance of the echo. Especially
relevant to the masked threshold are the works of Burgtorf (1961) and
Seraphim (1961, 1963). Figure 3.45 shows this threshold as a function
of the delay of the test reflection when there is one additional reflection.
Different curves are obtained in connection with other levels and directions of sound incidence. It should be recalled that the criterion that
determines the masked threshold is often an increase in the extent of
the auditory event, which is a spatial attribute. Even if the increase in
extent is not the criterion, it still occurs shortly after the masked threshold
has been passed; according to Seraphim (1961), it occurs 6 dB above
this threshold. The dependence of the echo threshold on additional
reflections is described by Ebata, Sone, and Nimura (1968a). Using an

impulse as the primary sound and a test reflection at the same level, they found the echo threshold to be 10 ms. When an additional reflection at the same level was inserted between these signals, the threshold was 20–30 ms; when the entire interval between the primary sound and the test reflection was filled up, the threshold was as great as 200 ms. Obviously the signals used to "fill up" the interval need not even be coherent with the primary sound. The effects of additional reflections on the threshold of equal loudness of the auditory event, on the echo threshold, and on the threshold of annoyance of the echo were investigated by Meyer and Schodder (1952), who confirmed that such reflections raise the threshold in these cases, too.

We now generalize our previous discussions of the inhibition of the primary sound, the influence of the degree of coherence on the position of the auditory event, and binaural signal detection to the case of multiple sound sources. It might be hypothesized that inhibition of the primary sound may occur in the general case in which there are several reflections with various delays. An example supporting this hypothesis will be mentioned below. An example of the influence of the degree of coherence k on the auditory events when there are several sound sources is given in figure 3.43a. When k is decreased, the locatedness of the auditory event becomes less precise and the auditory event becomes more extensive; when $k \approx 0.2$, the event fills almost the entire upper hemisphere. As k sinks even further, four separate auditory events can be expected (though these were not measured in the work cited). The influence of the degree of coherence is, then, basically the same as with two sound sources. It should be noted that in this example each signal has the same degree of coherence with respect to the other three signals, so that this is a special case.

The advantages of binaural over monaural signal detection are especially apparent in sound fields generated by multiple sound sources. The popular term "cocktail party effect" points to the great relevance of this phenomenon to hearing in daily life. No investigations, however, have yet gone beyond what was discussed in section 3.2.2.

At this point the following summary statement can be made. *All spatial hearing effects observed in connection with two sound sources can also occur in connection with multiple sound sources, though these effects are modified in some cases.* When there are only two sound sources, certain effects such as summing localization and the law of the

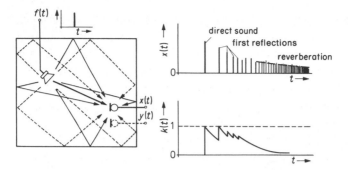

Figure 3.46
The impulse response of an acoustical transmission path in an enclosed space
(adapted from Danilenko 1969). Top right: Echogram. Bottom right: Correlation
echogram.

first wavefront cannot occur simultaneously. However, when multiple
sound sources can be arranged in any conceivable way in space and
can radiate any combination of identical or differing signals, these effects
can occur either successively or simultaneously. To this extent the case
in which there are multiple sound sources represents a generalization
of the case in which there are only two.

We now turn to spatial hearing in connection with the class of sound
fields with multiple sources that is of greatest practical importance:
sound fields in enclosed spaces (rooms).* As an introduction to this
subject we first consider qualitatively the impulse response of an acoustical transmission path inside a room with totally or partially reflecting
walls (figure 3.46). It will be assumed that a brief pressure impulse is
generated at some point inside the room. At the point where sound is
collected (in this case the microphone drawn with solid lines), an impulse
response such as the one shown at the upper right in the figure can be
observed. This is sometimes called an "echogram," and it is generated
in the following way. The primary sound (in this case a pressure impulse)
arrives first at the point of sound collection. It is followed by a series
of reflections that have only once encountered one of the walls enclosing
the room. Then, finally, reflections arrive at the point of sound collection
after encountering more than one wall. The density of the reflections

*The word "space" (Raum) takes on its common meaning here: a volume enclosed by
surfaces. This concept is not the same as the mathematical concept used, for example,
in the terms "spatial hearing" or "auditory space" (see section 1.1).

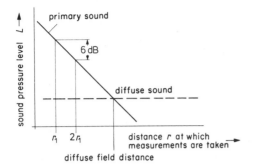

Figure 3.47
Representation of the sound field in an enclosed space produced by a stationary signal. The diffuse sound field consists of superposed reflections.

per unit of time increases as the square of the elapsed time after the sound source radiates the pulse or, as formulated by Cremer (1948),

$$\text{no. of reflections/s} = \frac{4\pi c^3}{V} t^2 , \tag{3.26}$$

where c is the speed of sound and V the room volume.

With time the reflections overlap each other to an increasing degree, and the resulting time function can be described only by means of statistical signal theory. This part of the echogram represents the reverberation of the room. The envelope of the reverberation approximates a decaying exponential function or, represented in terms of level, a downward-sloping straight line.

Echograms, the impulse responses of acoustical transmission paths in enclosed spaces, are different for each room and for each arrangement of the sound source and sound collection device. Thorough compilations of measured echograms, with information about the distribution of early reflections and their directions of incidence, are given by Meyer and Thiele (1956) and Schodder (1956a).

If, instead of an impulse, a signal that is constant over time, such as white noise, is introduced into a room, the sound field that develops is stationary over time. As long as the room does not have an extremely short reverberation time, it is possible to describe the sound approximately in terms of the relationships shown in figure 3.47. Throughout the entire room there exists a sound field that is largely diffuse with respect to the direction of sound incidence and of constant average energy density. This sound field is composed of the reflections. Only in the vicinity of the sound source does the level of the primary sound exceed that of the diffuse field. In conformity with the $1/r$ law, the level of the primary sound increases by 6 dB with each halving of the distance to the source, given a point source. The distance from the source at which the level of the primary sound and that of the diffuse sound field are equal is called the "diffuse field distance." When the sound radiated by the source is an impulse, the diffuse field distance is the distance from the source at which the energy of the primary sound is equal to that of the sum of all of the reflections.

One microphone in figure 3.46 is indicated by solid lines and a second by dashed lines. We now examine the degree of coherence k of the output signals of these two microphones when the sound source radiates a pressure impulse. Since the microphone output signals are not constant over time, we do not use k as it was defined in equation 3.11; instead we define a short-term degree of coherence $k(t)$, based on short-term correlation as defined in equations 3.21 and 3.22:

$$k(t) = \max_{\tau} |\Phi(t, \tau)|$$

$$\tag{3.27}$$

$$= \max_{\tau} \left| \frac{\int_{-\infty}^{t} x(\vartheta)y(\vartheta + \tau)G(t - \vartheta)\,d\vartheta}{\sqrt{\int_{-\infty}^{t} y^2(\vartheta)G(t - \vartheta)\,d\vartheta \int_{-\infty}^{t} x^2(\vartheta)G(t - \vartheta)\,d\vartheta}} \right| .$$

Here $G(s)$ is the weighting function defined in equation 3.23.

From measurements by Danilenko (1969) it can be determined that $k(t)$ for the given echogram is approximately as shown at the bottom in figure 3.46. Its numerical value reaches unity as the primary sound arrives. The first reflections cause a few more peaks; with the onset of the reverberation that can be described only statistically, it quickly falls toward zero. To a first approximation $k(t)$ for the ear input signals of a subject at the position of the microphones would have a similar time function.

Given these preliminary remarks, we are in a position to describe the basic principles of spatial hearing in enclosed spaces. If we stay at

first with the example of the impulse sound source, we may describe
the situation as follows. The primary sound arrives first at the position
of the subject, generating a primary auditory event. The primary sound
also elicits an inhibitory effect, in conformity with the law of the first
wavefront. For a certain length of time the forming of further auditory
events is suppressed. After a time interval corresponding to the echo
threshold, either a strong reflection leads to the forming of an echo and
to further inhibition, or else the intervening reverberation has been
strong enough that a precisely located auditory event is no longer formed.
Instead the largely incoherent ear input signals resulting from the reverberation generate a diffusely located auditory event whose components more or less fill the subject's entire auditory space. The primary
auditory event merges into the reverberant auditory event in such a
way that the primary event appears to disperse spatially. The resulting
diffusely located reverberant auditory event then decays more or less
rapidly, depending on the reverberation time of the room. If one or
more echoes appear after the primary auditory event, these also merge
into a diffuse reverberant auditory event.

   If the sound source in the room radiates a signal that is stationary
over time, the ear input signals are also stationary if the head is held
still. Their degree of coherence is a function of the levels of the primary
sound and of the diffuse field. The higher the level of the primary sound
in comparison with that of the diffuse field, the more precisely located
is the primary auditory event. If the level of the diffuse field is over-
whelmingly higher than that of the primary sound, there is no primary
auditory event but only a diffusely located reverberant auditory event.
The primary event is in this case backward-masked by the reverberant
sound. This case can, indeed, be considered an example of inhibition
of the primary sound. Figure 3.43b shows the directions of the auditory
events that resulted under a specific set of experimental conditions
when a primary sound and a simulated reverberant sound field were
presented. The parameter varied between the different diagrams is the
level of the reverberation relative to that of the primary sound. When
the relative level of the reverberant sound is $+3$ dB, no primary auditory
event is heard. Further data on the masking effect of diffuse sound
fields are given by Burgtorf and Wagener (1967/68), among others.

   The closer a person approaches a sound source in an enclosed space,
the stronger the component of the primary field in comparison with

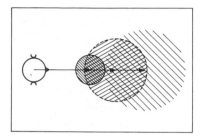

Figure 3.48
In enclosed spaces the extent and localization blur of the primary auditory event increase with its distance.

that of the diffuse field (figure 3.48). The difference between the levels of the primary and the reflected sound furnishes information to the auditory system about the distance of the sound source. The auditory system takes this information into consideration in forming the distance of the auditory event. This relationship has been described many times (see, e.g., von Hornbostel 1926, Maxfield 1933, Steinberg and Snow 1934, von Békésy 1938, Eargle 1960, Lerche and Plath 1961, Gardner 1969a,b, Kuhl 1969). The degree of coherence of the ear input signals becomes smaller as the component of reflected sound increases, so that the primary auditory event appears more diffuse and more spatially extended with a more distant source. This effect is especially noticeable at distances near the diffuse field distance. Plenge (personal correspondence 1972) has measured the just-noticeable difference of sound-source distance in enclosed spaces. Thresholds are in the range of 2–3 percent, considerably lower than localization blur in a free sound field (see section 2.3.2).

It must be pointed out that the meager statements about spatial hearing in enclosed spaces up to this point are only valid as general rules. Departures from these rules and additional effects can occur in connection with rooms of specific shapes, with particular sound sources, and with specific types of signals. An especially interesting and frequently mentioned phenomenon of this sort is the so-called Franssen effect (Kietz 1959, Franssen 1959, 1960, 1963). Two loudspeakers are placed in an enclosed space, with a subject at some distance in front of them (figure 3.49). One loudspeaker is driven with a sinusoidal signal of several seconds' duration, with exponential onset and decay curves;

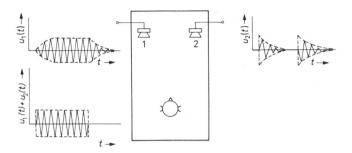

Figure 3.49
Signals used to drive the loudspeakers in demonstrations of the Franssen effect.

this is the signal $u_1(t)$. The other loudspeaker is driven with a signal $u_2(t)$ such that the sum of $u_1(t)$ and $u_2(t)$ is a rectangular tone, that is, a sinusoid modulated in amplitude by a rectangular pulse. Loudspeaker 2, then, mostly transmits switching transients, while loudspeaker 1 radiates a signal that rises and falls slowly and is of constant amplitude in between. The interesting feature of this experiment is that the subject has the impression that only loudspeaker 2 is in operation. Only by switching off loudspeaker 1 is it possible to convince the subject that the sustained part of the signal is not radiated by loudspeaker 2.

The law of the first wavefront has often been brought into play to explain this effect. The switching transient radiated by loudspeaker 2 is first to reach the subject and determines the direction of the auditory event. The subject consequently gains the impression that loudspeaker 2 is the sound source. What is remarkable is that this impression is maintained for a time interval of seconds or longer. In the comparable case illustrated in figure 3.21c a change in the direction of the auditory event was noticed after only 180 ms. In fact, a subject who listens carefully to Franssen's experiment will notice that the auditory event of a "click," which is at first precisely located, dissolves quickly into a diffusely located auditory event of a "sustained tone." Nonetheless the impression is not overturned that the loudspeaker at the position of the click is the only sound source. This case is a particularly telling example of how subjects use different criteria in accomplishing the task defined as "identifying the sound source" and that defined as "determining the position of the auditory event."

When a sound field such as that in an enclosed space is presented to a subject, the subject spontaneously arrives at a conceptual image of the type, size, and properties of the actual or supposed room. This conceptual image is called, somewhat inaccurately, the "spatial impression." The spatial impression occurring in any actual case is bound up very closely with the specific spatial, temporal, and qualitative attributes of the auditory events heard in that actual case. Reichardt and Schmidt (1966) simulated the sound field of a room, varying the difference between the levels of the primary sound and the diffuse field. They were able to generate all conditions along the continuum between a pure, reverberation-free primary sound and a pure diffuse field (pure reverberation). The subjects could distinguish 14 intermediate steps between these extremes. Reichardt and Schmidt (1966) regarded these as the steps of a scale of spatial impressions, even though they were aware that only one particular aspect of the spatial impression could be measured according to this scale. Important parameters in establishing specific impressions of rooms, such as the spectrum and specific temporal behavior of the reverberation and the number, level, and directions of incidence of early reflections, were not varied in the process used to establish this scale. The auditory system is, for example, particularly sensitive to changes in the parameters of the reverberant field that have been mentioned (see, e.g., Plenge 1971a).

It has been found that a sufficient number of early reflections from sideward directions (so-called lateral reflections) is necessary to obtain a spatial impression desirable in "good acoustics" in rooms designed for musical performances (Somerville et al. 1966, Schroeder et al. 1966, Marshall 1967, de Keet 1968, Barron 1971). These lateral reflections are automatically achieved by the "shoe-box" form of classical concert halls, whereas some modern fan-shaped or arena-shaped halls show a distinct lack of lateral reflections. The psychoacoustical effect of lateral reflections is a spatial broadening of the auditory events.

A question of particular importance to communications engineers is the technical feasibility of transmitting a particular spatial impression as faithfully as possible across a distance of space and time. The purely acoustical or electroacoustical part of this task is identical with the task of reproducing exactly at the listener's position in the playback room the spatial, temporal, qualitative constellation of auditory events that occurred in another space or position and at another point in time.

In principle two approaches to solving this problem are possible. One consists of generating a sound field in the playback room that corresponds largely to that in the recording room. Such an electroacoustically generated sound field is called a "synthetic sound field." The second approach proceeds from the assumption that an optimal acoustical reproduction is attained if the subject's ear input signals are identical to the ear input signals that would be generated at the position and time of sound collection. To this end, ear input signals are collected, transmitted, and reproduced. Processes employing this technique are called binaural or "head-related" since a head, usually a dummy head, is used in collecting the ear input signals (see figure 2.11).

We shall first examine the processes using synthetic sound fields. In order to simulate the sound field as it existed in the space where the transmission or recording originated, it is in principle necessary to imitate the primary sound, all individual reflections, and the reverberant field. It is clear that this task is not achievable using practical means; at least not with reference to the sound field of the entire room in which the transmission or recording originated. It is possible, however, to simulate with sufficient accuracy the sound field at one particular position in the room in which the sound is collected—for example, at a specific location in a concert hall. To achieve this goal many loudspeakers are used in the playback room (an anechoic chamber is best suited to the task). These loudspeakers are positioned in the directions of incidence of the most important reflections, with reference to the position of the subject; a number of additional loudspeakers radiate the diffuse, reverberant field. The loudspeakers are driven individually or in groups by circuits containing filters, level controls, delay units, and reverberation devices. Probably the most versatile apparatus for generating synthetic sound fields is the one shown in figure 3.50. The experimental results shown in figures 3.28 and 3.43, among others, were obtained using this apparatus.

The synthesis technique allows quite faithful imitation of sound fields and consequently makes possible a number of investigations that would be impossible in the original sound fields. For example, synthetic sound fields differing in ways that serve particular experimental goals can be presented rapidly, one after another, so that the subject can compare them directly. Manipulation of the sound field in the room where the sound is collected—in terms of diffuseness and reverberation time perhaps—is another possible application of the technique of sound-field

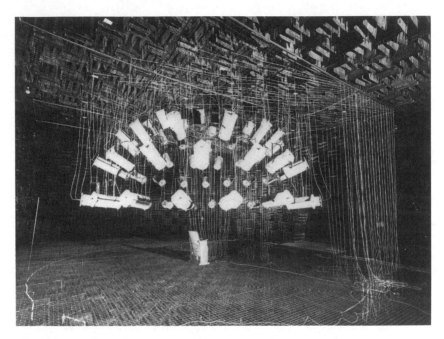

Figure 3.50
An apparatus for imitating sound fields electroacoustically, at the Third Physical Institute of the University of Göttingen; 65 loudspeakers surround the subject (after Meyer, Burgtorf, and Damaske 1965).

synthesis (Knowles 1954, Kleis 1955, Vermeulen 1956, 1958, Meyer and Kuttruff 1964).

A relatively large number of electroacoustic channels (more than about 20) is necessary in order to reproduce sound fields faithfully using sound-field synthesis. A considerable technical effort is also necessary to measure the primary sound, reflections, and reverberant field in the room where the sound is collected. In practical applications, such as the reproduction of sound for entertainment purposes, the process is consequently not practical in its exact form. It can, however, be simplified, albeit with some loss in accuracy of reproduction.

An apparatus that requires a very much less complex sound collection procedure, and many fewer transmission channels, has been suggested by Aschoff (1960) and Wendt (1960b). In the room in which sound is collected, one microphone is placed at a distance that is short in com-

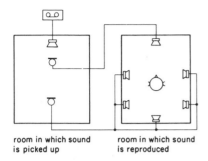

room in which sound   room in which sound
is picked up   is reproduced

Figure 3.51
A simple arrangement to transmit spatial information about a room (after Aschoff 1960, Wendt 1960b).

parison with that of the diffuse field distance, and another at a long distance. One microphone receives mostly the primary sound, and the other mostly the reverberation. Reproduction of the primary sound is over a single loudspeaker, and reproduction of the reverberation is over several loudspeakers connected together and positioned around the room. This apparatus can generate a spatial impression somewhat similar to that in the room in which sound is collected. Information about the direction of the sound sources is not transmitted. One disadvantage of this procedure is that only one reverberant signal, reproduced over several loudspeakers connected together, cannot generate a sufficiently diffuse reverberant field. Under some conditions summing localization can occur; that is, the auditory event of the reverberation can appear relatively precisely located (e.g., above the head). This difficulty can be avoided to some degree by connecting some of the loudspeakers out of phase. Keibs (1965) describes an apparatus with two transmission channels and four loudspeakers that conveys more information about the direction of sound sources than does the process illustrated in figure 3.51.

The entertainment industry has for some time tried to promote a transmission technique using four loudspeakers and four transmission channels, called "quadrophony." Such an arrangement, along with one of the sound-collection procedures suited to it, is illustrated in figure 3.52. Quadrophony can transmit information about both the direction of sound incidence and the reverberant sound field. Directions of sound incidence in broad parts of the horizontal plane (especially the frontal

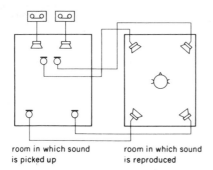

room in which sound   room in which sound
is picked up   is reproduced

Figure 3.52
Four-channel arrangement for the collection, transmission, and reproduction of sound
fields (quadrophony).

and rear sectors, though not the lateral sectors) are transmitted more
or less precisely. However, four loudspeakers and four transmission
channels fall far short of synthesizing the sound field at one position
in a concert hall faithfully enough so that an attentive listener cannot
notice considerable differences in comparison with the original sound
field.

The binaural or "head-related" process, on the other hand, allows
nearly perfect reproduction of the auditory events in the room in which
sound is collected. Moreover, the technical means are simple. The
principle of a head-related transmission system was illustrated in figure
2.11. A device called a dummy head is used; it includes external ears
that imitate very closely those of a human being (see on this subject
especially Damaske and Wagener 1969, Kürer, Plenge, and Wilkens
1969, Wilkens 1972). The sound signals at the "eardrums" or other
suitable pick-up points of the dummy head are collected and presented
to subject over headphones. Ideally the transmission channels generate
the same sound signals at the subject's eardrums as if the subject were
at the position of the dummy head.

The signals from the eardrums of the dummy head can be presented
to the subject over loudspeakers instead of headphones by means of
a process suggested by Bauer (1961b) and Atal and Schroeder (1966),
and realized in practice by Damaske and Mellert (1969/70, 1971) and
Damaske (1971). Using this so-called TRADIS (True Reproduction of
All Directional Information by Sterophony) process, it is possible to

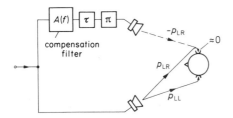

Figure 3.53
The principle according to which head-related two-channel signals can be reproduced over loudspeakers: the TRADIS process of Damaske and Mellert (1969/70, 1971). Only the apparatus used in presenting one of the two signals (p_{LL}) is shown.

present sound selectively to each ear, that is, to eliminate the cross-talk from one ear to the other that normally occurs in a free sound field. The principles behind the procedure are shown in figure 3.53. The signal p_{LL} is intended to be presented to the left ear. But then an unwanted signal component p_{LR} reaches the right ear. A compensatory signal $-p_{LR}$ is radiated by a second loudspeaker. The component of the compensatory signal that again reaches the left ear is, without further processing, sufficently attenuated as to be masked by p_{LL}. When signals generated by means of a dummy head are reproduced using the TRADIS process with two loudspeakers, the subject must take a precisely determined position in a largely anechoic environment. For a process similar to TRADIS, see Wilkens, Plenge, and Kürer (1971).

4 Progress and Trends since 1972

4.1 Preliminary Remarks

In the foregoing chapters an attempt has been made to present the material in as broad and comprehensive a manner as possible. The intent was to allow readers to survey the subject without having to make frequent excursions to the original literature. The present chapter is structured differently. It does not give a general overview but instead deals with a few selected problem areas that have especially occupied the author's attention in the past few years, and in some of which he and his co-workers have made contributions.

Section 4.2 focuses on the physics of the external ear. Special emphasis is given to the transfer characteristics for sound signals, since these characteristics play an essential role in forming the input signals of the human auditory system. Sections 4.3 and 4.4 discuss the processing of these input signals by the auditory system in connection with the forming of the position and extent of auditory events. These sections present the results of psychoacoustic experiments as well as models of signal processing. Section 4.5, finally, explores practical applications of knowledge about spatial hearing in the fields of architectural acoustics and communications electroacoustics.

Physiological considerations related to spatial hearing will, as before, be discussed marginally if at all; interested readers are referred to Erulkar (1972) and to the book by Altman (1972/78). We precede our own discussion with references to the following selected surveys of spatial hearing: on the physics of the external ear, Shaw (1974a, 1980); on the psychoacoustics of spatial hearing and on models of signal processing, Durlach and Colburn (1978) and Colburn and Durlach (1978); on practical applications, Cremer and Müller (1978/82), Ahnert and Reichardt (1981), and Blauert et al. (1978). Brief, summary descriptions of spatial hearing from the point of view of psychoacoustics may be found in many textbooks on the psychology of hearing (e.g., Green 1976, Moore 1977). A collection of relevant articles from the viewpoints of physics, physiology, psychology, and engineering has been edited by Gatehouse (1981).

4.2 The Physics of the External Ear

From the point of view of spatial hearing, it has already been noted that the sound pressure signals at the eardrums of an experimental subject are the most significant acoustical input signals to the auditory system. It has nonetheless been hypothesized repeatedly that bone-conducted sound, generated by air-conducted sound and passing through the skull, might play a supplemental role. In light of the fact that the threshold of hearing for bone-conducted sound in a free sound field lies some 50 dB above that for air-conducted sound (Blauert et al. 1980), it can be stated with great confidence that bone-conducted sound plays no part in spatial hearing under normal conditions.

In order to make the signals at the eardrums available for experimental purposes, and in order to describe these signals, it is necessary either to measure them directly or to calculate them using what is known about the transfer characteristics of the external ear. These characteristics can be described quantitatively by means of transfer functions. In the past few years, great progress has been made in the techniques for the measurement and evaluation of these transfer functions; only a few of the more important developments will be reported here.

The acoustical termination of the external ear can be described quantitatively by the so-called eardrum impedance (see section 2.2.1). New methods allow measurement of eardrum impedances throughout the frequency range of human hearing. These methods permit a simultaneous measurement of the cross-sectional area of the ear canal, which changes along the course between its entrance and the plane of the eardrum.

Important progress has been made recently in understanding the physical basis of the external-ear transfer functions. For one thing, it can now be confirmed that the dependence of the transfer functions on the direction and distance of the sound source, which comprise "the spatial characteristic" of the external ear, is unaffected by the eardrum impedance in the normal spectral band of hearing.

4.2.1 Measurement and interpretation of the transfer functions of the external ear

In recent years there has been considerable improvement in available techniques for measuring the transfer functions of the external ear. Such measurements may now be carried out routinely (for comprehensive data see Shaw 1974b, Mehrgardt and Mellert 1973, 1977). Progress has been due both to the development of improved microphones for taking measurements inside the ear canal and to the increased availability of computers for use in processing data. Probe microphones, described in section 1.3.3, have two important disadvantages: a poor signal-to-noise ratio, particularly at high frequencies, and a high sensitivity to mechanically induced noise. Platte et al. (1975) and Platte (1979) have described a means of overcoming both of these disadvantages by careful design of the acoustical coupling element between the probe tube and the microphone capsule, and by an increase in the polarizing voltage. They were able to construct microphones with probe tubes 54 mm long and 2 mm in diameter which, after electronic equalization, displayed a flat frequency response (± 2 dB) up to 12 kHz and a weighted signal-to-noise level difference of 58 dB when measured according to the German standards DIN 45590/91 (1974). This signal-to-noise level difference is equivalent to a noise level of 36 phon at the microphone.

Whenever it is not necessary to take measurements directly before the eardrum, subminiature electret microphones may be used in place of probe microphones. Such microphones (e.g., Knowles type BT 1759), currently mass-produced for use in hearing aids, are so small (approximately $10 \times 4 \times 2.5$ mm^3) that they may be inserted directly into the ear canal without difficulty. Their frequency response and signal-to-noise ratio are acceptably good. To be sure, the sound field in the ear canal is disturbed more by a subminiature electret microphone than by a probe microphone; but it can be shown that this is of no importance if we are concerned only with the spatial characteristic of the external ear. (On the subject of systematic error in measurements using probe microphones see Platte (1979) and Hudde and Lackmann (1981), which contains references to additional literature.)

We have already shown that the transfer functions of the external ear can be measured using broadband, brief sound-pressure impulses whose amplitude spectrum does not fall to zero anywhere in the frequency range of interest. Methods of measurement using impulses have now become standard in measuring the properties of the transfer functions of the external ear; and the use of computers has considerably simplified the process of carrying out such measurements (Platte et al. 1973, Blauert et al. 1974, Mellert et al. 1974, Mehrgardt and Mellert 1977). The primary advantages of computer-based methods are short measurement times, with consequent minimal disturbance to the subjects, automatic generation of the test signal, and automatic registration and evaluation of measured results.

Unfortunately, methods using single impulses as test signals have two fundamental disadvantages. First, because of the brief duration of the test impulses, the signals to be measured decay rapidly. Consequently, the signal-to-noise ratio is poor during most of the time interval when the measurement is taken, and the accuracy of measurement is reduced. The second disadvantage is the "picket-fence effect," a spectral periodicity that occurs in discrete Fourier transforms of signals that were originally nonperiodic and of limited extent in time. Spectral interpolation is necessary to smooth the Fourier transforms (see Mehrgardt and Mellert 1977). The necessity for interpolation also limits the accuracy of measurement.

A modified impulse method described by Hudde (1978b, 1980a) eliminates both disadvantages. In the modified method, the test signals are periodic impulse trains whose instantaneous power is almost constant as a function of time. Measurements are taken under steady-state conditions. Appropriate adaptation of the amplitude spectrum of the test signals to the particular system being measured allows equal accuracy of measurement across the entire range of frequencies of interest.

Improved microphones and computer-aided test procedures have eliminated all fundamental problems in measuring the transfer functions of the external ear. Such problems do arise, however, when we come to the task of meaningfully correlating the results of multiple measurements of the same type (e.g., measurements made on different subjects). As shown in section 2.2.3, it is possible to average the results independently and linearly for each frequency at which measurements are taken. However, the measured results are complex numbers and can be represented in different ways (real and imaginary parts, magnitude and phase, level and group delay). The "average" transfer function of the external ear will be different for each representation. Which rep-

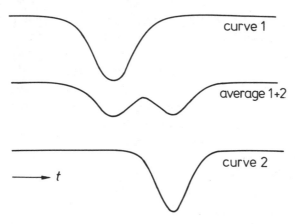

Figure 4.1
Attenuation of the structural attribute "dip" when the values of the function are averaged independently at each frequency.

resentation is most "meaningful" must be determined according to the particular experimental task at hand.

All averaging methods that regard measured values for different frequencies as being independent from one another have a fundamental disadvantage: They tend to flatten out the structural features of the transfer functions (e.g., peaks and dips in the plot of level against frequency). This is shown in figure 4.1. So-called structural averaging procedures have been applied in an attempt to reduce this disadvantage (Mellert 1971, Mehrgardt and Mellert 1977, Platte 1979). The fundamental idea behind structural averaging procedures is as follows: Two or more real functions of frequency whose plots are similar are to be averaged. Before the actual averaging of values, each curve, perhaps after being smoothed, is subjected to a nonlinear transformation of the abscissa—a "warping"—so as to construct a new, common frequency axis that results in maximum similarity of the curves in terms of certain prescribed criteria. It is immediately clear from this description that how the warping procedure is carried out depends fundamentally on how the similarity between the curves is defined. This definition depends in turn on which structural attributes of the frequency plot are held to be most significant.

Mellert (1971) uses the cross-correlation function as the index of similarity. By shifting, compressing, and extending the curves along the

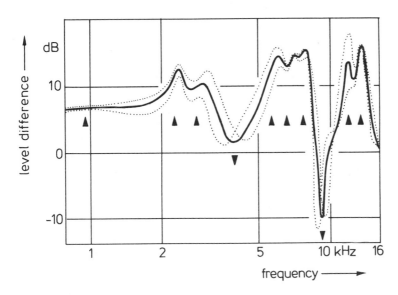

Figure 4.2
Two individual, smoothed external-ear transfer functions and structurally averaged curve (after Platte 1979). The resonances and antiresonances are indicated.

logarithmic frequency axis, a maximal cross-correlation is achieved; the curves are then averaged. Platte (1979) starts with a model that regards each transfer function of the external ear as representing a finite number of resonances and antiresonances. In each particular case, the curves are approximated by a rational function, $W(f) = Z_S(f)/Z_H(f)$, so as to reduce average quadratic error to a minimum. Here $Z_S(f)$ and $Z_H(f)$ are the impedances of passive one-port filters, which in each case represent a finite number of parallel series-resonant circuits and a resistive shunt; $|Z_S(f)|$ corresponds to the resonant peaks in the curve and $|Z_H(f)|$ to the dips. Each peak and each dip, then, can be represented in terms of the characteristic parameters of a particular resonant circuit. The actual structural averaging is performed by geometrically averaging the numerical data for the resonant circuits representing corresponding peaks and valleys of the different curves. The result is an averaged curve $\bar{W}(f)$ with the same number of resonant peaks and dips as appeared in the original curves. Figure 4.2 shows two individual curves and the curve derived from them by structural averaging. Figure 4.3 shows that Platte's method preserves the form

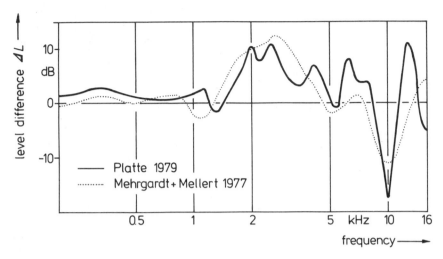

Figure 4.3
Structurally averaged free-field external-ear transfer function for sound incident from
the front (solid line: after Platte 1979, 6 subjects; dotted line: after Mehrgardt and
Mellert 1977, 20 subjects). Points of measurement 2 mm and 4 mm inside the
entrances of the auditory canals.

of the resonances of the curves better than does Mellert's. Structural
averaging can certainly be further improved by making the underlying
model for describing the curves correspond better to physical reality.

Another possible way of evaluating the results of measurements of
more than one subject is to choose from the ensemble of individual
curves the ones that are most representative or typical with respect to
given structural criteria. The result obtained in this way is an actually
measured, natural transfer function. One use of this method is in choosing a "typical" natural external ear, for example in order to pour a
mold to be used in preparing a dummy head (see section 4.5.2).

Figures 4.4a and 4.4b show monaural and interaural level difference
functions for the typical pair of ears of the commercial dummy head
preferred by German radio stations (Hudde and Schröter 1981). This
was chosen as the pair whose measured data differed least from an
average over all directions of sound incidence of an ensemble of measured pairs of ears. Frequency ranges in which large variations among
individuals occur were consequently taken into account less than frequency ranges in which these variations were small.

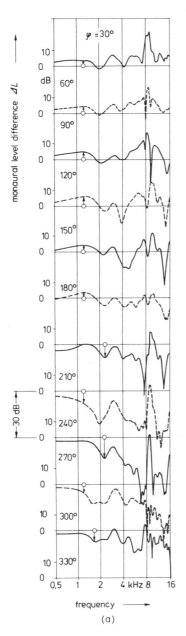

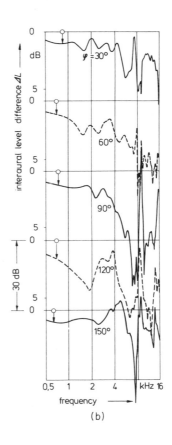

Figure 4.4
a: Level differences of the monaural transfer functions of the external ears in the horizontal plane for a "typical" pair of ears (Schröter 1980). b: Level differences of the interaural external-ear transfer functions in the horizontal plane of a "typical" pair of ears (Schröter 1980).

4.2.2 Area function and termination of the ear canal

In order to analyze the sound field in the external ear mathematically, one must know the terminating impedance of the ear canal in a given reference plane. If a plane at right angles to the axis of the ear canal is chosen, intersecting the eardrum or very close to it, the impedance is called, simplifying somewhat, the "eardrum impedance" (see equation 2.6).

In section 2.2.1 we discussed the "classical" methods for measuring the eardrum impedance and also some of the resultant data. None of the classical methods give reliable results at frequencies above 5 kHz, and some fail at frequencies as low as 2 kHz. Unavoidable systematic errors associated with each method are to blame for the failure. This objection holds even for the results of several recent measurements made using classical methods (Platte and Laws 1976, Laws 1978, Stirnemann 1978). Recently developed methods of measurement, however, allow measurement of the eardrum impedance at frequencies as high as 20 kHz.

The first of the new methods that we shall discuss is based on a phenomenon well known in the theory of waveguides and transmission lines: In an acoustically narrow tube in which waves can propagate only in the direction of the axis (i.e., a one-dimensional waveguide), the relative distributions of sound pressure and sound velocity depend only on the properties of the tube (dimensions and impedance of the lining) and on the terminating impedance. Consequently, if the properties of the tube are known, it is possible to calculate the terminating impedance from the transfer function between any two points inside the tube. Thus, in measuring eardrum impedances, the ear canal itself is used as a measuring tube, and the transfer function between at least two points inside the ear canal is determined, usually by means of the impulse method.

In the earliest measurements using this procedure (Blauert 1974a, Blauert and Platte 1976, Mehrgardt and Mellert 1977) the ear canal was assumed, for purposes of modeling, to be a tube with a constant cross section A_0 and with walls of infinite impedance. In this case,

$$Z_{\text{Tr}}(f) = \frac{jZ_{\text{w}} \cdot \cos \beta l}{H(f)^{-1} - \cos \beta l}, \quad \text{with} \quad Z_{\text{w}} = \frac{\rho \cdot c}{A_0}, \tag{4.1}$$

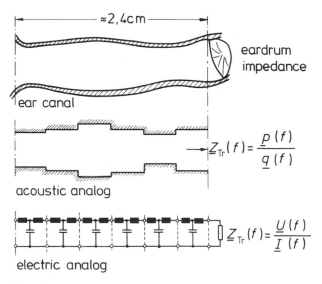

Figure 4.5
Analog representations of the ear canal that take into account the variation of the
cross section along its length.

where $\underline{Z}_{Tr}(f)$ is the impedance in the reference plane near the eardrum
and $\underline{H}(f)$ is the transfer function of sound pressure between this reference
plane and another plane at the distance l. In carrying out the measurement, it is important for the microphone probe to be at least 3
mm away from the eardrum; at the eardrum itself, dispersion occurs,
so that the sound wave is no longer one-dimensional there (Schröter
1976).

Hudde (1976) was able to show that the assumption of a constant
cross section for the ear canal leads to serious errors in calculation,
since in fact the cross-sectional area of the ear canal varies along its
length. The ear canal may be more accurately approximated as a series
of cylindrical sections of tubing of differing cross-sectional areas (figure
4.5). It might be assumed, then, that the transfer function of each of
these sections of tubing would have to be measured in order to determine
the impedance of the termination. Hudde (1978a, 1980a,b), however,
has proven that it is sufficient to measure only two transfer functions,
for example, by means of broadband sound pressure measurements at
three points inside the ear canal. These three measurements make it

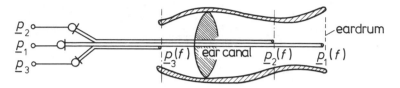

Figure 4.6
Measurement of the cross-sectional area of the ear canal and of the impedance of the
eardrum (after Hudde 1978a,b, 1980a,b).

possible to determine the cross-sectional area of the ear canal as a
function of distance along the canal and hence to calculate the eardrum
impedance. Specifically, the propagation of sound in the ear canal at
frequencies up to approximately 23 kHz may be calculated using Webster's differential equation

$$\frac{\delta^2 p}{\delta l^2} + \frac{1}{A(l)} \cdot \frac{\delta[A(l)]}{\delta l} \cdot \frac{\delta p}{\delta x} + \left(\frac{2\pi f}{c}\right)^2 p = 0, \tag{4.2}$$

where $A(l)$ is the cross-sectional area function. Two boundary conditions
(e.g., sound pressure at the entrance to the ear canal and directly before
the eardrum) must be known in order to solve this second-order differential equation. If a third measurement is taken, for example halfway
along the tube between these two points, it becomes possible to estimate
$A(l)$. The eardrum impedance may then be calculated. Figure 4.6 is a
diagram of the measuring apparatus.

Joswig and Hudde (1978) and Joswig (1981) have devised another
method of measurement for determining the area function and the
eardrum impedance, based on an idea first put forth by Sondhi and
Gopinath (1971). Figure 4.7 illustrates the method. An additional measuring tube containing an impulse sound source is placed at the entrance
to the ear canal. The sound source radiates a brief test impulse, which
reaches the ear canal and is reflected by the changes in cross-sectional
area and by the eardrum impedance. It can be shown that the necessary
information about the area function and about the eardrum impedance
is contained in the first- and higher-order reflections from the ear canal.
These reflections can be picked up by a microphone. Evaluation requires
the solution of an integral equation, which can be done using a laboratory
computer. In figure 4.8, other results from the literature are compared

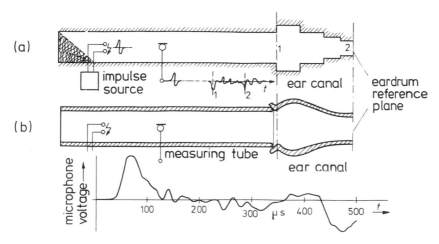

Figure 4.7
Measurement of the cross-sectional area of the ear canal and of the impedance of the eardrum (after Joswig and Hudde 1978, Joswig 1981). a: Schematic. b: A realistic example.

with measured results for human eardrum impedances obtained by means of the two methods just described.

Hudde (1980a) has noted that better agreement between measurements of different individuals is obtained if the eardrum impedances $Z_{Tr}(f)$ are recalculated as coefficients of reflection (reflectances) $r_{Tr}(f)$, according to the equation

$$r_{Tr}(f) = \frac{[Z_{Tr}(f)/Z_w(l = 0)] - 1}{[Z_{Tr}(f)/Z_w(l = 0)] + 1}, \quad \text{with} \quad Z_w = \frac{\rho \cdot c}{A(l = 0)}. \tag{4.3}$$

The representation in terms of reflectances is better adapted to describing wave behavior at higher frequencies. Figure 4.9 compares the results of Hudde (1980a) for structurally averaged eardrum reflectances with other authors' results.

The area functions measured by Joswig and by Hudde differ markedly from one individual to another. They are in basic agreement, however, with the area functions that Johansen (1975) obtained by measuring molds of cadaver ears.

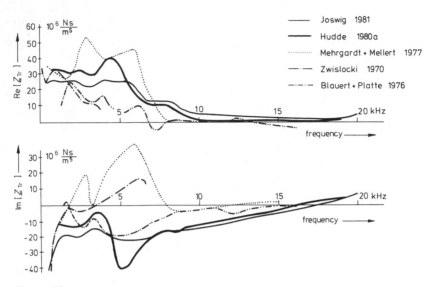

Figure 4.8
Human eardrum impedance as measured by various authors. The results of Hudde
(1980a) and of Joswig (1981) are structurally averaged.

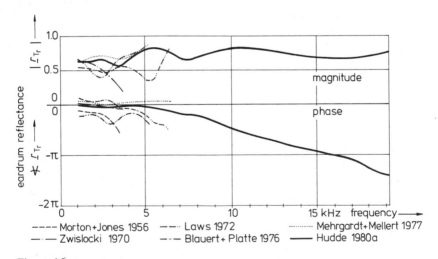

Figure 4.9
Human eardrum reflectance as measured by various authors. The results of Hudde
(1980a) are structurally averaged.

4.2.3 Analysis of the transfer characteristics of the external ear

On its path from the sound source to the eardrums of a listener, the sound signal undergoes linear distortions; that is, its magnitude and phase spectrum are altered. These linear distortions can be described by the transfer functions of the external ear and are due to the following physical effects: shadowing, reflection, and diffraction by the head and partly also by the torso; reflection, dispersion, and diffraction by the pinnae; and resonances in the system composed of each pinna, ear canal, and eardrum. Given the dimensions of the head (diameter approximately 18.5 cm), pinna (greatest linear dimension approximately 6 cm), and ear canal (length approximately 2.5 cm), it can be seen that the head causes significant linear distortions for frequencies above approximately 500 Hz, the pinna for frequencies above approximately 1,500 Hz, and the ear canal as coupled to the pinna for frequencies above approximately 3,000 Hz.

Several recent investigations have attempted a more precise determination of the role of different parts of the external ear in shaping the transfer function. We shall start here by discussing the sound transmission path from the entrance of the ear canal to the eardrum. This is distinguished from the other parts of the sound transmission path in that its transfer function is independent of the distance and direction of the sound source since only one-dimensional sound propagation occurs in the ear canal up to about 23 kHz.

Shaw (1977, 1980) and Rabinowitz (1977) have attempted to explain the eardrum impedance in terms of models that describe the acoustical characteristics of the middle ear and its coupling to the eardrum. Most models consist of networks of lumped elements, and their validity is limited to the frequency range below approximately 5 or 6 kHz. No satisfactory models have yet been developed for higher frequencies. It is interesting that the eardrum impedance becomes more and more independent of the eardrum and the ossicles in the frequency range above 8 kHz, as shown by the data in figures 4.8 and 4.9. In this range the eardrum impedance may possibly be substantially determined by reflections from the rear wall of the middle ear cavity. The influence of reflections from the end of the wedge-shaped cavity formed by the eardrum as it lies obliquely within the ear canal is another possibility. Models that attempt to describe the eardrum impedance above 5 kHz must include dispersed transmission-line elements. Work is presently in progress to develop such models.

There is unity of opinion that models of the ear canal for frequencies above 5 kHz must take its varying cross-sectional area into account. Now that appropriate methods of measurement for the area function are available, experimental technique is up to the level of theory on this point. Models that are to be very precise must also take into account propagation losses in the ear canal.

The pinna, the head, and the torso—the parts of the external ear system whose transfer function depends on the distance and direction of the sound source—are interposed ahead of the entrance to the ear canal. The external ear transfer functions as a whole are therefore dependent on the distance and direction of the sound sources. This specific dependence is called the "spatial characteristic" of the external ears. The spatial characteristic is particularly important in the study of spatial hearing.

We now consider the question of whether the spatial characteristic of the external ears depends in any way on the acoustic impedance at the entrance to the ear canal and thus on the shape of the ear canal and on the eardrum impedance. The path between the sound source and the entrance to the ear canal constitutes a two-port system. Since the transfer characteristics of a two-port system depend, in general, on its quantitative characteristics and on its terminating impedances, such a dependence of the spatial characteristic has been hypothesized several times; some authors have confirmed these hypotheses by measurement (Laws and Platte 1978, Kleiner 1978, Mellert 1978). Others have not found such a dependence, or have found only a slight dependence (Morimoto et al. 1975, Shaw 1974c). Hudde and Schröter (1980) have been able to resolve this problem (see also Fukudome 1980a,b). Their line of reasoning is most easily understood with the aid of the reciprocity principle. We undertake a thought experiment in which we conceive of the external ear as an acoustical radiator driven by the outer end of the ear canal. As every communications engineer knows, the spatial characteristic of a radiator is independent of the source impedance. In conformity with the reciprocity principle, the same is true of the external ear considered as a receiving antenna. The spatial characteristic of the external ear (i.e., the dependence of the transfer characteristic on the direction and distance of the sound source) is thus independent of the shape and terminating impedance of the ear canal. This is true for frequencies up to approximatly 23 kHz, for which the sound waves at the entrance to the ear canal may be assumed to be plane waves.*

A number of investigations of the head and the pinna have attempted to establish the details of the dependence of the transfer function of the external ear on the direction and distance of the sound source. As noted in section 2.2.2, the effect of the pinna may, for example, be explained in terms of either the time domain or the frequency domain. Although in principle time-domain and frequency-domain descriptions are equivalent, since they are linked by the (linear) Fourier transform, pinna models based on the two descriptions are different, since different simplifications are made.

Watkins (1978, 1979), working in the time domain and building on the work of Batteau (1967, 1968), sees the transfer function of the external ear as being synthesized by a delay-and-add system with one direct path and two delayed paths; the output signals of the three branches are added together (figure 2.19b). The delays (0–80 μs and 100–300 μs) are explained as being due to reflections from different parts of the pinna. Shaw (1974c, 1980) has undertaken the most significant research in the frequency domain, based in part on the pioneering work of Shaw and Teranishi (1968). Shaw is now able to construct mechanoacoustical models of the pinna that accurately reproduce the resonances of the pinna–ear canal–eardrum system up to 13 kHz and also the dependence of the response of this system on direction and distance. Figure 4.10 shows such a model; the dependence of its transfer function on direction and distance corresponds quite accurately to the dependence exhibited by typical natural pinnae. It should be emphasized that this model includes no superfluous details: every cavity and every barrier has its specific acoustical function.

It has often been stated in the literature that the distance- and direction-dependent effects of the external ear are caused primarily by the pinna, so that no strong dependence of the transfer characteristic on distance and direction should be expected at low frequencies (below approximately 2 kHz). Such an interpretation considerably underrates

---

*The fact that the spatial characteristic is independent of the shape of the ear canal and the eardrum impedance does not imply that such independence holds for the external-ear transfer functions as a whole. These are dependent on both the shape and termination of the ear canal.

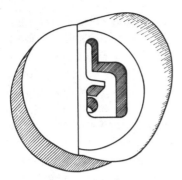

Figure 4.10
Acoustomechanical model of a human external ear (adapted from Shaw 1974c, 1975).

the diffraction effects of the head (see figures 2.23–2.26). As an example, a decrease in sound pressure of about 3 dB may be observed at 1.5 kHz, and an increase of about 3 dB may be observed at 300 Hz, when the direction of sound incidence is shifted from the front ($\varphi = 0°$, $\delta = 0°$) to the rear ($\varphi = 180°$, $\delta = 0°$) (see figure 2.49). The difference is due primarily to diffraction effects around the head; reflections at the torso (shoulder bounces) may also play a role.

When the head is approximated by a rigid sphere in modeling diffraction effects, it is important that the ear points on the sphere not be positioned in a plane of symmetry of the sphere at 90° from the front (Woodworth and Schlosberg 1954, Kuhn 1977). The ear points must be positioned approximately 100° from the front. Modeling the head as an ellipsoid conforms even better to nature (Mellert 1978).

4.3 Evaluation of Monaural Attributes of the Ear Input Signals

Monaural attributes of the ear input signals are those for whose reception one ear is sufficient; interaural attributes are those for whose reception two functioning ears are necessary (see section 2.3). There is no doubt that monaural attributes play a role in forming the position of the auditory event by the hearing apparatus. As noted in sections 2.3.1 and 2.3.2, most researchers accept the conclusion that monaural attributes of the ear input signals provide the most significant cues in forming the distance and elevation angle of the auditory event and in differentiating auditory events at the front from those at the rear.

A question addressed in several recent investigations is whether in a free sound field a person with normal hearing sometimes solely relies on monaural attributes—for example, when forming the position of the auditory event in the median plane (see, e.g., Gardner 1973, Hebrank and Wright 1974a, Searle et al. 1975, Hebrank 1976). This question, however, is imprecisely formulated, since a person with two normally functioning ears can never have solely monaural attributes available for evaluation. Even in the hypothetical case of a head symmetrical about the median plane and a sound source in the median plane, so that both ear input signals are identical, there is an important interaural attribute, namely that the difference between the ear input signals is zero. Consequently, when the ear input signals are identical, the auditory event appears in the median plane or close to it (see also Gardner 1973).

A related problem is the following: Since actual heads are not ideally symmetrical about the median plane, the ear input signals differ even when the sound source is in the median plane. These differences between the ear input signals are at least partially above thresholds of perceptibility (figure 2.39). They depend on the angle of elevation δ and on whether the sound source is in the front or rear hemisphere; the differences vary among individuals (Searle et al. 1975, Shelton & Searle 1978). The question, then, is whether these particular differences between the ear input signals play a role in directional hearing in the median plane. It is not possible to answer this question by comparing errors in the evaluation of the direction of the sound source in the median plane when one ear is plugged against errors for normal, two-eared hearing (Bothe and Elfner 1972, Hebrank and Wright 1974a). Since all auditory events are strongly lateralized to the side of the open ear when one ear is plugged, we must conclude that subjects in this situation tend to rely on attributes of the auditory event other than its position to estimate the direction of the sound source. It is somewhat better to suppress the natural monaural attributes at only one of the two ears, which can be done by filling the cavities of one pinna (except for the entrance to the ear canal) with putty or by inserting into the ear canal a small tube that bypasses the pinna (Gardner 1973). The ear otherwise remains functional. These approaches retain the "centering" effect of interaural phase delay, whereas natural monaural attributes are for the most part available only at the unmodified ear.

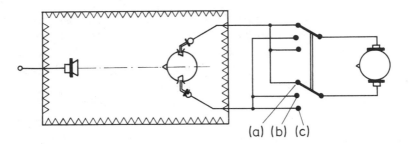

Figure 4.11
Diotic and dichotic sound presentation with ear input signals simulating those from sound sources in the median plane (after Platte 1979).

It is possible, however, to conceive of an experiment addressing the present question against which no theoretical objection can be advanced. This experiment is carried out as follows: Sound signals are picked up at the entrance to one of a subject's ear canals while sound is presented from different directions in the median plane. Later these signals are played back diotically to the same subject, equalized carefully so that the signals in the ear canals are identical to those recorded earlier. When this experiment is carried out, the directions of auditory events are essentially the same as in the case of direct hearing in a free sound field (Blauert 1969a, 1969/70, Platte 1979). One clear conclusion of this experiment is that "correct" localization in the median plane is possible when the ear input signals are identical.

What happens when "natural" interaural attributes, as would be present in the case of normal hearing with the sound source in the median plane, are reintroduced? Platte (1979) addressed this question with the experiment illustrated in figure 4.11. Signals picked up in the ear canals of one subject are played back to another subject either diotically (left or right signal to both ears) or dichotically (left signal to the left ear and right signal to the right ear). As has already been noted, localization can be largely "correct" when the presentation is diotic. Distinct differences in tone color are noted between diotic presentation of the left and of the right ear input signal; careful alignment of the head of the subject whose ear input signals are being recorded cannot eliminate these differences. When the presentation is switched from diotic to dichotic, two auditory events appear for a short while—one near the left ear and one near the right ear. Then, after a few seconds, these fuse into a single auditory event in the median plane which generally seems "more natural" than the corresponding auditory event when sound is presented diotically. (Regarding the necessary "adaptation time" of hearing in tasks of this sort see Plenge 1972, 1974.)

It can, then, be taken as established that monaural attributes of the ear input signals play an important role even when clear interaural differences between the ear input signals are present, as, for example, when the sound source is displaced laterally from the median plane (Bloom 1977b, Watkins 1978, 1979). In any case of spatial hearing in a free sound field with two functioning ears, monaural and interaural attributes of the ear input signals are present simultaneously.

Consequently, several attempts have been made to determine the relative importance of monaural as compared to interaural attributes in localization. The technique has generally been to alter monaural or interaural attributes independently of each other (Bothe and Elfner 1972, Gardner 1973, Hebrank and Wright 1974a, and all works that investigate only lateralization; see sections 2.4.1–2.4.3 and 4.4.1). In drawing conclusions from such experiments, it has generally been assumed, either implicitly or explicitly, that the attributes of the ear input signals that are varied cooperate independently in forming the auditory event (e.g., that they combine additively). A few researchers have raised doubts as to whether this modeling assumption is accurate. Plenge (1972, 1973, 1974), for example, proceeds from the assumption that unnatural (non-ear-adequate) combinations of monaural and interaural attributes of the ear input signals can lead to the auditory event's appearing inside the head (see also Theile 1980, 1981c).

The dependence of monaural attributes of the ear input signals on the direction of sound incidence has been investigated thoroughly in recent years (Gardner 1973, Bloom 1977a,b; see also the works cited in section 4.2). It may be asked which particular properties of monaural ear input signals are used by the hearing apparatus as cues in forming the direction of the auditory event. This question has been investigated mainly for the case of directional hearing in the median plane. New conclusions have been drawn and older ones confirmed as follows.

The distortions of the arriving sound signal by the pinnae play a dominant role in directional hearing in the median plane. If the pinna is altered (e.g., by filling its cavities with putty), then directional hearing in the median plane is disturbed (Gardner and Gardner 1973, Gardner

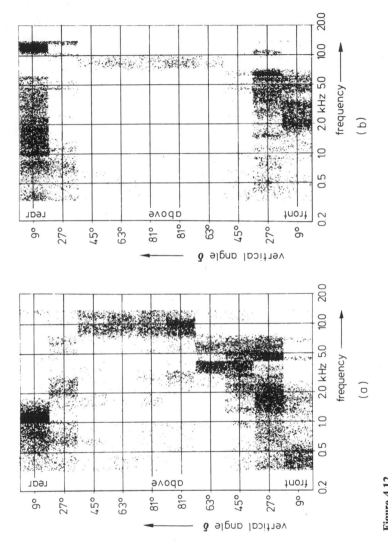

Figure 4.12
Directions of auditory events when narrow-band signals are presented from various directions in the median plane (after Mellert 1971). a: Sinusoidal signals. b: 1/12-octave noise. The directions of the auditory events are categorized into sectors whose width is $\Delta\delta = 18°$. The degree of shading is proportional to the relative number of auditory events in the corresponding sector.

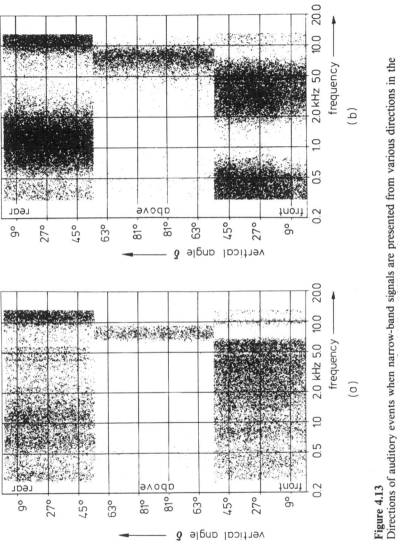

Figure 4.13
Directions of auditory events when narrow-band signals are presented from various directions in the median plane. a: 1/12-octave noise (after Mellert 1971). b: 1/3-octave noise (after Blauert 1969a). The auditory events are categorized into three sectors. The degree of shading is proportional to the relative number of auditory events in the corresponding sector.

1973). The agreement between the direction of sound incidence and the direction of the auditory event improves when the signal contains high-frequency components above 4 or 5 kHz (Gardner 1973, Wettschurek 1973, Belendiuk and Butler 1975). On the other hand, there is much evidence that the frequency range from approximately 500 Hz to 4 kHz is not entirely without importance (Blauert 1969a, Mellert 1971, Gardner 1973, Wettschureck 1973).

Wettschurek (1973) carefully remeasured localization blur in the median plane. He found it to be approximately ±4° for white noise in the forward direction increasing to ±10° directly overhead. These values are as much as doubled for low-pass filtered noise with an upper frequency limit of 4 kHz and a 30 dB per octave cutoff slope.

One question to which there is not yet a clear answer is whether the overall intensity of the ear input signals plays a role in forming the direction of the auditory event in the median plane. Most authors have been unable to confirm such an effect (Davis and Stephens 1974, Harkness 1974, Hebrank and Wright 1975; see also figure 2.46).

There have been several recent attempts to determine which specific spectral attributes of the ear input signals establish the direction of the auditory event in the median plane (Mellert 1971, 1972, Wright et al. 1974, Hebrank and Wright 1974b, Bloom 1977, Butler and Belendiuk 1977, Watkins 1978, 1979, Rodgers 1981). Like Blauert (1969a, 1969/70), Mellert presented narrow-band signals to his subjects from various directions in the median plane, categorizing auditory events in segments spanning 18°. Figure 4.12 shows the results for sinusoidal tones and for 1/12-octave noise signals. (See also figure 2.6.) Figure 4.13 shows the results for the 1/12-octave noise signal for three sectors of the median plane, in a representation similar to that in figure 2.45b. Also included for comparison are the results of Blauert (1969a) for 1/3-octave noise (see figure 2.46). It can be seen that finer distinctions are made in connection with sinusoidal signals and 1/12-octave noise signals than in connection with 1/3-octave noise signals.

Blauert (1972a) and Mellert (1972) had hypothesized that notches in the spectra of the ear input signals, as well as peaks, are important cues in forming the direction of the auditory event. In particular, the notch that varies between 6 and 10 kHz according to the angle of elevation of the sound source (Shaw and Teranishi 1968) was shown to be important by Blauert (1972a), Bloom (1977b), and Butler and Belendiuk (1977).

Hebrank and Wright (1974b) and Watkins (1978, 1979) regard it as proven that a particular combination of spectral peaks and notches determines the direction of the auditory event in each specific case. According to Hebrank and Wright, the following monaural attributes are important for directional hearing in the median plane: for the forward direction, a one-octave notch, having a lower cutoff frequency between 4 and 8 kHz and increased energy above 13 kHz; for the upward direction, a 1/4-octave peak between 7 and 9 kHz; for the backward direction, a small peak between 10 and 12 kHz with a decrease of energy above and below the peak. These results agree with the "directional bands" shown in figures 2.47–2.53.

Watkins has investigated the forming of the angle of elevation of lateral auditory events using synthesized signals modeled on Batteau's (1967, 1968) system with one direct branch and two delayed branches ("two-delay-and-add system"), illustrated in figure 2.19b. When white noise was used as the original signal, the result was a test signal containing specific notches whose position along the frequency axis was determined by the settings of the two delay units. The test signal was, so to speak, comb-filtered white noise. The task of the subjects was to report the path of the angle of elevation of the auditory event as the setting of one of the two delay units was continuously changed. It is of particular interest that multiple auditory events appeared under these conditions; for example, one auditory event might move downward and become more prominent while another simultaneously moved upward and became less prominent. Such multiple auditory events had previously been observed by Blauert (1971). It must be concluded from this phenomenon that the hearing apparatus is able to recognize more than one pattern of monaural attributes simultaneously in the same pair of ear input signals.

Up to the present, most authors have preferred to discuss the monaural cues as being spectral cues; that is, they have preferred to use frequency-domain descriptions. Since frequency-domain and time-domain descriptions are basically equivalent, time-domain descriptions would also be possible. However, when interpreting the time structure of the ear input signals, one should remember that the hearing apparatus works mainly on the signal's fine structure for components below about

1.5 kHz but on the envelopes only for components above this approximate limit (see section 2.4.1).

Finally, we note an observation made by Butler and Belenduik (1977) that the pinnae of certain individuals are particularly good at generating the patterns of monaural attributes necessary for directional hearing in the median plane. Subjects can sometimes hear directions in the median plane better using these pinnae than using their own (see also Morimoto and Ando 1977, 1982). This observation points to the conclusion that the evaluation of monaural attributes of the ear input signals cannot be explained simply as a learning process in which the central nervous system adapts to the pinnae.

4.4 Evaluation of Interaural Attributes of the Ear Input Signals

In the preceding section it was shown that monaural and interaural attributes of the ear input signals never occur separately for a person with normal hearing under "natural" conditions, that is, for example, with two functioning ears in an free sound field. The monaural and interaural attributes always occur together in specific combinations.

Under certain experimental conditions, however, only the monaural or the interaural attributes are varied, while the attributes of the other class are held constant. Such conditions lead inevitably to more or less "unnatural" patterns of ear input signals. The possibility must not be disregarded that the hearing apparatus undertakes evaluation in a very different way when the ear input signals are highly unnatural (Plenge and Romahn 1972, Plenge 1973, 1974, Theile 1980, 1981a,b,c).

This caution is especially to be applied to so-called lateralization experiments (see section 2.4). In such experiments, sound is presented dichotically to subjects, using headphones. In this type of sound presentation, monaural attributes are, as a rule, strongly attenuated or completely absent. As a result, there is considerable controversy as to whether the results of many lateralization experiments are relevant to "normal" spatial hearing. Generalizations must be cautious as long as no definitive answer to this question is available.

By means of dummy heads and electronic filters that simulate natural external-ear transfer functions (see section 4.5.2), it is now possible to generate largely natural ear input signals even when sound is presented over headphones. It is to be hoped that a few crucial lateralization experiments will be repeated using such ear input signals. But even in this case, the objection may be raised that isolated manipulation of the interaural attributes must lead to unnatural patterns of ear input signals. Still, the extent of the unnaturalness would be very much smaller than has been the case with lateralization experiments carried out up to the present.

We shall report here on new results that are related to the interpretation of interaural attributes and that have been published since approximately 1972. The cautions about unnatural signal combinations in the preceding paragraphs are applicable to section 4.4.1, whose exclusive subject is lateralization experiments. Section 4.4.2 reports phenomena observed when there are more than two sound sources radiating largely coherent signals. In this case, the evaluation of interaural attributes plays a dominant role. Section 4.4.3 discusses binaural localization in the presence of interfering noise signals and binaural detection and recognition of desired signals in the presence of interfering noise. In section 4.4.4, finally, are to be found some fundamental considerations of models of binaural signal processing; the general outline of one such model is discussed in terms of its relevance to spatial hearing.

4.4.1 Lateralization and multiple auditory events

Lateralization experiments have been used to determine which interaural attributes of the ear input signals lead to lateral displacements of auditory events. A detailed discussion of this question was given in section 2.4. The relevant attributes are interaural level differences throughout the frequency range of human hearing, interaural time differences of the fine structure of the signals in the frequency range up to approximately 1.5 kHz, and interaural time differences between the envelopes of the signals up to the high-frequency limit of hearing. The literature on lateralization continues to be large, due in part to the relatively simple experimental apparatus needed to conduct such experiments.

It has been conclusively proven that the evaluation of interaural signal attributes is frequency-selective; that is, the auditory system first dissects the ear input signals into narrow-band components and then separately examines the interaural signal differences in each frequency range. As of 1972 the bandwidth of the filters that undertake the running spectral analysis had not yet been determined. Scharf (1974a), Scharf and Florentine (1975), and Scharf et al. (1976) have carried out ex-

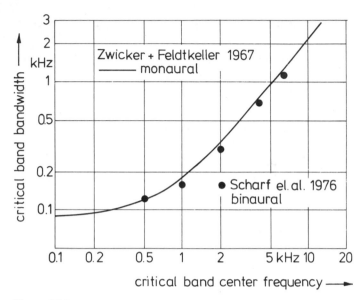

Figure 4.14
Critical bands observed in monaural and binaural experiments (after Scharf et al. 1976, Zwicker and Feldtkeller 1967).

periments relevant to this question. Using tone bursts, they measured the minimal interaural time difference between onset slopes of tone bursts that led to a lateral displacement of the auditory event (τ_*) as a function of the difference between the carrier frequencies of the tone bursts (Δf). They determined that τ_* is constant if Δf is below a certain value, and that when Δf increases beyond that value, τ_* also increases. The critical frequency difference Δf beyond which τ_* increases, and its dependence on the frequency range of hearing in which it is measured, agree with the critical bands that have been measured in monaural experiments involving the peripheral selectivity of the hearing apparatus (Zwicker and Feldtkeller 1967; for a survey of such experiments see Scharf 1970).

Figure 4.14 compares the results of monaural and binaural experiments. The comparison makes it clear that peripheral frequency selectivity has the same effect in both monaural and binaural signal processing. Any other result would have been very unlikely, given what we know of the physiology of the inner ear and the subsequent signal-processing steps. However, it is not at all the case that this binaural frequency selectivity manifests itself in the same way in all experiments. For example, in experiments on binaural masking, the critical bands were found to be slightly broader if the masker and the test tone were 180° out of phase (Sever and Small 1979). Other experiments also lead to somewhat different values for the binaural critical bands (Robinson 1971, Henning 1974a, Nuetzel and Hafter 1976, 1981, Canévet et al. 1980). However, in monaural experiments the critical bandwidth also depends to some degree on, among other things, the test signals used and the experimental procedure.

The peripheral running frequency analysis that precedes binaural signal processing does not, in principle, make it impossible for a higher level of the nervous system to recombine information from different critical bands. Relatively broad bands for binaural interaction, as observed, for example, by Kronberg (1975, 1976) when measuring dichotic pulsation thresholds, might possibly be explained in this way.

When the frequency ranges of the signals at the right and left ears differ greatly, no fusion occurs; instead, two distinct auditory events appear, one at the left ear and one at the right. The range in which a transition occurs between fusion and separate auditory events is interesting: here the same signals presented to the same subject may lead to a single auditory event one time and to separate auditory events another time. The distance between the two auditory events can change. Clearly "pulling effects" occur, of the type described in another context by Butler and Naunton (1964). The relation of the phenomena observed in such experiments and in other similar experiments to musical pitch is examined by Van den Brink et al. (1976); see also Durlach and Colburn (1978, p. 395).

We shall begin here by discussing signals all of whose frequency components lie within a binaural critical band, such as sinusoidal tones, tone bursts, narrow-band noise, and similar signals. Recent measurements of the sensitivity of the hearing apparatus to interaural attributes of such signals have shown that binaural interaction occurs even when the interaural level difference ΔL is 45–50 dB (Hafter and Kimball 1980). When there are no interaural time differences τ, the lateralization blur $\Delta(\Delta L)_{min}$ depends less on ΔL than was previously believed to be the case (see section 2.4.2, Wallerus 1977, Hafter et al. 1977). Also, and in agreement with this new result, the lateralization blur $\Delta\tau_{min}$

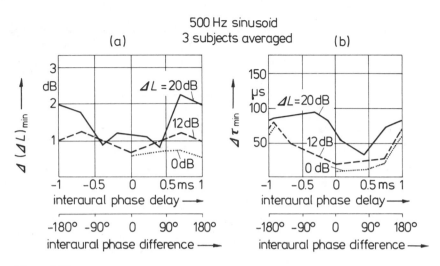

Figure 4.15
Lateralization blur of a 500 Hz sinusoid (3 subjects, averaged, sound pressure level approximately 55 dB). a: $\Delta(\Delta L)_{\text{min}}$ as a function of τ and ΔL. b: $\Delta\tau_{\text{min}}$ as a function of τ and ΔL (after Domnitz and Colburn 1977).

changes only slightly as τ is changed if the time difference $|\tau| \leq 500$ μs, the signals are below 1.5 kHz, and there is no interaural level difference (Hafter and de Maio 1975, Yost 1974). However, if either $\Delta(\Delta L)_{\text{min}}$ or $\Delta\tau_{\text{min}}$ is observed as a function of τ and ΔL, the relationships are as shown in figure 4.15 (Domnitz 1973, Domnitz and Colburn 1977). Also, when τ and ΔL are changed, not only the lateral displacement but also the spatial extent of the auditory event may change; the auditory event may also split up into multiple components.

For signal components above 1.5 kHz, $\Delta\tau_{\text{min}}$ depends on τ for any interaural level difference; in fact, it increases at a rapid rate as τ is increased (Hafter and de Maio 1975). This is the frequency range in which the auditory system evaluates the interaural attributes of the envelopes of the signals, rather than the fine structure of the signals themselves.

Although the fundamental relationships underlying the evaluation of the envelopes in binaural signal processing were known in 1972 (see section 2.4.1), much research on this question has been undertaken in recent years (Young and Carhart 1974, Raatgever 1974, Henning 1974a,b, 1980, 1981, McFadden and Pasanen 1976, Yost 1976, Nuetzel

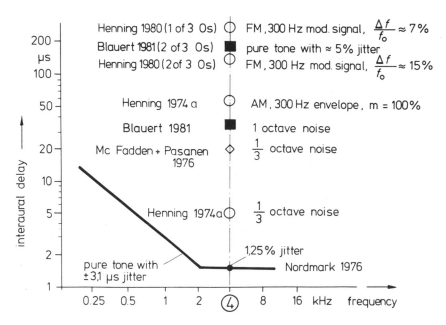

Figure 4.16
Lateralization blur $\Delta(\tau = 0)_{min}$ for narrow-band signals centered at 4 kHz (several authors' results).

and Hafter 1976, 1981, McFadden and Moffitt 1977, Bloom and Jones 1978, Henning and Ashton 1981, Hafter et al. 1981, Jones and Williams 1981; see also Tobias 1972). It has been found that, under appropriate conditions, about the same small lateralization blurs can be observed in connection with the evaluation of envelope time differences above 1.5 kHz as are observed in connection with differences in the fine structure of signals below 1.5 kHz (figure 4.16). In connection with brief signals (clicks) containing no components below 1.5 kHz, the lowest values of lateralization blur are attained after several repetitions. In connection with amplitude-modulated sinusoidal signals with sinusoidal envelopes, the lowest values of lateralization blur were observed in connection with envelope frequencies between approximately 150 and 400 Hz and carrier frequencies in the range of approximately 3–5 kHz. High-pass filtered noise signals, even uncorrelated ones, produced

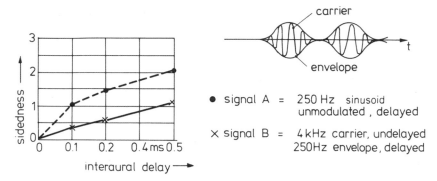

Figure 4.17
Lateral displacement for the same interaural time difference for a 250 Hz sinusoid
and for a 250 Hz envelope on a 4 kHz carrier (Blauert 1982a).

a fused auditory event as long as the envelopes of the two ear input
signals were the same.

When a low-frequency signal is presented to both ears, the lateral
displacements correspond differently to interaural time differences than
when modulated high-frequency carriers with the same modulation
frequency as the previous low-frequency signal are presented (figure
4.17). Blauert (1982a) notes in this context that a low-frequency signal
undergoes a sort of half-wave-rectification during the signal processing
in the inner ear, while the envelope of a high-frequency carrier is maintained as a full-wave signal. A half-wave-rectified signal may provide
more distinct time cues than a full-wave signal, due to its transient
features. Figure 4.18 shows the lateral displacement of a noise signal
one critical band wide as a function of the center frequency (Blauert
1978). The lateral displacement decreases as the center frequency is
increased.

Frequency-modulated signals above 1.5 kHz also lead to laterally
displaced auditory events (Bielek 1975, Nordmark 1976, Henning 1980;
figure 4.16). One possible explanation is that the inner ear's bandpass
filter characteristics transform frequency modulation into amplitude
modulation (Blauert 1980c, 1981), as in electronic FM detector circuits.
This explanation cannot account for the extremely low values of lateralization blur measured by Nordmark (1976), but no other authors
have yet found such low values.

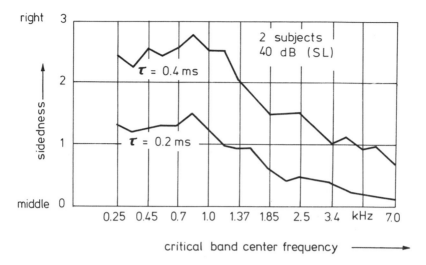

Figure 4.18
Lateral displacement of noise signals one critical band wide as a function of the center frequency for a fixed interaural time difference τ (Blauert 1978; two experienced subjects, 40 dBSL).

If signals whose spectrum is more than one critical band wide are presented to a subject, multiple auditory events may occur (Sayers 1964, Toole and Sayers 1965a). Figures 4.19 and 4.20 show two examples of this phenomenon that are of interest in connection with the evaluation of envelope curves (Blauert 1978, 1982a). Both were obtained using experienced subjects. Figure 4.19 shows the results of an auditory experiment in which an interaural time difference was generated in one critical bandwidth of a broadband noise signal, while the interaural time difference for the rest of the signal was zero. As a rule, the subjects perceived two components of auditory events: one in the median plane, the other laterally displaced and corresponding to the frequency band containing the time difference. When the center frequency of the band containing the time difference was raised above 1.5 kHz, the lateral displacement of the corresponding auditory event became smaller and smaller. When the center frequency was above 2.5 kHz, generally only one auditory event was perceived. Figure 4.20 illustrates an experiment in which the signal consisted of three components, each of which was a critical band wide. The center frequencies of the first two components were 540 and 840 Hz. The center frequency of the third component

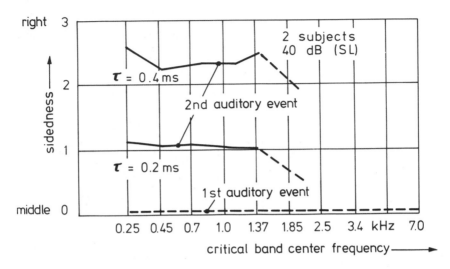

Figure 4.19
Lateral displacement of broadband noise a critical-band-wide component of which is
presented with an interaural time difference $\tau \neq 0$; for the rest of the signal $\tau = 0$
(two experienced subjects, 40 dBSL).

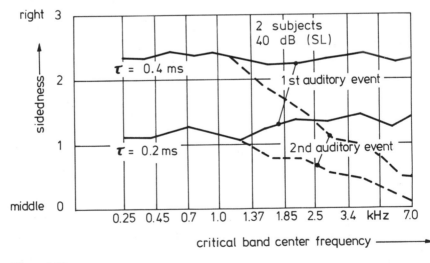

Figure 4.20
Lateral displacement of a signal with three components, each of which is one critical
band wide. Center frequencies: $f_1 = 540$ Hz, $f_2 = 840$ Hz, f_3 variable (abscissa). Two
experienced subjects, 40 dBSL.

was variable. The same interaural time difference τ was used for each of the three components. As soon as the variable component lay above 1.5 kHz, a separate component of the auditory event was heard that was less displaced than the main component.

Inexperienced subjects as a rule do not recognize any separate components of auditory events in the experiments illustrated in figures 4.19 and 4.20. Instead they describe a single, spatially extended auditory event for which they can give an average displacement; this could be called the displacement of the "center of gravity" of the auditory event. The question immediately arises as to whether all frequency components contribute equally to the judgment, or whether certain frequency components are particularly effective in determining the lateral displacement of the auditory event. What is known at this time is that the lateral displacement of the auditory event and its lateralization blur are primarily determined by the signal components below 1.5 kHz if only pure time differences exist between the signals (Yost et al. 1971, Blauert 1978, 1982). The frequency range around 600 Hz is, in this case, dominant (Bilsen and Raatgever 1973, Raatgever 1974, 1976, 1980a, Bilsen 1977). Under free-field conditions (i.e., when there are simultaneous level and time differences such as to produce lateral displacements in the same direction), localization blur $\Delta(\varphi = 0)_{\text{min}}$ is also smallest if the signal includes components below 1.5 kHz (Banks and Green 1973). On the basis of results from the literature, Blauert (1972b) formulated a hypothesis according to which the signal components above 1.5 kHz would be of pronounced importance under the conditions of daily life; however, no experimental confirmation of this hypothesis is available at this time. (It should be noted in this context that the level of the frequency range around 2–3 kHz is raised very considerably in a free sound field, due to the effect of the pinna and ear canal.)

A favored experimental method for comparing different types of interaural attributes with respect to their potency in effecting lateral displacements of auditory events is "trading" (see section 2.4.3). In an experiment using this method, the auditory event is displaced laterally by means of an interaural attribute of a single type (e.g., a time difference); then the lateral displacement is compensated for by an opposite interaural attribute of another type (e.g., a level difference), so that the auditory event regains its original position. This method has been applied in many investigations in recent years (e.g., Babkoff et al. 1973, Young and Carhart 1974, Ruotolo et al. 1979; see also Molino 1974), although for some time there has been fundamental doubt as to its validity (Hershkowitz and Durlach 1969b, Hafter and Carrier 1972). Doubt arises because multiple auditory events with differing lateral displacements can occur in trading experiments; this difficulty can arise even when the ear input signals are less than one critical band wide.

It has long been known that multiple auditory events can occur in connection with narrow-band signals (see sections 2.4.1 and 2.4.2 and figure 2.72; for recent reconfirmation see Yost 1981). Whitworth and Jeffress (1961) observed two components of the auditory event. One could be displaced laterally only by interaural time differences (the "time image"); the other could be displaced by both interaural time differences and interaural level differences (the "intensity image"). Other authors, including Ruotolo et al. (1979) and Blauert, found it difficult to identify just these two components, although they did observe multiple auditory events—however, at least the time image has been reinvestigated recently by a some authors (e.g., Hafter 1977, and, in the context of binaural pitch phenomena, Raatgever 1980a, b).

Trading experiments, then, may lead to uncertainty as to whether the subject is describing the position of one of the multiple auditory events—and of which one—or is describing some sort of a spatial average or "center of gravity." For this reason the present author believes that all results of trading experiments must be regarded with great skepticism. This is especially so when the subject's task is to judge only the lateral displacement of the auditory event, disregarding other spatial attributes such as its extent.

A primary goal of future investigations, especially those aimed at developing a model of binaural signal processing (see section 4.4.4), must be to identify the individual components of multiple auditory events and to analyze their behavior under varying conditions. Training of the subjects and details of the experimental procedure (e.g., in directing the subjects' attention toward specific components of the auditory event) will be of particular importance. In this author's opinion, trading experiments are not appropriate for such investigations. Much better are the mapping methods (see Guttman 1962, Domnitz and Colburn 1977, but also Chernyak and Dubrowsky 1968, Damaske 1967/68, Wagener 1971, and others), in which the position and extent of the auditory events are described directly. Tracking techniques (Damper 1976) may also be appropriate.

In recent years there has been great interest in the perception of moving auditory events (Briggs and Perrott 1972, Huggins 1974, Altman and Viskov 1977, Perrott and Musicant 1977a,b, Deutsch 1978, Pollack 1978, Grantham and Wightman 1978, 1979, Perrott 1979). The results of experiments in this area allow conclusions to be drawn about the integration times of the auditory system and therefore about the persistence of the spatial properties of auditory events as a function of time.

We have already addressed the question of spatial persistence in previous chapters (e.g., in sections 2.1 and 2.4.3; see also Aschoff 1963, Plath et al. 1970, Blauert 1970a, and the references to the literature on binaural beats in section 2.4.1). If, for example, equidistant sound impulses are presented alternately to the right and left ear of a subject, then—if the time interval between impulses, T, is great enough—a single auditory event appears, jumping from the right ear to the left and back again in time with the presentation of the impulses. But as T is decreased, a threshold is reached beyond which the auditory event no longer jumps back and forth but remains for a while at one ear, perhaps then jumping to the other. It dissociates into primary auditory events and echoes. As T is decreased still further, there finally appears— though there is no precise threshold—a single diffusely localized auditory event in the middle of the head.

The threshold T_2 beyond which the auditory event no longer jumps back and forth between the ears in time with the impulses, is called the "threshold for the perceptibility of directional changes." This threshold has been measured for a great variety of signals and types of sound presentation both under free-field conditions and using headphones. Despite these significant differences, the measured values all lie in the range of approximately $T_2 = 100$–200 ms. This range of values agrees with that for similar thresholds observed in experiments with binaural beats or experiments in which the intelligibility of dichotically alternating speech was measured. The range of time intervals in which the law of the first wavefront takes effect is also similar. It is thus not wide off the mark to regard a time constant of 100–200 ms as typical for the persistence of the spatial properties of auditory events.

Pollack (1977, 1978) reported a psychoacoustic experiment from which he concluded that an additional, much smaller time constant T_1 exists in connection with binaural signal processing in spatial hearing (in this context see also von Wedel 1979, 1981). Pollack's experimental conditions are as follows: a pseudonoise signal consisting of a train of brief impulses whose phase angle varies randomly between 0° and 180° is presented to the left ear. The same signal is presented to the right ear, but by way of a "polarity switch" that periodically reverses the phase angle. The right ear input signal, then, alternates periodically between being in phase and being 180° out of phase with the left ear input signal. If the switching interval is long ($T \geq T_2$), then the subjects hear a sharply localized and a diffusely localized auditory event following one another periodically. But if the switching interval is made shorter, only a single unified auditory event is perceived, and its spatial extent increases as T decreases. When T becomes very short, the auditory event is, finally, completely diffusely localized. What is measured in the experiment is the value T_1 of the switching interval at which the subject perceives a just-noticeable decrease in the spatial extent of the fully diffuse auditory event. When signal parameters are appropriate, T_1 is no greater than 1.5–3.5 ms.

Pollack's interpretation of his results is based on the hypothesis that T_1 represents the minimum time interval needed by the auditory system in order to establish that the ear input signals contain components that are interaurally in phase. This hypothesis needs further experimental confirmation. It is attractive insofar as it emphasizes that the persistence of hearing in evaluating interaural signal attributes cannot be represented by a single time constant. Neither can the evaluation of monaural signal attributes such as, for example, loudness (Zwicker 1968, 1977, Green 1973, Vogel 1975). One possible speculation is as follows: The shorter time constant T_1 could be a property of relatively peripheral evaluative mechanisms, perhaps of the duration of the impulse response of the peripheral band filters. The longer time constant T_2 could be related to a more central evaluative mechanism (see section 4.4.4).

4.4.2 Summing localization and the law of the first wavefront

In this section we report some new results related to these topics, which were previously discussed in sections 3.1 and 3.3.

When two or more sound sources radiate coherent or partially coherent signals, only one auditory event may appear, with its spatial attributes depending on the positions of all of the contributing sound sources and on the signals they radiate. Even sounds that reach the listener's ears up to 50 ms later than the first arriving sound may take part in this "summing localization," provided that their level is adjusted adequately (Barron 1971, 1974). The main application of this phenomenon is in stereophonic reproduction processes. Questions about this application have led to new investigations by Matsudaira and Fukami (1973), Gaskell (1976, 1978), Theile and Plenge (1977), Theile (1978, 1980), and Gotoh et al. (1980) (see also Damaske and Ando 1972).

One important recent result is the fact that the position of the auditory event can be well controlled when the loudspeakers are placed in front of the listener in the standard stereophonic arrangement (figure 3.1), but not when the loudspeakers are placed at the side of the listener. Figure 4.21 shows the dependence of the azimuth of the auditory event on the level difference between the loudspeaker signals when the loudspeakers are at the side. One clear inference is that it is not possible to generate precise auditory events in directions to the side using four loudspeakers, as is common in quadraphonic sound systems (figure 3.52). At least six loudspeakers are necessary for a reasonably precise representation of all azimuths around the listener.

Gaskell (1976, 1978) added further evidence to the hypothesis that summing localization is based on interaural differences of the ear input signals as produced by linear (running) superposition of the signal components stemming from different sound sources. However, her results have been rendered by a lateralization paradigm, thus being subject to the warning expressed at the beginning of this section (p. 312).

Theile studied the following phenomenon: In summing localization, each ear input signal is derived from at least two loudspeaker signals that are displaced in time with respect to each other. Consequently each ear input signal shows strong comb-filter effects (see figure 3.10, top). The auditory event, however, has almost the same timbre as if only one of the two loudspeakers were driven; that is, it has the same timbre as if no superposition of differently delayed signals occurred. Moreover, the timbre of the auditory event changes but little when the listener's head turns with respect to the loudspeaker arrangement. On

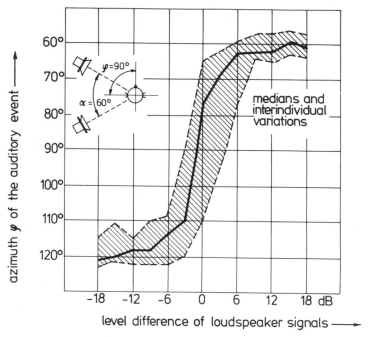

Figure 4.21
Azimuth of the auditory event as a function of the level difference ΔL between the loudspeaker signals when the loudspeakers are at the side. The signals are coherent broadband noise impulses and speech (after Theile and Plenge 1977). Shown are medians and quartiles of the directions reported by the subjects.

the other hand, whether there are one or two loudspeakers, a listener with one ear plugged perceives distinct colorations of timbre that depend on the direction of sound incidence. Early reflections from rigid surfaces such as tabletops and walls can also lead to strong colorations of timbre ("hollowness") in monaural listening; but this phenomenon is less noticeable, and sometimes not at all noticed, in binaural hearing (Koenig 1950, Zurek 1976, 1979).*

Clearly, then, the auditory system possesses the ability, in binaural hearing, to disregard certain linear distortions of the ear input signals in forming the timbre of the auditory event. The auditory system might,

---

*Monophonic (single-channel) electroacoustical transmission corresponds to monaural listening. Consequently, in monophonic transmission, colorations of timbre due to early reflections occur frequently.

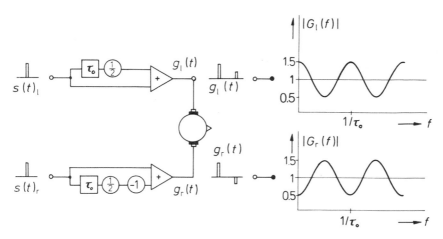

Figure 4.22
Inhibition of the effect of comb-filter distortions of the ear input signals on timbre in binaural hearing (after Zurek 1976, 1979).

for example, compensate the ear input signals by means of appropriate inverse filtering (Batteau 1967, Zurek 1976, 1979, Allen et al. 1977, Theile 1978, 1980, Platte 1979). Theile suggests that, under certain conditions, the auditory system recognizes the positions of all of the sound sources that contribute to summing localization and undertakes appropriate inverse filtering based on this information. This hypothesis is not without its opponents (e.g., Platte and Genuit 1980). Furthermore, it does not by itself explain how a binaural suppression of comb-filter effects comes about in connection with ear input signals that cannot be generated by the external ear, such as those shown in figure 4.22. There is as yet no comprehensive theory of the binaural suppression of colorations of timbre.

Like summing localization, the "law of the first wavefront" is a highly important psychoacoustical effect that occurs in connection with multiple sound sources radiating coherent or partially coherent signals. This law describes the cases in which a single auditory event appears whose position is determined solely by the first wavefront reaching the listener. Recent publications on or related to this subject are those of Scharf (1974), Perrott and Baars (1974), Blauert and Cobben (1978), Hafter et al. (1979), Zurek (1980), and Kunov and Abel (1981).

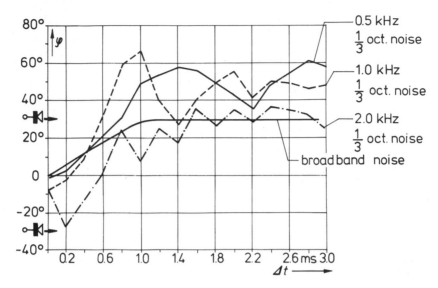

Figure 4.23
The azimuth of the auditory event as a function of the delay Δt of the left loudspeaker signal. Standard stereophonic loudspeaker arrangement in an anechoic chamber. Average values of answers given by 10 subjects with normal hearing. Signals:
1/3-octave pulses (center frequency 0.5 kHz, 1.0 kHz, and 2.0 kHz) and broadband
impulses (Blauert and Cobben 1978).

The law of the first wavefront functions in such a way that the direction
of the auditory event coincides with that of the sound source radiating
the first wavefront, but only if the signals are sufficiently broadband.
If narrow-band test signals are used, other relationships may occur,
such as those shown in figure 4.23. The plot of the azimuth of the
auditory event can be explained in terms of the interaural time difference
between the ear input signals. In each particular case this difference
results from superposition of the components originating at the two
loudspeakers (Blauert and Cobben 1978).

If instantaneously switched signals are presented over the two loudspeakers, the position of the auditory event is determined for approximately 100–200 ms by the arrival time difference between the onset
slopes of the ear input signals (figure 3.21; see Ebata et al. 1968a, Perrott
and Baars 1974, Hafter et al. 1979, Kunov and Abel 1981 in this
context, and also figure 3.49). This is true even when the the tones are
below 1.5 kHz and the time difference of the fine structure does not

correspond to that of the onset slopes. Even when the frequencies of the signals radiated by the two loudspeakers differ, the onset slopes determine the position of the auditory event for a certain length of time (Scharf 1974).

Section 3.1.2 mentioned the usual assumption behind attempts to explain the law of the first wavefront: that both ipsilateral and contralateral inhibition (postmasking) are at work. Zurek (1980) has carried out several interesting experiments that cast further light on binaural signal processing in the context of the law of the first wavefront. Using lateralization experiments, he investigated, among other topics, the lateralization blur of a simulated reflection as a function of the delay of this reflection with respect to a simulated first wavefront. The signals were brief impulses of broadband noise. Figure 4.24 shows typical results. It can be seen that the lateralization blurs $\Delta(\Delta L = 0)_{min}$ and $\Delta(\tau = 0)_{min}$ are distinctly increased, with a maximum in the range between 2 and 3 ms after the arrival of the first wavefront. In other words, the ability of the auditory system to recognize that reflected sound comes from a direction other than that of the primary sound is distinctly reduced immediately after the arrival of the first wavefront.

Section 3.1.2 stressed that the law of the first wavefront states only that a single auditory event appears, not that the reflected sound cannot be perceived. The fact is that the masked threshold for reflections lies at a lower level than the echo threshold (figure 3.13). The subject may recognize that reflected sound below the echo threshold is present not only on the basis of changes in loudness and timbre, but also on the basis that the auditory event is "more spacious" when reflected sound is present than when it is not. The degree of the increase in the spatial extent of the auditory event due to reflected sound is largely independent of the delay of the reflected sound. The level difference (or, described in another way, the energy ratio) between the first wavefront and the reflected sound has a much greater effect (Barron 1971, 1974a,b; Reichardt and Lehmann 1978a,b). This increased spaciousness of the auditory event when reflected sound is present plays an important role in architectural acoustics in the design of rooms for the performance and reproduction of music. We shall deal with this effect in more detail in section 4.5.1.

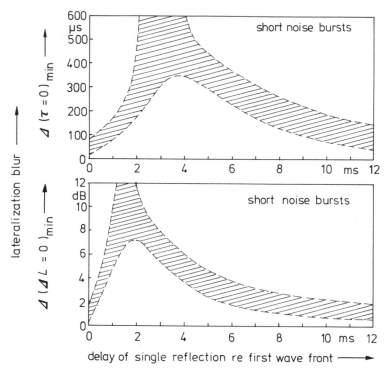

Figure 4.24
Lateralization blurs $\Delta(\tau = 0)_{min}$ and $\Delta(\Delta L = 0)_{min}$ of a simulated reflection as a function of the time interval after the simulated first wavefront (after Zurek 1980, schematized).

4.4.3 Binaural localization, signal detection, and speech recognition in the presence of interfering noise

The study of localization in the presence of interfering noise takes in a broad range of topics. One reason for this is that the definition of the desired sound and the interfering noise may differ greatly depending on the situation or on the conditions of an experiment. For example, it is often the case that several sound sources are radiating incoherent signals, but that only the signal radiated by one of the sources is regarded as the desired sound. The sound source radiating the desired signal can change, for example, during a conversation among several persons. When multiple sources are radiating coherent or partially coherent signals (e.g., in multiple-channel electroacoustic transmission), the interfering noise may be generated by these sources themselves (amplifier noise or hum) or by additional sources. Even when a single sound source radiates a noise-free signal, interfering noise may exist in the form of reflections such as occur in enclosed rooms. Depending on the circumstances, the reflected sound may be, to varying degrees, counted as part of the desired sound or regarded as interfering noise. For example, in rooms for the reproduction of music, early reflections up to approximately 80 ms after the primary sound are regarded as desirable; late, single, strong reflections are interfering noise, since they are audible as echoes. A reverberant sound field perceived as desirable in music reproduction can interfere with the reproduction of speech. This series of examples could be extended.

Very few works come to grips with the practical applications of localization in the presence of interfering noise, even though this is how localization mostly occurs in daily life. Experiments on lateralization in the presence of interfering noise are somewhat more numerous.

A closely related topic is signal detection in the presence of interfering noise (see section 3.2.2), since the capacity for both localization and signal detection is based on binaural signal processing. Recent surveys of work on signal detection in the presence of interfering noise include those of Durlach and Colburn (1978) and Colburn (1977a). We limit ourselves here to a few works dealing with specific questions of interest.

Jacobsen (1976) made a direct attempt to investigate the impairment of localization by interfering noise (see also King and Laird 1930). Localization blur $\Delta(\varphi = 0)_{min}$ in the forward direction was measured.

The interfering noise, a homogeneous mix of sounds of automotive traffic at a level of 30 sone, was presented from the front. The result was that as long as the level of the test signals was about 10–15 dB above their masked threshold, localization blur was no greater than when no interfering noise was present. With 500 Hz sinusoidal signals at 3 dBSL (i.e., only 3 dB over the masked threshold), localization blur was hardly greater than when the SL was more than 10 dB. With 3,000 Hz signals, on the other hand, the localization blur increased to over 5 times as great at 3 dBSL as at 10 dBSL.

The investigation of whether intensity stereophony or delay stereophony is more resistant to interfering signals began quite a few years ago. Intensity stereophony makes use of pure intensity differences, and delay stereophony makes use of pure delay differences, between the loudspeaker signals. Among the first investigators were Leakey and Cherry (1957), who found delay stereophony to be highly susceptible to interfering noises. For similar reasons, Schirmer (1966a) recommends intensity stereophony as the better of the two encoding schemes. Scherer (1959) asserts that delay stereophony is totally unsuited to the transmission of directional information in reverberant rooms. In a few pilot experiments, this author has been able to establish that no significant degradation of directional imaging occurs with either intensity stereophony or delay stereophony if the level of superimposed, interchannel-uncorrelated noise is 8 dB or more below that of the desired signal (music, speech, or noise). Houtgast and Plomp (1968) report that lateralization blur reaches its minimum value if the level of interfering noise is 15 dB or more below that of the signal.

If noise is superimposed on the desired signal in only one ear in a lateralization experiment, then the auditory event corresponding to the desired signal generally shifts toward the ear to which the interfering noise is not presented (von Békésy 1933, Sayers and Cherry 1957); the extent of the shift depends on the relationship between the desired and interfering signals. This effect is useful in the study of the "internal representation" of the magnitude and phase of the monaural interfering signal in the hearing apparatus (for descriptions of this and similar experimental methods see Houtgast 1977, Sieben and Gerlach 1980).

Recent investigations using a variety of methods have dealt with lateralization blur in the presence of interfering noise (Robinson and Egan 1974, Henning 1974b, Yost 1975, Gaskell 1978, Gaskell and

Henning 1979, 1981). It appears to have been conclusively proven that the mechanism that evaluates interaural envelope time differences is significantly more susceptible to noise than is the mechanism that evaluates interaural time differences in the fine structure of the signals. On the other hand, taking broadband pulses disrupted by broadband noise, lateralization based on interaural level differences seems to be more robust than that based on time differences. It is not yet clear how all this fits together.

McFadden (1969), McFadden and Pasanen (1978), Ito et al. (1979), and Cohen (1978, 1981) have reported interesting results pertaining to both lateralization blur and binaural signal detection. They used interfering noise signals with various interaural phase relationships (e.g., N_0, in phase; N_π, out of phase; N_t, interaurally delayed) or interaurally uncorrelated noise (N_u). The desired signal was a 250 Hz tone burst or narrow-band noise with a center frequency of 500 Hz or 4 kHz. In each case the masked threshold—allowing the binaural masking level difference (BMLD, see section 3.2.2) to be determined—and the lateralization blur were measured. The results at first seem surprising: The conditions under which lateralization blur is greatest are those under which the signal is most easily detected, and vice versa. For example, lateralization blur is least for N_0, greater for N_u, and greatest for N_π. Figure 4.25 shows the relationship especially clearly; lateralization performance is always poorest in the presence of interfering noise when the interaural time difference of the signal leads to a minimum of the interaural cross-correlation of the signal, that is, when the fine structure of the signal is interaurrally out of phase.

Colburn (1977b), Cohen (1978), and McFadden and Pasanen (1978) found an explanation for this relationship (see also Hafter 1971 in this context). Since both the signal and the interfering noise are narrowband noise signals, they interfere with each other. Because they are statistically independent of each other, the phase angle between them varies over time. At some times they cancel; at others they reinforce each other. If the fine structure of the noise is interaurally out of phase, then one ear input signal is always intensified when the other is attenuated, and vice versa. Consequently interaural level differences are generated whose direction is constantly changing. (An equivalent effect, by the way, happens with regard to interaural time differences.) Therefore

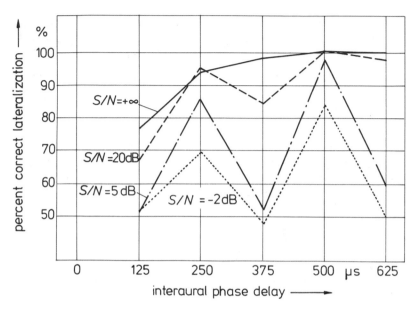

Figure 4.25
Lateralization "performance" as a function of the interaural time difference of the signal. Signal: Narrow-band signal at 4,000 Hz ± 25 Hz. Noise: Narrow-band noise at 4,000 Hz ± 25 Hz (N_0), independent of the signal. The parameter is the S/N ratio (adapted from McFadden and Pasanen 1978).

the lateral displacement of the auditory event changes stochastically. This aids in signal detection but worsens the lateralization blur.

An effect that is of practical importance and related to binaural signal detection is binaural suppression of reverberation. Many years have passed since von Békésy (1931) and Koenig (1950) first pointed out that an acoustical presentation in a room sounds less reverberant when a person listens with both ears than when one ear is plugged. This implies that in two-eared hearing the interaurally correlated primary sound is more easily recognized in the presence of interaurally uncorrelated interfering noise (the reverberant signal) than it is with one ear plugged. Danilenko (1967, 1969) gave a vivid experimental demonstration of the effect (see figure 4.26). Broadband noise, amplitude-modulated to give a sinusoidal envelope, is introduced into a room and listened to via a monophonic (one-channel) transmission system or, alternatively, via direct two-eared hearing. The smallest modulation

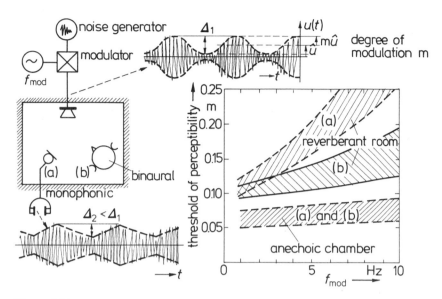

Figure 4.26
Inhibition of reverberation in binaural hearing (after Danilenko 1967, 1969).

index m is measured at which an oscillation of the noise can be perceived auditorily. It can be seen that a significantly lower modulation index can be perceived using binaural hearing in a reverberant room than over a monophonic channel. The "slurring effect" of the reverberation is, then, less noticeable in binaural hearing. Reverberant sound is binaurally uncorrelated; the expected BMLD of 3 dB for uncorrelated noise can, to be sure, partly explain binaural suppression of reverberation (Koenig et al. 1977). It is certain that the time sequence of the primary signal and the reverberation also plays a role (Zurek 1976, 1979). In this connection, the results for binaural forward masking must also be taken into consideration (Yost and Walton 1977; for further references see Durlach and Colburn 1978).

In the last decade a number of papers on speech recognition in the presence of interfering noise have appeared (e.g., Quante 1973, Plomp 1976; Lazarus-Mainka and Lazarus 1976, vom Hövel 1981). Some of these results deserve to be repeated here because they are related to binaural hearing and are of great practical importance. The characteristic variable measured is the BILD or MILD (binaural or monaural intel-

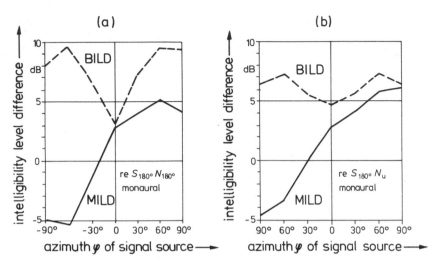

Figure 4.27
a: BILD and MILD for a source of interfering noise behind the subject. b: BILD and MILD for six uncorrelated sources of interfering noise distributed evenly around the horizontal plane. Signal: Groups of three identical monosyllables each. Noise: Noise simulating speech (65 dBA). Criterion: 50 percent intelligibility level. Approximately 10 subjects, BILD with two ears, MILD with one ear (adapted from vom Hövel and Platte 1980).

ligibility level difference; see section 3.2.2). The BILD or MILD represents the amount by which the signal-to-noise ratio can be degraded with respect to a reference condition when the only requirement is that a constant degree of intelligibility be maintained.

Figure 4.27 shows results for the horizontal plane with one source of interfering noise behind the subject (N_{180}) or with six uncorrelated sources of interfering noise distributed evenly around the horizontal plane (N_u). The interfering noise was random noise simulating speech (SPL = 65 dBA). The reference condition was for the target speech source to be behind the subject (S_{180}) and monaural listening, so the reference conditions of the two experiments were $(S_{180}N_{180})_{\text{monaural}}$ and $(S_{180}N_u)_{\text{monaural}}$, respectively. The figure shows results for positions of the target speech source in the forward part of the horizontal plane (cf. figure 3.41).

Figure 4.28 shows the dependence of the plot of the BILD on the reverberation time of the room in which the sound is reproduced. In this experiment the reference condition was $(S_0N_0)_{\text{binaural}}$; in other

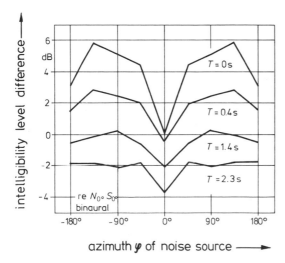

azimuth φ of noise source ⟶

Figure 4.28
The BILD as a function of the reverberation time of the room in which sound is re-produced. Distance of the sound source is 10 m; 10 subjects, binaural hearing. Noise: Noise simulating speech, SPL = 55 dB. Signal: Speech, connected discourse. Criterion: Threshold between intelligible and unintelligible (adapted from Plomp 1976).

words, the target speech sound source and the source of interfering noise were both located directly in front of the subject. The maximum values of the BILD decrease as the reverberation time increases; yet a BILD of about 1.5 dB remains even if the sound field is largely diffuse, as long as the angle $\Delta\varphi$ between the target speech signal sound source and the source of interfering noise is more than 45°.

4.4.4 Models of binaural signal processing

Historically, a great number of experiments have been carried out to develop functional models of binaural signal processing. Section 3.2.1 included a description of the principles of a functional model capable of evaluating interaural time differences and identifying coherent components of the two ear input signals (see figures 3.32 and 3.34). This is called the "coincidence or cross-correlation model." Four further models of binaural signal recognition were mentioned in section 3.2.2: the vector model, the equalization and cancellation model, the accumulation model, and a particular correlation model.

There are other models yet, including the group of "count comparison models" (von Békésy 1930a, Matzker 1958, van Bergeijk 1962, Hall

1965); we mentioned these only in passing. There is also the purely mathematical model of Searle et al. (1976), which is based entirely on statistical decision theory. Colburn and Durlach (1978) give an exhaustive summary and analysis of works on binaural signal processing models published up to approximately 1974.

Given what we assume today, any model that is to describe binaural signal processing in the most comprehensive way possible—at least with respect to binaural localization and binaural signal recognition— must include the following six functional elements (figure 4.29):

A. Filters that simulate the transfer functions of the external ear.
B. Filters that simulate the transfer behavior of the middle ear.
C. Functional elements that simulate the functions of the inner ear (cochlea), especially its frequency selectivity and its transformation of deterministic acoustical-hydromechanical "analog" signals into probabilistic "digital" nerve signals, that is, into nerve firing patterns.
D. A functional element that simulates the evaluation of interaural time differences and the identification of interaurally coherent signal components.
E. A functional element that accounts for the evaluation of interaural level differences.
F. A functional element in which the information derived by way of elements D and E is comprehensively evaluated, and in which binaural localization (i.e., the correlation of positions and extents of auditory events) or binaural signal detection (i.e., the decision "signal present or not") takes place.

If it is taken into account that spatial hearing occurs even when sound is presented only to one ear (there is no such thing as "nonspatial" hearing!), then additional functional elements for monaural signal processing must be assumed (see section 3.2.1 and Stern and Colburn 1978). It is in any case more appropriate to start with the assumption that, even when sound is presented to both ears, monaural as well as binaural signal processing always takes place. We shall not, however, explore monaural signal processing any more deeply in what follows. Instead, in order to avoid misunderstandings, we emphatically note that we do not represent our given general outline of a signal-processing model as a universal one that encompasses all aspects of auditory signal processing. For example, the model does not exclude the existence of

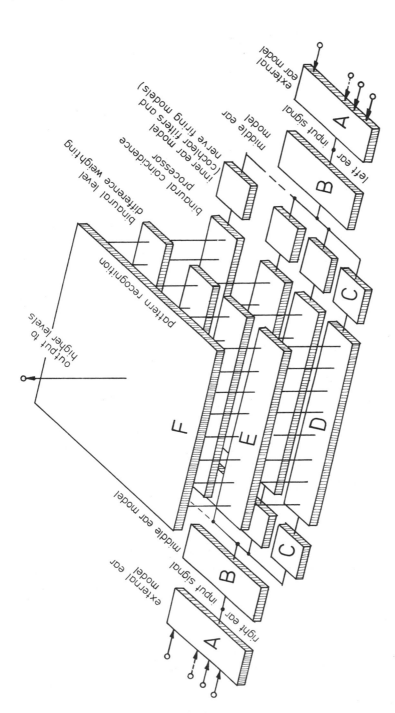

Figure 4.29
Functional diagram of a model of signal processing in binaural localization and binaural signal detection.

other processing steps for auditory signals, parallel to the steps we have described, and also furnishing information to the central nervous system.

In what follows we shall give a brief sketch of the current state of development of models corresponding to the individual functional elements in figure 4.29.

Element A   The transfer functions of the external ear are known, or are easily measured and simulated (section 4.2.1), yet they have only rarely been taken into account in developing models of binaural signal processing (Damaske 1969/70, Blauert 1973, Blauert and Cobben 1978, Lindemann 1982).

Element B   The transfer behavior of the middle ear has not yet been incorporated into models of binaural signal processing, although it would in principle seem to be of great importance.

Element C   A simulation of signal processing in the inner ear in model form is assumed in all relevent work in this subject area. The simplest case is for the frequency selectivity of the inner ear to be simulated by a bank of adjacent bandpass filters with rectangular or trapezoidal pass curves; the bandwidth of each filter might correspond to a "critical band." More precise models simulate the frequency selectivity for each point on the basilar membrane, by means of approximations of the impulse response of the basilar membrane (Blauert 1973, Colburn 1973, Blauert and Cobben 1978) or by finite-element mapped solutions of systems of differential equations that describe the motions of the basilar membrane in detail (for an example of a "computer-friendly" algorithm see Schlichthärle 1978, 1981).

A precise simulation of actual physiological conditions requires that the model include an algorithm that converts movements of the basilar membrane into nerve firing patterns. These patterns are sample functions of stochastic point processes; that is, they consist of a stochastic series of individual nerve impulses (spikes). Once the necessary physiological and mathematical prerequisites for such patterns had been reported in the pioneering works of Kiang et al. (1965) and Siebert (1968), such an algorithm was in fact included in several models (Duifhuis 1972, Blauert and Cobben 1978, but especially Colburn 1969, 1973, 1977a, Stern 1976, Colburn and Latimer 1978, Stern and Colburn 1978). Including this element made the models considerably more accurate, especially in simulating binaural signal detection.

As long as the main interest is in binaural localization, that is, in the positions and extents of auditory events, it is often possible to do without the simulation of individual nerve impulses. Instead, one can generate deterministic signals that represent the time function of the firing probability of auditory nerve fibers or bundles of them (Bilsen 1977, Raatgever and Bilsen 1977, Blauert and Cobben 1978, Raatgever 1980a). In some simple models the probability of firing is assumed to be proportional to (positive) displacements of the basilar membrane; that is, saturation effects observable in the nerve firing patterns are not taken into account. To the extent that the ear input signals include components above approximately 1.5 kHz, it must be assumed that the probability of firing corresponds more and more at higher frequencies to the envelope of the movements of the basilar membrane and not to the fine structure (Kiang et al. 1965, Russell and Sellick 1978). This phenomenon can be approximated by half-wave rectification followed by an RC lowpass filter of the first order with $\tau = 1.25$ ms (see figure 3.34).

Interactions between neighboring points on the basilar membrane can be observed, for example, as the frequency-selectivity-increasing effect of lateral inhibition. Such interactions have, however, not been included in binaural signal-processing models. In the future they may be expected to be. Appropriate algorithms for the modeling of such phenomena are known (e.g., Schlichthärle 1981).

Element D The task of this element is to identify and separate components that are present in both ear input signals (i.e., the ones that are interaurally coherent) and to report the interaural time differences of these components. We described the fundamental principles of this element in section 3.2.1 (figures 3.32–3.34). These principles are based on the coincidence model of Jeffress (1948), whose functioning we here assume to be well-known; however, for further clarification we illustrate the model in a somewhat different form in figure 4.30. The input signals are the nerve firing patterns, that is, the specific series of spikes that arrive from the two inner ears. Nerve signals arriving from points representing the same critical frequency in the two inner ears are interpreted in the same coincidence detector. The result of this evaluation is a running three-dimensional activity pattern over a frequency-delay plane, that is, a running coincidence pattern.

The following additional assumptions are needed to make the co-

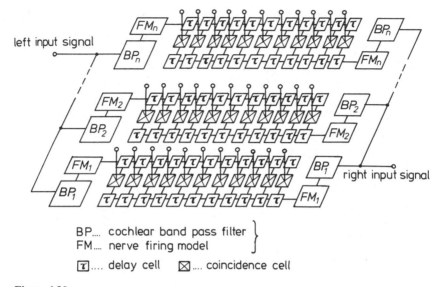

left input signal

right input signal

BP.... cochlear band pass filter ⎫
FM.... nerve firing model   ⎬
                                    ⎭

⊡ .... delay cell   ⊠ .... coincidence cell

Figure 4.30
A diagram of functional elements for the identification of interaurally coherent components of the ear input signals and for the measurement of interaural time differences (a so-called coincidence model).

incidence model conform to psychoacoustical data. First, the coincidence of two nerve impulses is assumed when they both arrive at a multiplier cell within a coincidence interval of approximately 50–150 μs. Second, there are many coincidence detectors in each frequency range, but those corresponding to longer delays are less numerous than those corresponding to shorter ones. The activity of the coincidence pattern is consequently subjected to a "fundamental attenuation" that increases monotonically with the interaural delay. Third, interaural delays of more than 1 or 2 ms may play no role.

A binaural coincidence model in the detailed form illustrated, that is, as an "auditory-nerve-based model," has been developed above all by Colburn and his co-workers and tentatively also by Blauert (1973) and Blauert and Cobben (1978). Most model builders still use deterministic input signals that are intended to represent the probability of firing of nerve fibers (Sayers and Cherry 1957, Licklider 1959, Osman 1971, Durlach 1972, Blauert 1973, Bilsen 1977, Raatgever and Bilsen

1977, Blauert and Cobben 1978, Raatgever 1980a, Lindemann 1982).*
If this assumption is made, then a running, appropriately normalized
interaural cross-correlation function must be generated, replacing the
running coincidence pattern and representing its basic features in the
frequency-delay plane.

Element E   This element accounts for the influence of interaural level
differences. Without additional assumptions, a binaural coincidence or
correlation algorithm such as is described in element D cannot evaluate
interaural level differences of the ear input signals. Early investigators
tried to solve this problem by postulating a supplementary peripheral
mechanism that transforms level differences into time differences (e.g.,
a latency mechanism such as the one illustrated symbolically in figure
2.88a). However, we have already shown in section 2.4.3 that a latency
mechanism is not sufficient to explain the existing psychoacoustical
data.

   More recent models of binaural signal processing account for interaural
level differences by means of a special interpretive weighting function
applied to the binaural coincidence or correlation patterns derived by
element D (Stern and Colburn 1978, Blauert 1980b, Lindemann 1982).
The position of the maximum of this weighting function along the delay
axis depends on the interaural level difference. The weighting function
falls off monotonically on either side of the maximum. Figure 4.31
gives examples of interaural cross-correlatograms for certain specific
frequencies, weighted in this way according to level differences. Figure
4.32 depicts two complete, instantaneous, weighted cross-correlation
patterns of the type that would be observed in connection with the
sound of an orchestral chord.

   Various algorithms have been suggested for implementing the
weighting that corresponds to interaural level difference. Blauert (1980b)

---

*Instead of a running cross-correlation (equation 3.21), Raatgever (1980a) used a delay-
and-add power function which, in each band, may be written as

$$P_{xy}(t, \tau) = \int_{-\infty}^{t} [y(\vartheta) + x(\vartheta - \tau)]^2 \, G(t - \vartheta) \, d\vartheta$$

$$= \int_{-\infty}^{t} y^2(\vartheta) \, G(t - \vartheta) \, d\vartheta + \int_{-\infty}^{t} x^2(\vartheta - \tau) \, G(t - \vartheta) \, d\vartheta + 2\Psi_{xy}(t, \tau),$$

thus including monaural information in the binaural activity pattern.

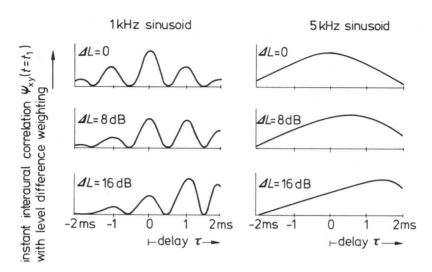

Figure 4.31
Interaural instantaneous cross-correlatograms for two specific frequencies (1 kHz, 5 kHz), after weighting corresponding to interaural level differences $\Delta L = 0$ dB, 8 dB, and 16 dB (after Blauert 1982b).

achieves the desired effect by means of an appropriate modification of the binaural coincidence detector. Colburn and Hausler (1980) and Colburn and Moss (1981) proceed from the assumption that a separate evaluative mechanism processes interaural level differences.

Element F   In this element the running interaural coincidence patterns, weighted according to level, are evaluated. So far this element has been defined quantitatively only for binaural signal detection and for simple tasks of lateralization. In experiments on binaural signal detection, one goal was to determine whether two distinct coincidence patterns could in any way be distinguished from one another (Colburn 1977a, Colburn and Latimer 1978, Raatgever 1980a). In simple lateralization tasks in which judgments are made about only a single auditory event, the lateral displacement of the auditory event is assumed, for example, to be proportional to the shift in the center of gravity of the coincidence pattern relative to the point on the delay axis representing zero delay (Stern and Colburn 1978; similar experiments had been conducted by Sayers and Cherry 1957).

In principle, all higher functions of the central nervous system that play a role in binaural signal processing must be included under element

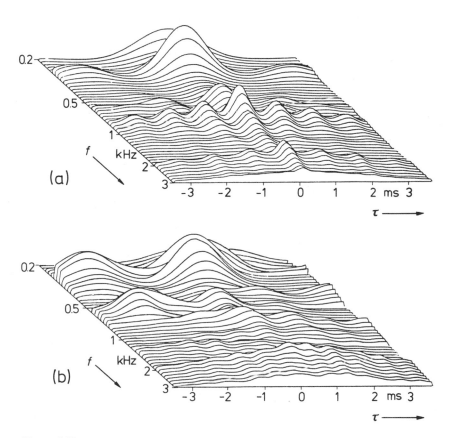

Figure 4.32
Interaural instantaneous correlatograms. a: Diotic presentation of a musical chord.
b: Musical chord, direct frontal sound plus one delayed reflection of the same strength
from the right and another from the left.

F. This element therefore represents a type of "multipurpose computer," and the human brain is in fact such a computer. To be sure, it is appropriate to assume that the coincidence pattern that exists at any one time is subjected to pattern-recognition processes—that a comparison occurs with stored (e.g., learned) patterns (see figure 3.34).

Models of binaural signal processing whose structure conforms to the plan shown in figure 4.29—or which at least include a coincidence detector or correlation detector corresponding to element D—have proven extraordinarily successful. Almost all data on binaural signal detection can today be explained quantitatively by means of such models, as can most data on lateralization blur and on the lateral displacements of auditory events that occur in simple lateralization experiments (see especially the works of Colburn and his co-workers). These models also explain dichotic pitch phenomena assuming a specific strategy in element F (Raatgever 1980a).

The fundamental concept underlying the model in figure 4.29 has other significant applications. For example, it has been speculated that this concept explains the appearance of multiple auditory events if it is assumed that individual peaks of the coincidence pattern indicate individual components of the auditory event that under certain conditions can be "separated" by experienced subjects. The position of each peak along the delay axis may, then, represent the lateral displacement of each corresponding component of the auditory event. Despite the existence of coincidence patterns with more than one peak, less-experienced subjects have only a single, less sharply localized auditory event whose lateral displacement they may possibly judge on the basis of the position of the center of gravity of the coincidence pattern. Furthermore, spatially extended auditory events may appear under the following conditions: (1) when the position of the relevant coincidence peaks is different from one frequency range to another ("spectral incoherence"); (2) when the position of the coincidence peaks shifts as a function of time ("temporal incoherence") (see Blauert 1982a).

Further binaural effects arguably lie within the scope of explanations furnished by the modeling concept: for example, summing localization (Theile 1980), the law of the first wavefront (Blauert and Cobben 1978), binaural suppression of reverberation (Danilenko 1967, Allen et al. 1977), what is called "spaciousness" (see section 4.5.1 and Lindemann 1982), the echo threshold, and more.

Particular problems, such as the quantitative description of the law of the first wavefront, would seem to require further refinement of some elements of the model. Other future model-building tasks proceed above all from the need to conceptualize and quantify appropriate procedures for the evaluation of the interaural, running, level-weighted coincidence pattern. We draw attention in this context to the concluding remarks of section 4.4.1, in which we noted that lateralization experiments support the assumptions of at least two time constants of the auditory system. The longer of these two ($T_2 = 100-200$ ms) might possibly be attributed to the central evaluative functions. We also draw attention to the hypothesis of Damaske (1971a), according to which the instantaneous function of loudness can furnish criteria for the recognition of echoes (figure 3.15). In recent years, functional models of monaural signal processing for forming instantaneous loudness have undergone considerable refinement (Zwicker 1977). Some of the relationships discovered in the course of this work may play a role in the evaluation of running interaural signal patterns.

4.5 Examples of Applications

This concluding section will offer two examples of application of knowledge about spatial hearing. Section 4.5.1 deals with a listener's "auditory spatial impression." This term refers to the part of the total impression of the space that is conveyed by means of hearing alone—for example, in a concert hall or any other place where people congregate. The auditory spatial impression is of great importance in determining whether a particular space is suitable for acoustical presentations. Architects must consequently be able to foresee and carefully control the auditory spatial impression. We shall devote particular attention to one component of the auditory spatial impression that relates to spatial hearing, namely "spaciousness."

Section 4.5.2 describes an electroacoustical process that leads to faithful ("authentic") reproduction. The auditory events of a person listening to the reproduced sound correspond very well to those the same listener would have at the place where the sound is picked up; that is, the qualitative, temporal, and spatial attributes of the auditory events are all very similar in the playback situation relative to the pickup situation. The transmission process uses dummy-head stereophony

in which a head replica equipped with microphones is used to pick up
the sound. Dummy-head stereophony is not new (see sections 2.2 and
2.3), but there has been considerable progress recently, particularly in
rendering this type of stereophony compatible with the more usual
technique of intensity stereophony.

4.5.1 The auditory spatial impression

Section 3.3 described how a subject, presented with a sound field,
spontaneously arrives at a concept of the type and size of an actual or
simulated space. We called this concept the "spatial impression."

One factor that contributes to the spatial impression is the characteristic temporal slurring of auditory events that results from late reflections and reverberation. There is also an auditory effect called
"spaciousness" (Eyshold et al. 1975, Kuhl 1977, 1978, Reichardt and
Lehmann 1978a, Schmidt 1978), which denotes a characteristic spatial
spreading of the auditory events, namely that they fill a larger amount
of space than is defined by the visual contours of an ensemble of sound
sources, such as an orchestra (Kuhl 1977). In other words, the extents
of the auditory events are more spacious than in a free sound field
under comparable conditions.*

It has long been known that persons listening to musical presentations
prefer sound fields that are perceived as spacious. So-called pseudo-
stereophonic processes (see figure 3.30) are a direct application of the
effect of spaciousness. A number of recent investigations have attempted
to identify the auditory components that determine how listeners judge
the quality of concert halls. These investigations also showed more or
less explicitly that spaciousness contributes to a positive judgment of
a concert hall (Siebrasse 1973, Wilkens 1975, Eyshold 1976, Lehmann
1976). For surveys of the subject see Schroeder et al. (1974), Plenge
et al. (1975), Cremer and Müller (1978/82), Schroeder (1980a,b), and
Lehmann and Wilkens (1980).

Spaciousness means that auditory events, in a characteristic way, are
themselves perceived as being spread out in an extended region of
space. This may be described phenomenologically in terms of either

---

*Many English-speaking authors use the term "spatial impression" not as a comprehensive
term but with the same meaning as "spaciousness" (in German, Räumlichkeit). The
same or similar meanings are given to terms such as "spatial responsiveness," "ambiance,"
"apparent source width," "subjective diffusion," "feeling of envelopment," and so forth.

individual auditory events of large spatial extent or multiple, distinguishable components of auditory events, each of small extent and occurring simultaneously or one after another within a region of space.

We know from sections 3.2.1 and 3.3 that the region of space occupied by auditory events depends on the interaural degree of coherence k (equations 3.1, 3.2, and 3.11). Weakly correlated ear input signals can lead, in the limiting case, to the listener's feeling completely enveloped by auditory events. In section 4.4.1 we also mentioned that extensive and diffusely located auditory events can appear when sound sources move so rapidly that the auditory evaluative system, with its characteristic time constant, cannot follow the rapid variations in interaural time and level differences. When this is the case, the auditory system perceives the ear input signals as uncorrelated.

It is appropriate at this point to consider how sound presented to a listener in an enclosed space can be made to lead to a lack of correlation of the ear input signals. This lack of correlation is, as we have already noted, a prerequisite of spaciousness. Sound fields in enclosed spaces are distinguished from free sound fields in that reflected as well as direct sound arrives at the ears of the listener (figure 3.46).

We shall first consider as an example the very simple case in which direct sound from the front is accompanied by a single reflection from the side. Figure 4.33 shows an interaural transfer function corresponding to one such case. The typical features of the transfer function of a comb filter are evident. We assume that the sound source radiates a sustained musical chord. The strong frequency dependence of the interaural attributes of the ear input signals may be called "spectral incoherence." This effect leads to different components of auditory events in the different frequency ranges. These components have different positions in auditory space, though the positions are constant over time.

In actual musical signals, long chords are rare. Real musical signals have a "running" spectrum of amplitude and phase that changes constantly. In other words, the level and phase differences between the direct frontal sound and the reflected component of each ear input signal vary over time. The variation is different for each ear, so the interaural time and level differences change constantly as a function of time. The result may be called "temporal incoherence." The listener perceives a fluctuation in the lateral displacement of auditory events or else spatially broad, diffusely located auditory events.

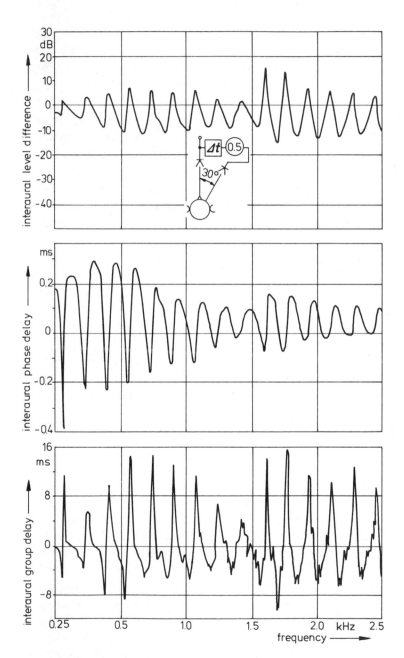

Figure 4.33
Interaural transfer function. Level difference, phase delay, and group delay for direct
sound plus one lateral reflection of equal strength. Delay of the reflection $\Delta t = 6$ ms.

In terms of the models described in section 4.4.4, spectral and temporal incoherence of the ear input signals has the effect that the functional elements D and E of figure 4.29 produce a binaural correlation pattern in which the position of the peaks varies from one frequency range to another and from on moment in time to another. Figures 4.31a and 4.31b, as an example, show two instantaneous correlatograms weighted according to level difference. These were derived from an orchestral chord for two differing cases: (1) direct sound alone, from the front; (2) direct sound from the front plus two lateral reflections, one from the left and one from the right. A comparison of the two cases reveals a clear frequency-dependent shift in the correlation peaks (Lindemann 1982).

Various investigators have attempted to define an index of spaciousness as a function of objective parameters of the sound field (Keet 1968, Barron 1971, 1974b, Gottlob 1973, Conant 1976, Lehmann 1976, Reichardt and Lehmann 1976, 1978a,b, Schmidt 1978, Jordan 1980, Barron and Marshall 1981). The index depends on either the interaural degreee of coherence k or the ratio of lateral sound energy arriving at the listener to frontal or total energy.

Even the early investigations of Chernyak and Dubrovsky (1968), Keet (1968), and Damaske (1967/68) led to the conclusion that the angular extent of the space occupied by auditory events at the position of the listener is approximately proportional to the interaural "incoherence" $1 - k$. Barron (1971, 1974b) and Barron and Marshall (1981) were able to show that this interaural incoherence $1 - k$ is proportional, given certain simplifying assumptions, to what may be called the "lateral energy fraction" E'_{lat}. Simplifying assumptions are as follows:

1. The sound energy arriving at the listener's position can be analyzed into a frontal (not lateral) component and a component that comes horizontally from the left and right (the lateral component).
2. Each ear is equally sensitive to frontal energy and to lateral energy from its side.

A formula for the lateral energy fraction is

$$E'_{lat} = \frac{\displaystyle\sum_{i=1}^{n} w_i(t_i)\cos \alpha_i}{\displaystyle\sum_{k=1}^{m} w_k(t_k)},$$

(4.4)

where 5 ms $\leq t_i \leq \tau_1$ and $0 \leq t_k \leq \tau_1$. It is assumed in this equation that a sound source at the front radiates a brief impulse of sound pressure. The $w_i(t_i)\cos \alpha_i$ are the energies of the reflections that arrive at the observer in the interval 5 ms $\leq t_i \leq \tau_1$ after the direct sound, with each reflection weighted by the cosine of the angle of incidence α relative to the ear axis. The $w_k(t_k)$ are the energies of the direct sound and all reflections in the interval $0 \leq t_k \leq \tau_1$ after the arrival of the direct sound. Barron chooses τ_1 such that only the early reflections are included in the equation (e.g., $\tau_1 = 80$ ms).

According to Barron and Marshall (1981),

$$E'_{lat} \sim 1 - k_{\tau_1} \sim \text{``amount of spaciousness,''}$$

(4.5)

where $\sim$ indicates proportionality. The index τ_1 signifies that the integration to calculate the degree of coherence should take in the same time interval as the integration to determine E'_{lat}. Figure 4.34 shows the relationship in equation 4.5 graphically.

The index of spaciousness of Barron and Marshall takes in only early reflections. Gottlob et al. (1975), Schmidt (1978), and Reichardt and Lehmann (1976, 1978a,b, 1981) also include the energy of the reverberant sound, which reaches the listener so late that it is for all practical purposes uncorrelated with the direct sound. The effect of the reverberant sound on the spatial attributes of auditory events is thus distinctly different from that of earlier lateral reflections. For example, reverberation results in an increase of the distance of the primary auditory events from the listener (see figure 3.48 and the literature cited in the accompanying text; also Sakamoto et al. 1976, 1977). Furthermore, when the pitch or loudness at the sound source changes, or when the sound ceases abruptly, the listener becomes aware of characteristic, decaying components of auditory events that are of great spatial extent (Reichardt and Lehmann 1978a, Kuhl 1978, Marshall 1979). It is debatable whether this latter effect can be included within the category

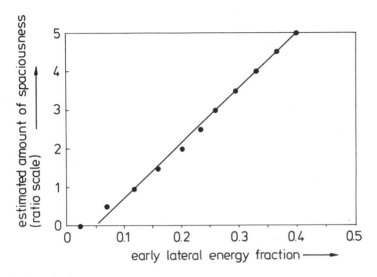

Figure 4.34
Estimated amount of spaciousness as a function of the early lateral energy fraction
E'_{lat} (after Barron and Marshall 1981).

of spaciousness. Nonetheless, the auditory effects of the reverberant sound certainly contribute to the total spatial impression.

The dependence of spaciousness on the parameters of the early lateral reflections should also be discussed here. Such parameters include delay time, level, angle of incidence, and spectrum. Also, the overall level of the direct sound and of the reflections is of central importance. The following statements are based above all on the works of Schubert (1966), Barron (1971, 1974b), Conant (1976), Kuhl (1978), and Barron and Marshall (1981) (see also Wettschurek 1976).

Figure 4.35 shows the range of levels and delays in which Barron (1971) found the effect of spaciousness to be pleasing in connection with musical signals. There was one early lateral reflection in this experiment. A pleasing effect of spaciousness occurs immediately at the masked threshold and becomes stronger as the level of the reflection is increased. The range of pleasing spaciousness is limited at high levels of the reflection by "image shifts"; in other words, summing localization occurs. It may occur in connection with delay times of up to 50 ms. The limit of the range of desirable spaciousness for longer delay times is set by the disturbing effect of the resultant echo. Changes in tonal

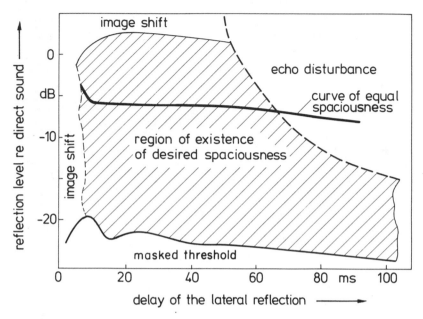

Figure 4.35
The region of existence of desirable spaciousness and a curve of equal spaciousness
(adapted from Barron 1971). Direct sound plus one echo from $\varphi = 40°$, $\delta = 16°$,
musical signal, total level of the direct sound plus the reflection constant at approximately 75 dBSPL.

color are observable in the range of delays between 10 and 50 ms. The
figure shows a line of equal spaciousness as evaluated by paired comparison with a reference condition (reflection at 40 ms and -6 dB).
The combined level of the direct sound and the reflection is held constant
at approximately 75 dBSPL.

The limit curves given for the range of "desirable" spaciousness
correspond only qualitatively with the curves in figure 3.13, in terms
of their definition as masked threshold, limit of image shift, and limit
of echo nisturbance. Further experiments are clearly necessary to resolve
this discrepancy. This author has nevertheless been able to convince
himself, through a few simple experiments, that figure 4.35 in principle
correctly represents the effects that occur in connection with one early
lateral reflection.

One especially important discovery is that the degree of spaciousness
generated by a single reflection is largely independent of the delay time

over a large range (5 ms $< \tau <$ 80 ms). Barron and Marshall (1981) were able to confirm this independence with two reflections, one from the left and the other from the right, for two musical phrases of different tempi.* Furthermore, spaciousness is clearly not significantly affected by whether the lateral energy stems from one reflection or from multiple reflections. Rather, what is important is E'_{l}: the ratio of the energy arriving from lateral directions to the total energy.

A number of hypotheses have been proposed to answer the question of whether certain frequency components of the reflections are of particular importance to spaciousness. Some authors consider the components below 1.5 kHz to be especially important (Barron 1974b, Wettschurek 1976, Blauert 1978, 1982a, Barron and Marshall 1981). This hypothesis is in agreement with the observation that the spatial extent of the auditory event in connection with low-pass-filtered signals (direct sound and lateral energy each limited to 1.5 kHz) is considerably greater than in connection with high-pass-filtered signals with the same frequency limit.

The dependence of the extent of spaciousness on the angle of sound incidence is shown in figure 4.36. It conforms well to the function cos α, where α is the angle of sound incidence relative to the axis of the ears (Barron 1974b, Alrutz and Gottlob 1978, Barron and Marshall 1981).

The fact that spaciousness is largely independent of the arrival time of lateral energy and is dependent in a characteristic way on the angle of incidence of the reflection has led to the development of the index of spaciousness described by equation 4.4. However, this equation leaves out one very important point, namely, that spaciousness increases markedly along with the overall sound level (Marshall 1967, Keet 1968, Wettschurek 1976, Conant 1976, Kuhl 1978, Barron and Marshall 1981). This dependence has not yet been investigated quantitatively enough to be included in the index of spaciousness.

One plausible attempt to explain the level dependence of spaciousness is based on the curves of equal loudness level (figure 2.54) (Wettschurek 1976, Conant 1976, Blauert 1982a); as the level increases, the low-

---

*On the other hand, Ando (1977, 1978) found preferred delay times that depended on the musical motifs. However, he used as his criterion for judgment not spaciousness per se but the "degree of subjective preference" as compared with the direct sound alone. There is a relationship between the length of the autocorrelation function of the musical motif and the preferred delay time.

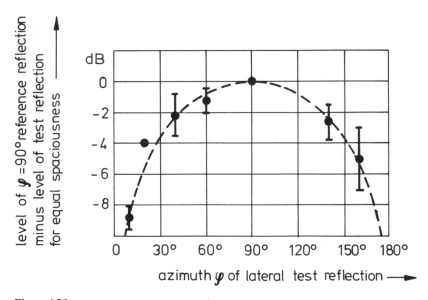

Figure 4.36
The level difference one reflection precisely from the side ($\varphi = 90°$, $\delta = 0°$) must have with respect to a reflection from another direction in the horizontal plane in order to generate equal spaciousness (Barron and Marshall 1981).

frequency components of the signal that are above threshold become relatively stronger as compared to the whole signal. Additionally, when there are many reflections attenuated to different degrees with respect to the direct sound, more and more of these reflections rise above the threshold as the overall level is increased. A further reason for the increase of spaciousness with rising level can be found, following Cremer and Müller (1978/82), in the nonlinear relationship between loudness and sound pressure level (see, e.g., Zwicker and Feldtkeller 1976).

In order to achieve "desirable" spaciousness in a concert hall, care must be taken that enough early lateral energy reaches the listeners. On the other hand, concert halls must have a certain minimum cubic volume (which depends on the number of seats) in order to attain the preferred reverberation time of approximately 2 s. In concert halls of traditional rectangular shape, lateral reflections are achieved by means of parallel side walls not too widely spaced from one another—25 m at the most. The ceilings are very high to make the cubic volume sufficiently great (West 1966, Marshall 1967, Barron 1974a).

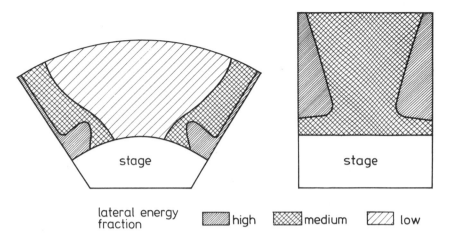

Figure 4.37
Early lateral energy fraction in fan-shaped and rectangular concert halls (after Fasbender 1981).

It is possible to pack more spectators closer to the stage in fan-shaped and arena-shaped concert halls. For this reason many concert halls of other than rectangular shape have been built in recent years. Their acoustic quality has often been disappointing, though, apparently because very little lateral energy reaches the listeners in large portions of the halls (figure 4.37). Large, appropriately dimensioned and positioned sound reflectors can solve these problems by directing sufficient lateral energy to the seating areas (Marshall 1979, Marshall and Hyde 1979). This approach allows more freedom in providing the necessary reverberation than in a rectangular hall. It should, however, be recalled in this context that spaciousness is dependent on sound level. As the volume of a hall with a given reverberation time increases, the sound level in the seating areas may decrease, given that the acoustical power output of the orchestra remains constant.

There are other possibilities besides purely acoustical ones for generating sound fields that lead to a pleasant spatial impression for the listeners. Modern electroacoustic processes allow the spatial impression to be manipulated with almost complete freedom (Gardner 1969, Kuhl and Plantz 1976, Chaudiere 1980, Ahnert and Reichardt 1981). Such processes are already in widespread use in consumer electronics and in the production techniques of popular music. There are serious acousticians as well who believe that electroacoustic aids will find increased application in concert halls in the future. Damaske and Ando (1972) investigated how loudspeakers might be arranged in space to achieve minimum interaural coherence of the listener's ear input signals.

4.5.2 Dummy-head stereophony

In section 2.2 we described an experiment in which probe microphones in the ear canals of a subject were used to pick up sound-pressure signals. The sound fields presented to the subject could be chosen at will. Subsequently, the signals from the probe microphones were played back to the same subject binaurally over appropriately equalized headphones (figure 2.11a). If the reproduced signals in the ear canals correspond exactly to those during recording, the spatial attributes of the auditory events also correspond exactly to those of the auditory events that the subject had during the recording. An "authentic" spatial reproduction thus takes place.

When the author first carried out this experiment (Blauert 1969a), the only available probe microphones had relatively high internal noise (figure 1.19). Platte et al. (1975), Laws and Platte (1975), and Platte and Laws (1976b) have since succeeded in building what they call an "apparatus for the exact reproduction of ear input signals," which incorporates better microphones. They have used it to conduct thorough tests of the reproduction of spatial attributes of auditory events, confirming once again that authentic reproduction is attainable if the equalization of the transmission path is undertaken with sufficient care.* The subjects were just as successful as in natural hearing, even when faced with difficult tasks such as distinguishing between sounds at the front and the rear. This was the case even though reproduction took place with the head immobilized and without any supplementary information such as visual cues or bone-conducted sound. Other, nonspatial properties of the auditory events such as timbre and reverberance were reproduced authentically as well (see also Plenge and Romann 1972).

It is easy to get a rough impression of the auditory authenticity of this type of binaural reproduction by placing two subminiature electret

---

*The magnitude of the transfer function must be accurate within approximately ± 1 dB. As long as they are the same for both ears, the following errors may remain uncorrected: frequency-independent delay, and frequency-dependent group-delay variations such as those based on the all-pass characteristics of the headphones, the latter up to approximately ± 400 μs (Blauert and Laws 1978).

microphones (e.g., Knowles type BT 1759) inside one's own ear canals. The tip of each microphone should be inserted approximately 1 cm. The signals from the microphones are subsequently played back over headphones equalized to free field. Although considerable errors of equalization go uncorrected, leading to audible distortions in tone color, the reproduction of spatial attributes of auditory events is of surprising fidelity.

In most applications of the binaural technique it is impractical to pick up the ear input signals using living subjects. For this reason dummy heads (Kunstkopf) are used, with or without a torso. The basic elements of a dummy-head reproduction system are shown in figure 2.11b. In what follows here, only dummy heads for binaural reproduction of sound are discussed. Others, some of them of considerably different construction, are used for various acoustical applications, such as the measurement of the properties of hearing aids and headphones (Burkhardt and Sachs 1975); the measurement of attenuation by personal ear protectors (Schröter and Els 1980a,b, Blauert et al. 1980); the carrying out of measurements on architectural scale models (Ruhr-Universität Bochum, unpublished).

A comparison of dummy-head systems with other electroacoustical sound-reproduction systems (Blauert 1974b, Kuhl and Plantz 1975) shows that the dummy-head systems achieve the most authentic auditory reproduction and that the apparatus required is relatively simple. For this reason dummy-head systems have been used routinely for many years in scientific investigations for which auditory authenticity is needed (see Gottlob 1978). Many of the investigations of concert halls cited in section 4.5.1 were carried out using dummy heads. Other applications include the preparation of transcripts of conferences and teleconferencing.

In the broadcast and recording industries the dummy-head technique, under the name of "Kunstkopf stereophony" or "binaural sound" has not yet achieved decisive acceptance, though there were a few hopeful attempts in the early 1970s. Industry spokespersons offer two reasons for the commercial failure of the dummy-head technique. The first is the less-than-optimal design of dummy heads available to professional audio engineers. Many listeners experience "forward-to-backward confusion"; that is, untrained listeners especially heard auditory events behind them when these were intended to be exactly in front of them.

This problem raises the question of exactly how the "ears" of a dummy head should be constructed so that the largest possible number of listeners hear as authentically as possible. In section 4.2.1 we discussed recent methods for the selection of "average" and "typical" external-ear transfer functions. However, even when the construction of the acoustically relevant parts of the dummy heads is "optimal," there remain unavoidable errors, since each listener's head is unique. To a certain limited degree, these errors can be corrected for each individual at the playback end of the electroacoustical transmission chain. Also, there is a more radical solution to the problem of front-to-rear confusion: an apparatus with adjustable equalizers (Boerger and Kaps 1973, Boerger et al. 1977). This alters the ear input signals as the head is moved, approximately as if the original sound source were in front of the listener (see section 2.5.1).

Errors in reproduction are not, however, the primary reason for the broadcast and recording industries' failure to adopt Kunstkopf stereophony. The primary reason is the incompatibility of signals from dummy heads with reproduction over loudspeakers (Plenge 1978). When played back over loudspeakers, the signals lead to auditory events whose tone color is unnatural; and, for consumers, loudspeaker reproduction is still the most common type. Methods have been known for quite some time that allow the correct reproduction of dummy-head signals over loudspeakers (such as the TRADIS process described in section 3.3, developed further by Sakamoto et al. 1978; see also Schöne 1981), but these require special equipment at the listener's end and/or at the originating end of the system. Moreover, these processes function correctly only if the room in which sound is played back has highly sound-absorbing walls and the listener is in a predetermined position. The head must also be held as still as possible.

Theile (1981a,b,c) has recently managed to achieve compatibility between the Kunstkopf sound-collecting technique and loudspeaker reproduction, avoiding the difficulties just mentioned. One prerequisite for success was the relaxation of the goals of this compatibility. Previously the goal had been for the listener to achieve the same authenticity of reproduction when listening to dummy-head signals over loudspeakers as when listening to them over headphones. The new, less demanding goal is that the dummy-head signals, presented over loudspeakers, be at least of comparable quality to signals used in the ordinary intensity

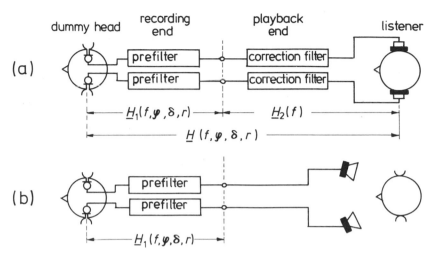

Figure 4.38
Separation of an overall transfer function $\underline{H}(f, \varphi, \delta, r)$ of a dummy-head reproduction system into a component at the originating end, $\underline{H}_1(f, \varphi, \delta, r)$, and one at the playback end, $\underline{H}_2(f)$. a: Connection for headphone playback. b: Connection for loudspeaker playback.

stereophony technique. Quality should be comparable for the direction as well as the tone color of the auditory events.

The solution is sketched in figure 4.38a, which is a somewhat altered version of figure 2.11b. The equalizer has been separated into two parts. The division between the originating and reproducing ends of the system is at the point shown. It can be seen immediately that the overall transfer function $\underline{H}(f, \varphi, \delta, r)$ is divided between the originating and reproducing ends of the system. The transfer functions at the originating and reproducing ends may be chosen at will, subject only to technical limitations, as long as $\underline{H}(f, \varphi, \delta, r) = \underline{H}_1(f, \varphi, \delta, r) \times \underline{H}_2(f)$ (Laws et al. 1976/77). The dependence of the transfer function on the position of the sound sources, that is, the spatial characteristic of the system, must naturally be defined at the originating end if the dividing point is to be one port only, as shown in the sketch.

The question, then, is whether it is possible to choose the dividing point of the system such that the output signals from the originating end can be played back over loudspeakers in the standard stereophonic arrangement without any additional apparatus. Different suggestions have been made as to the definition of the dividing point, based on different aspects of the problem (Mellert 1975, 1976, Weber and Mellert 1978, Kleiner 1978, Killion 1979, Tsujimoto 1980, Hudde and Schröter 1980, Fukudome 1980a, Schöne 1980b, Gotoh et al. 1981). Some examples are the following:

1. The most common suggestion is based on the usual conditions of headphone reproduction. Headphones are usually "equalized to a free field"; in other words, their transfer function ideally corresponds to that of a typical external ear when sound is presented in a free sound field directly from the front and from a considerable distance ($r \gg 25$ cm). If such headphones are used without equalization at the reproducing end of the system, then the transfer function at the originating end must be $H_1(f, \varphi = 0, \delta = 0, r \gg 25$ cm$) = 1$, given frontal sound incidence.

2. Another suggestion is that the left channel of the originating end be equalized to a "flat" frequency response for the direction of sound incidence $\varphi = +30°$, $\delta = 0$; in other words, $H_{1,\text{left}}(f, \varphi = +30°, \delta = 0, r \gg 25$ cm$) = 1$. The right channel is equalized the same way for the direction of sound incidence $\varphi = -30°$, $\delta = 0$. One factor that helps to shape this suggestion is the position of the loudspeakers in the standard stereophonic arrangement at $\varphi = \pm 30°$, $\delta = 0$ relative to the listener.

3. A further suggestion would make the equalization of the left channel at the originating end such that the average of the transfer functions for all directions of sound incidence $0 \leq \varphi \leq 90°$, $\delta = 0$ is 1; in other words, $\bar{H}_{1,\text{left}}(f, 0 \leq \varphi \leq 90°, \delta = 0, r \gg 25$ cm$) = 1$. The right channel is equalized the same way for the directions $0 \geq \varphi \geq -90°$, $\delta = 0$.

Without analyzing these suggestions in detail, we can still state the following. Suggestion 1 is not appropriate for loudspeaker reproduction. Suggestions 2 and 3, which, by the way, can be realized by means of almost identical equalizers at the originating end (Mellert 1978), do not lead to fully satisfactory reproduction over loudspeakers; distortions of tone color are clearly audible. The basic concept of these suggestions, that of "flattening" the spectrum of the dummy-head ear input signals for the most important directions of sound incidence, is, however, a step in the right direction.

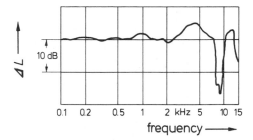

Figure 4.39
Level difference curve of the frequency response of a dummy-head system equalized to a diffuse field minus the frequency response of a system equalized for frontal sound incidence.

The following general solution to the problem of choosing the dividing point was produced by Theile (1981a,b,c). Since the dummy-head signals should lead to auditory events in loudspeaker reproduction comparable with those of conventional intensity stereophony, the dummy-head apparatus must be equalized to a studio microphone used in intensity stereophony. A good studio microphone, however, is "equalized to a diffuse field"; that is, its average transfer function over all directions of sound incidence is 1: $H_{1,\text{diffuse}} = \bar{H}_1(f, 0° \leq \varphi \leq 360°, 0° \leq \delta \leq 90°, r \gg 25\text{ cm}) = 1$. It has long been known in practice that the tone color in loudspeaker reproduction—and also in headphone reproduction—depends not only on the direct sound arriving at the microphone, but also on the reflections and reverberation, which arrive from many directions. Correct reproduction of tone color is, then, assured by "diffuse field equalization" of the microphone. Figure 4.39 shows the frequency response of a dummy-head system equalized to a diffuse field, compared with the frequency response of a system equalized for the forward direction as in suggestion 1. The same curves apply to the left and right channels.

The Institut für Rundfunktechnik in Munich has carried out extensive auditory experiments with dummy-head systems equalized to a diffuse field. Recordings of concerts were the preferred signals. When these signals were reproduced over loudspeakers in the standard stereophonic arrangement, the tone color of the auditory events was largely authentic, and their localization and localization blur corresponded for the most part to that of intensity stereophony. As with intensity stereophony, the auditory events appeared in the sector between the two loudspeakers. Thus dummy-head systems equalized to the diffuse field can be used to originate signals in the same way as traditional microphones used in intensity stereophony. The desired compatibility between Kunstkopf stereophony and traditional intensity stereophony for loudspeaker reproduction has been attained.

In order to obtain the authentic reproduction of Kunstkopf stereophony from dummy-head signals equalized to a diffuse field, it is, however, necessary to use appropriately equalized headphones (or an appropriately equalized TRADIS system; see figure 3.53). When a diffuse sound field is presented to the dummy, the ideal headphone transfer function generates the same ear input signals as if the listener were at the position of the dummy and the same diffuse sound field were presented. The transfer function of such headphones, equalized to a diffuse field, is different from that of the usual headphones equalized to a free field in the forward direction. Listening tests have shown, however, that headphones equalized to a diffuse field are more pleasing than the usual headphones even for the reproduction of intensity stereophony signals (Theile 1981b).

It is to be expected that the developments just mentioned will lead to more widespread application of Kunstkopf stereophony in the future. We shall therefore close this section with some details on practical problems in the construction of dummy heads for Kunstkopf stereophony, and also some details of the processing of dummy-head signals and conventional microphone signals.

In designing and building dummy heads one must choose the appropriate shape for the head, the pinnae, and other parts; the terminating impedance of the ear canal, the microphone capsule, and the coupling of this capsule to the dummy head must also be appropriate. The range of choice is bounded by the following conditions as determined by Hudde and Schröter (1980; see also section 4.2.3):

1. The spatial characteristic of the external ear does not depend on the shape of the auditory canal or on the eardrum impedance. For this reason it is unnecessary to reproduce these parts of the outer ear accurately more than about 4 mm beyond the entrance of the ear canal.
2. Although the transfer functions do indeed depend on the shape of the ear canal and on the eardrum impedance, the influence of these

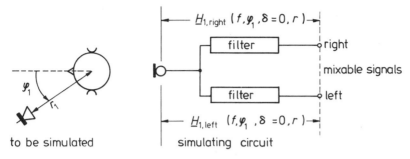

Figure 4.40
Conversion of conventional microphone signals into signals mixable with dummy-head signals.

parts on the transfer function can be simulated by an appropriate two-port linear equalizer. In principle, the appropriate transfer function of the equalizer depends on the particular geometry of the sound field.* However, measurements have shown that the equalization for a free sound field is in fact satisfactory in most applications.

The most successful dummy heads result when no attempt is made to duplicate the ear canal and the eardrum impedance exactly but, rather, the coupling of the microphone capsules to the entrance of the ear canals is designed so as to achieve the highest possible signal-to-noise ratio (Kleiner 1978, Schöne 1980a,b). Furthermore, the coupling parts can be shaped in such a way that as much as possible of the equalization of the dummy head to a diffuse field takes place in the acoustical part of the system. In some cases it is then possible to do entirely without additional electronic filtering (Wollherr 1981).

If dummy heads are to be used in professional audio applications on exactly the same basis as conventional microphones, then it has to be possible to mix dummy-head signals with signals from conventional microphones. This is highly desirable, since as a rule several microphones are used at once in professional recording applications. However, the signals from a conventional microphone do not include the "spatial information" of dummy-head signals. Consequently, in the case of

*The "radiation" impedance at the plane of the entrance of the ear canal, as measured from the inside to the outside, depends on the geometry of the sound field. It can be altered noticeably if, for example, there are reflecting surfaces near the dummy head.

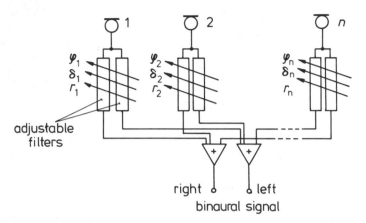

Figure 4.41
A binaural mixing console.

reproduction over headphones without additional, corrective measures, they lead to inside-the head locatedness (IHL) (see section 2.3.2).

If each conventional microphone picks up signals mostly from one particular sound source at one particular position (e.g., from one musical instrument), the mixing problem can be solved relatively simply. The signal from the microphone must in this case be passed through two filters that simulate a pair of external-ear transfer functions (in this and similar contexts see Bauer 1961b, Blauert 1972a, Blauert and Laws 1973, Platte and Laws 1978, Morimoto and Ando 1977, 1982). Appropriate selection of the external-ear transfer functions can generate two binaural signals from the microphone signals. The binaural signals can lead to an auditory event at any predetermined position (figure 4.40). These binaural signals can then be mixed with dummy-head signals.

Platte and Laws (1978) and Platte (1979) describe, along these lines, the laboratory prototype of a "binaural mixing console" (figure 4.41), with which they can process signals from conventional microphones in such a way as to generate auditory events in twelve directions in the horizontal plane over headphones. The distance of the auditory events could also be adjusted by mixing in appropriate binaural reflections and reverberation (Sakamoto et al. 1976, 1977, 1978). In principle, binaural mixing consoles pose the additional possibility of remixing the many multitrack recordings already in the libraries of the broadcast and recording industry into binaural, quasi-Kunstkopf versions. Such binaural versions would be compatible with loudspeaker reproduction if the dividing point defined above, equalized to the diffuse field, were used at the output of the binaural mixing console. In headphone reproduction a version remixed in this way could provide spatial effects far beyond those of conventional stereophony, since auditory events could in principle be generated at all positions in auditory space.

In closing, it should be noted once again that the external-ear transfer functions of an "average" or "typical" subject are used in designing a dummy head or the filters of a binaural mixing console. The binaural signals generated using these devices may show considerable discrepancies from those of an individual subject. Individual equalization at the reproducing end of the system is therefore a desirable feature. This equalization might, for example, be such that the critically important forward direction is reproduced correctly over headphones. Methods are conceivable in which adaptation to individuals would be achieved automatically by appropriate coupling of the listener's external ear to the electroacoustical transmission chain—for example, by placing the headphone transducers in the forward direction, in front of the pinnae, not on them (West et al. 1976). Research into such possibilities has not yet arrived at definitive solutions.

5 Progress and Trends since 1982

5.1 Preliminary Remarks

The last update to this book, chapter 4, was written in 1982 at a time when the first American edition was being prepared. Since then, a dramatic evolution has occurred in the field of spatial hearing.

The advent of microcomputers and, consequently, the availability of the necessary computational power for real-time processing of audio signals have initiated and fostered the development of a new technology, "binaural technology," which has established itself as an enabling technology in many fields of application, such as information and communication systems, measurement technology, hearing aids, speech technology, multimedia systems, and virtual reality.

Modern technology has also changed the way research in spatial hearing is performed. Sophisticated psychoacoustic experimental investigations into complex auditory environments, such as concert halls, has been facilitated by the advent of binaural technology and digital signal processing. One important outcome of this kind of research is an increased awareness among experts of the role of cognition in spatial hearing.

In this chapter I discuss recent trends in spatial hearing by presenting typical examples. I have cited some German work, which is less easily accessible to the international reader. For more detailed coverage of, and extensive references to, the current literature in spatial hearing, four books can particularly be recommended: Blauert (1992), Begault (1994), for 3-D sound and auditory virtual reality, and Yost and Gourevitch (1987) and Gilkey and Anderson (1996) for binaural and spatial hearing in general. The review articles of Wenzel (1992) and Wightman and Kistler (1993) are further suggestions for reading.

The following sections, 5.2, 5.3, and 5.4, each deal with one of the three steps of information processing in the course of spatial hearing, namely, the propagation of acoustical signals in the sound field, including the external ears; signal processing in the subcortical auditory system; and the involvement of the cortex in auditory perception and judgment (cognition). In other words, they deal, in sequence, with the physical, the psychophysical, and the psychological aspects of spatial hearing.

Section 5.2 is devoted to acoustical signals in the sound field up to their entrance into the auditory system. Binaural room simulation and auditory virtual reality are typical application areas attached to this part. Section 5.3 deals with binaural processing of auditory signals, the enhancement of speech under acoustically adverse conditions — the cocktail-party problems — being an exemplary application. Finally, section 5.4 reports on evidence for massive involvement of cognition in spatial hearing concluded from recent experimental results on the precedence effect (see section 3.1).

The line of thinking that led to this particular subdivision of the material in these three sections is outlined in the schematic model of auditory information processing shown in figure 5.1. As a matter of fact, this model is an extended version of the models depicted in figures 3.34 and 4.29.

The first step of the model represents the external ear. The input signals to the two ears, stemming from the sound field, are modified by the transfer functions of the external ears. The external ears are succeeded by the middle ears, which once more modify the incoming acoustical signals in a specific way. The external-ear and middle-ear modules together represent the physical aspect of auditory information processing within the model.

The output signals from the middle ears are delivered to the inner-ear modules (cochlea), where decomposition into spectral components and subsequent conversion into nervous signals in each of the spectral bands are performed. The nervous signals are then further processed physiologically, in connection with which it seems to be appropriate to assume monaural channels as well as binaural ones. In the binaural channel the signals from the two ears are combined in a sophisticated way.

The current model assumes at this point that as a result of both monaural and binaural processing some kind of a consolidated, running internal representation of the signals to the two ears has been established, here called the "binaural activity pattern." Up to this level the model shows a so-called bottom-up (signal-driven) architecture, which, among other things, means that all the auditory information

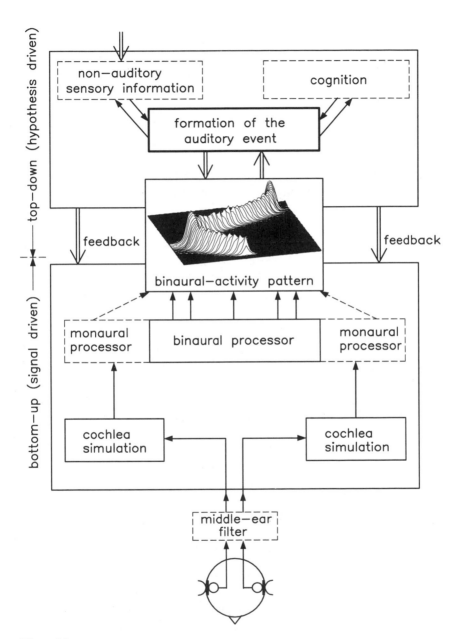

Figure 5.1
Schematic model of spatial hearing, comprising the physical, psychophysical, and psychological aspects of auditory information processing.

accessible to higher stages of the model is believed to be contained in the binaural activity pattern. The model components from the cochlea modules through the monaural and binaural channels up to the running binaural activity pattern represent the psychophysical aspect of the model.

The last stage of the model reflects on the psychological aspect of perception, including cognition and cross-modal interaction. From the point of view of the model architecture, the bottom-up, signal-driven approach has now been substituted by a top-down, hypothesis-driven mode of operation. The idea is that higher stages of the central nervous system set up a hypothesis as to what an appropriate percept could be in a certain situation. They then test this hypothesis – among other things on the evidence given by the binaural activity pattern – and accept or reject it. If a hypothesis is accepted, the formation of the respective percept will take place. If the hypothesis is rejected, a new hypothesis will most likely be set up. The setup process for hypotheses is thought of – at least partly – as a cognitive process. Apart from auditory sensory information, information from other modalities (visual, tactile, proprioceptive, etc.) and knowledge of the scenario and its history may play a role, as well as mental effects such as attention and expectation.

A conceptual model, shown in figure 5.1, definitely has to consider that feedback from higher to lower stages is likely to take place at different levels of the auditory system. As a matter of fact, there is some speculation that feedback takes place from the cognitive level down to the inner ears, in the sense that subjects can "sharpen their ears spectrally" when listening attentively to specific cues (see Scharf et al. 1987, Scharf 1995). That subjects can direct their heads to an optimal listening position is another and evident example of feedback, though a multimodal one.

5.2 Binaural Room Simulation and Auditory Virtual Reality

Sections 2.2 and 4.2 of this book deal in some length with the effects of the external ears (pinnae, head, and torso) on the sound signals propagating to the two main input ports of the auditory system, the two eardrums. It appears that these effects are purely physical.

In the static case, an external ear can be seen as a linear time-invariant system. The modification of signals passing through this system are fully characterized by the system's impulse response (in the time domain) or transfer function (in the frequency domain). Extensive measurements of external-ear transfer functions (now usually referred to in the literature as "head-related transfer functions," or HRTFs) have been carried out on a variety of subjects for various angles of incidence and source distances (Schröter et al. 1986, Pösselt 1987, Wightman 1989, Middlebrooks and Green 1990, Hammershøi et al. 1992, among others) using adequate measuring techniques (e.g., Xiang 1988, 1991, Abel and Foster 1994, Pralong and Carlile 1994, Hartung 1995).

As explained in previous chapters, it is assumed that the role of the external ears in the course of auditory signal processing is as follows. The external ears superimpose linear distortions on the incoming signals, which, in each case, are specific for the direction of incidence of the sound wave and the source distance. In this way, spatial information is encoded into the signals that are received by the eardrums. A further assumption is that the auditory system is capable of decoding this specific information and of making use of it in the process of forming auditory events in the subject's perceptual space.[*]

The knowledge of the role of the external ears in spatial hearing and the availability of quantitative data for modeling external ears paves the way for various applications, for example, creating auditory events at prescribed directions and distances in a subject's perceptual space. As a matter of fact, the modeling of the acoustic behavior of the external ears and the application of these models for practical purposes is fundamental to what is now called "binaural technology" (Møller 1992, Gierlich 1992, Blauert 1994, 1996).

One of the generic tasks of binaural technology (and of audio technology in general) is to authentically transmit and reproduce auditory percepts over space and time. Authenticity, in this context, means that the subjects at the receiving end do not sense a difference between their actual auditory events and those which they would have had at the recording position when the recording was made.

---

[*] Non-upright position of the head does not seem to hinder this process (Wolf et al. 1993).

An approach frequently used to achieve authentic auditory reproduction is based on the following assumption: If the same acoustical
signals are delivered to the subjects at the receiving end as were present
at the recording end, the auditory events at the recording and at the
receiving ends will also be the same.

This basic assumption, namely, that a subject will always hear the
same sound when exposed to identical sound signals, is obviously not
true in a strict sense. Cross-modal or cognitive effects are negated by
this assumption, for example. Nevertheless, as a working hypothesis,
this assumption has been in use for a long time. It has, among other
things, served as the initial design criterion for dummy-head stereophony (see figures 2.11 and 4.38)

Yet, as has been known since the early days of audio technology
(e.g., from public address systems, radio broadcasting, and phono-
graphic recordings), authentic reproduction is rarely required. More
often the technological task is to enhance or augment acoustical scenarios rather than to replicate them authentically. In public address
systems human voices are amplified to make them well understood
under acoustically adverse conditions; sound material on the radio
and on disk is processed in such a way as to achieve the optimal
auditory effect, for instance, from an artistic point of view.

To enhance or augment binaural signals requires signal processing
that takes account of HRTFs. A block diagram of a binaural system
that supports such manipulations is shown schematically in figure
5.2.

Binaural systems of this type, that is, with built-in signal processing
capability and memory, are important commercial products of the
binaural-technology industry (e.g., Genuit and Blauert 1992, Gierlich
1992). Such systems are, for example, widely used for analyzing and
designing industrial sounds. In the context of this section, the focus is
placed on the fact that, with the aid of such systems, auditory events
can be added to a perceptual scenario or can be removed from it. The
addition of auditory events is achieved with the algorithm described in
the context of binaural mixing consoles (see figures 4.40 and 4.41). The
removal of auditory events from the auditory scenario (e.g., to get rid
of the sound of a particularly annoying source while preserving the
rest of an auditory scenario) is not yet generally possible. More potent
algorithms for such a purpose, akin to the cocktail-party processor

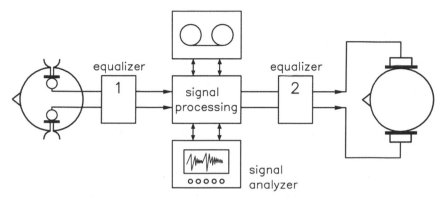

Figure 5.2
Schematic of a binaural system that, among other things, allows binaural signals to
be enhanced and augmented.

discussed in section 5.3, are, it is hoped, will become available in the
near future.

The mixing-console algorithm is based on the notion that the external ears are, acoustically speaking, linear time-invariant systems.
These systems act as linear filters. In real and in dummy heads these
filters are realized acoustically, that is, by the physical properties of
pinnae, head, and torso. In the mixing console, equivalent filters are
realized digitally.

It becomes apparent at this point that auditory scenarios can be
generated even without any recordings of real-head or dummy-head
signals in real scenarios. The binaural mixing-console algorithm can
be used to simulate binaural signals, such as those produced by direct
sound waves from one or multiple sound sources, as well as those
produced by accompanying reflections and reverberation, such as
those that can be observed in enclosed spaces.

Figure 5.3 gives an outline of the architecture of a binaural system
to simulate auditory scenarios as in enclosed spaces. Systems of this
kind can, for instance, be applied to the design of spaces for acoustical
performances (e.g., concert halls) as well as to designing sound systems
for such spaces. For example, the actual task may be to simulate the
auditory perception of a listener in a specific seat in a concert hall
when the music is playing — before this hall has actually been built.

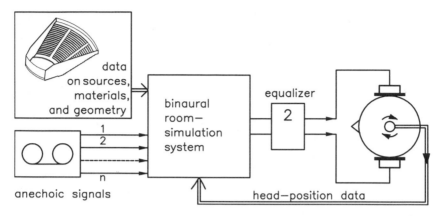

Figure 5.3
Outline of the architecture of systems for simulating auditory scenarios, such as in
enclosed spaces — binaural room simulation.

Simulation processes of this kind are referred to as "binaural room
simulation."

Binaural room simulation has been developed to a state of some
maturity and, hence, provides a sound basis for many binaural technology applications. A wide range of literature on the method is available from the Bochum laboratory (e.g., Pösselt et al. 1988a,b, Blauert
and Pösselt 1989a, Blauert and Lehnert 1992, Blauert et al. 1991a,b,
Lehnert and Blauert 1991a, 1992, Lehnert 1992a,b, 1993c, 1995; see
Blauert et al. 1991b for further references).

A binaural room simulation system needs the following initial input
data: positions, orientations, and directional characteristics of the
sound sources; positions and orientations of the listeners; positions,
dimensions, and orientations of walls and of other acoustically relevant objects (e.g., the audience); and the absorption or reflectance
characteristics, respectively, of the walls and other relevant objects
(figure 5.4).

On the basis of these data, a sound-field modeling module makes it
possible to calculate the sound propagation in the space to be simulated. As a result, components of the sound field that impinge upon
the listener's head, namely, direct sounds and reflections of different orders, are identified with respect to their direction of incidence
and arrival time. Furthermore, linear distortions, such as spectral

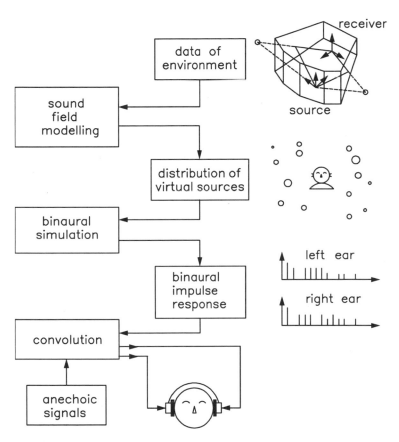

Figure 5.4
A more detailed block diagram of a binaural room simulation system.

modification, to which the sounds are subjected on their way from the source to the receiving point, are calculated.

Current sound-field models for binaural room simulation are usually based on geometric acoustics. Widely used algorithms are the so-called ray-tracing method and the mirror-image method, which may be combined for computational efficiency (Vorländer 1988a,b, Lehnert 1992a). In ray tracing the path of "sound particles" is traced along straight lines and reflected at walls and other reflected objects (figure 5.5a). In the mirror-image method, the sound sources are specularly mirrored in all reflecting surfaces, the result being presented as

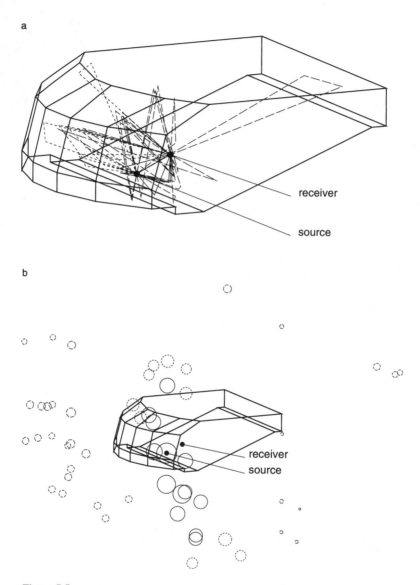

Figure 5.5
Ray tracing (a) and mirror imaging (b), two rough-and-ready methods often used for
sound-field modeling in binaural room simulation systems.

a cloud composed from those mirror-image sources, visible from the listener's position (figure 5.5b).

A typical output of the sound-field modeling process is a cloud of mirror-image sources that surround the space containing the original sound sources. This cloud of mirror images, presupposing that the geometric approximation holds to some degree, represents the complete information about the spatial and temporal structure of the sound field. As each image source can be further spectrally weighted, information on wall reflectances and source directivity can be included.

Since a space with reflecting walls is basically a linear system, its impulse response fully represents the transmission characteristics from the sources to the listeners. This impulse response is rendered by exciting the direct sound source and all its image sources simultaneously with a Dirac impulse and then collecting the incoming signals at the listener's position.

For binaural room simulation, in addition to the process described above, the acoustical characteristics of the listener's ears must be included. This is performed as follows. The signal component from each sound source, direct or mirrored, is convolved with the impulse response of the listener's ears for the specific direction of incidence of this particular component. Finally, the respective components from all the sources are added, and the so-called binaural impulse response of the room is obtained. This is in fact a set of two responses, as there is one impulse response for each of the listener's two ears.

The last step of binaural room simulation is called "auralization," that is, making audible. This step is conceptually obvious. Since binaural impulse responses represent linear time-invariant systems consisting of a sound source with specific directional characteristics in a space with a specific geometry containing specific absorptive materials, the output signal for any input signal to such a system can be obtained by convolving it with the impulse response of the system.

In binaural room simulation, signals like music or speech, which have preferably been recorded in an anechoic (acoustically dry) environment, are convolved with each of the two binaural impulse responses. The two resulting signals can then be delivered to the listeners via properly equalized and adjusted headphones. The listeners will have the auditory illusion of being auditorily displaced in the simulated space and of listening to the sound sources in it.

At this point a few remarks are necessary for clarification: Binaural room simulation usually assumes a static case, that is, fixed positions and orientations of sound sources and listeners. In the case of multiple sound sources the process as described above has to be performed for each sound source individually. Nevertheless, the signals can finally be summed up for auralization of the multiple source scenario. Ideally, for each listener, his or her individual external-ear impulse responses, or HRTFs, should be used. Ray tracing and mirror-imaging are approximate methods. They come in many varieties; some include a degree of diffuse reflection (e.g., Shao 1992, Heinz 1993).

Since binaural room simulation is an approximate method, especially in the light of the geometrical acoustics principles applied, perceptual validation is necessary. One way of doing this is auditory comparison of dummy-head recordings from an existing hall with binaural signals as rendered by the simulation algorithm. The work of Pompetzki follows this paradigm (Pompetzki 1993, Pompetzki and Blauert 1990, 1994).

An existing lecture hall of 1800 m³ was chosen for this purpose. The linear dimension of the hall and the reflectances of its wall elements were properly measured in situ. Then, speech samples from different male and female talkers were presented via a loudspeaker on the podium and were recorded with a dummy-head system at different audience positions. For comparison, three binaural room simulations of different detailedness were performed (figure 5.6a, b, c). The number of specified wall segments and other reflecting planes was 48, 126, and 238, in increasing order of the amount of added details. Seven thousand early reflections or mirror sources were considered in each case. Late reflections were simulated using a simplified reverberation algorithm. Diffusion was not included in the modeling process.

The results of auditory tests, in which the real and simulated binaural signals were compared, led to the following conclusions. Binaural room simulation is able to evoke auditory perceptions that are regarded as being authentic even by critical listeners. When authenticity of the created virtual auditory environment with respect to a real one is required, as in the planning of halls for acoustical performances, the following rules should be observed. Extreme care has to be taken with respect to the modeling of reflecting surfaces that are close to the sound sources. If these surfaces are large, it makes sense to implement

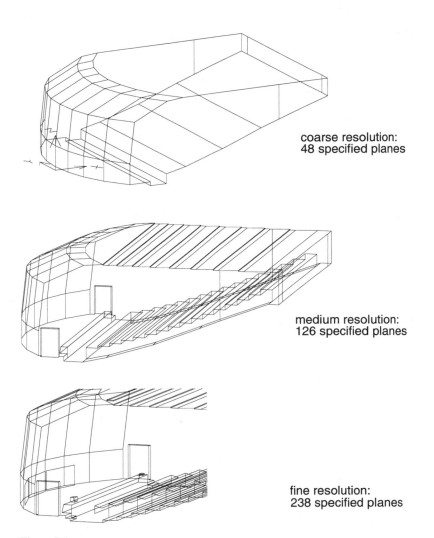

coarse resolution:
48 specified planes

medium resolution:
126 specified planes

fine resolution:
238 specified planes

Figure 5.6
Room simulation models of a lecture hall with a volume of 1800 m^3 in three different degrees of resolution.

their reflectances realistically. In general, however, it does not make sense to build highly detailed ray-tracing or image-source models. First, the reflectance of small wall elements (small when compared with the wavelength) cannot easily be specified. Second, the spatial and temporal selectivity of human hearing is limited. In the case reported here, an auditorium of about 1800 m^3, excited with speech, 238 specified planes and 7000 detected mirror-image sources led to reasonably authentic percepts.

It is worth mentioning in passing — now that computer-based binaural room simulation is on its way to being accepted as a standard tool for planning acoustic spaces and audio systems — that an alternative method exists which is also capable of providing realistic auralization. This method makes use of scaled-down physical models of the space to be constructed (usually at a scale of $1:10$ to $1:8$). These models are driven by ultrasonic sound. Recordings are made with scaled-down dummy heads. Given that the laws of modeling are properly observed (including an adequate selection of materials and of the model atmosphere), these physical models produce very realistic binaural impulse responses, which, after adequate frequency transformation, can be used for auralization, as in the method described above. The scale-model method is well developed. For details the reader is referred to the literature (e.g., Blauert 1984a, Els 1985, 1986, Els and Blauert 1985, 1986, Xiang 1989, 1990, 1991, Xiang and Kopatz 1989, Xiang and Blauert 1991a,b, 1992, 1993).*

Binaural room simulation, as well as the scale model technique, model the static case, that is, sound sources and listeners at fixed positions and orientations in a fixed space. This leads to an unrealistic effect for the listeners, which is also typical for dummy-head stereophony in general. When the listeners move their heads, the signals at their two ears do not vary the way they would with natural hearing. As has been emphasized in section 2.5.1, listeners use the specific variation of the signals at the two ears as strong cues for localization in conjunction with their awareness of head position, orientation, and movement. If these cues are not available or are distorted, localization errors may occur, such as front-back reversals (e.g., along a cone of

---

* It goes without saying that binaural impulse responses can also be obtained from real, existing halls, that is, $1:1$ models (Pösselt et al. 1988b, Tachibana et al. 1989)

confusion; see figure 2.94) and inside-the-head locatedness (section 2.3.2). Carefully measured external-ear transfer functions and individual adjustment to the specific listener reduce the problem, although they do not eradicate it completely. In cases where, because of a lack of individual adjustment, listeners are presented sound signals through somebody else's transfer functions (i.e., listening through somebody else's ears), the resulting localization errors sometimes seriously corrupt the auditory impression being aimed at.

Returning to figure 5.3, a possibility to resolve the problem emerges. As the auditory scene is generated by a computer rather than recorded by a dummy head, the actual computations can be performed for the actual head position and orientation. To this end, the current head position and orientation are tracked and the information is fed back into the computer. Position- and orientation-tracking sensors (six degrees of freedom) are readily available for this purpose, based on, for example, mechanical, optical, or magnetic principles (Meyer et al. 1992). If the adjustment of the input signals to the two ears of the listeners is performed in a realistic way, the localization errors clearly decrease, and individual adjustment of the external-ear transfer function may not be necessary in less critical applications. Furthermore, the perceptual space of the listener is now spatially fixed while the head is moving and no longer moves unrealistically in accordance with the head. This so-called perceptual space constancy provides the listeners with, among other things, an improved sense of involvement, as they now perceive themselves as moving in an otherwise fixed scenario.

As a matter of fact, the introduction of a head-tracking device into binaural systems is an important conceptual step in the development of binaural technology, as it introduces interaction of the system and the listener. By moving their heads, the subjects interactively control part of the simulation procedure. The introduction of interactivity into binaural simulation systems is actually an indispensable step to yet another branch of novel technology, namely, the field of so-called virtual reality. This widely used term, *virtual reality*, is obviously semantically inconsistent and, consequently, needs some explanation.

Virtual-reality technology aims to perceptually displace subjects into "virtual" environments which are different from the environments that they are actually exposed to. Ideally, the subjects feel "present" in the virtual environments and actually accept them as being real: virtual reality! For example, the subjects may behave intuitively in the way they would in corresponding real environments.

Technologically speaking, these perceptual illusions are achieved by presenting adequate, computer-controlled stimuli directly to the sensory inputs of the subjects. Virtual-reality systems are multimodal and interactive. The most important modalities are vision, audition, proprioception (position, orientation, force), and tactility. Interaction may include such things as head-position–orientation tracking, hand-position–orientation tracking, and gesture tracking, as well as possibilities for manipulating objects with regard to their spatial position, for instance, operating mechanical controls, and thereby sensing visual, auditory, tactile, and force feedback.

In the following some problems related to the auditory components of virtual-reality systems are discussed (see also Lehnert 1990, 1993a,b, 1994a,b, Blauert 1992, Blauert and Pompetzki 1992, Lehnert and Blauert 1991b, Blauert and Lehnert 1995a,b). As an introduction, the architecture of virtual-reality systems is illustrated by example of a bimodal (auditory-tactile) interactive system (Blauert and Lehnert 1993). This system has been designed as a research tool for psychophysical research. The definition of the experimental scenario is as follows: A subject is exposed to a virtual space with various (invisible) auditory-tactile objects distributed in it. He or she will localize and identify these virtual objects auditorily and be able to reach toward them and grasp them individually. Upon tactile contact, the contour, texture, and thermal attributes of the virtual objects will be perceived. It is the task of the subject to manually move the objects around, that is, to rearrange their spatial position and orientation according to an experimental plan. Auditory feedback is given.

The general structure of the system is illustrated in figure 5.7. A "virtual world" is implemented on a computer. This virtual world — actually a set of computer programs and databases — and the subject are considered as two nodes, connected by four pathways transferring information: two of them provide auditory and tactile stimuli to the subject, the other two collect information about the status of the subject at any given time. Figure 5.8 offers a more detailed view of the auditory part of the system. The upper left block encompasses the virtual world with its two prominent modules: a word model contain-

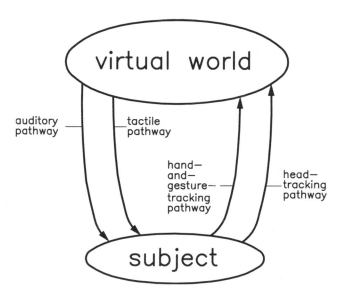

Figure 5.7
Global structure of a system for generating bimodal virtual environments.
Interactivity is provided via head-position, hand-position, and gesture trackers.

ing the definition of objects and their mutual relationships in specific applications, and a central controller which monitors the events happening, makes necessary decisions, and initiates appropriate actions. The world model draws upon a built-in database which contains data on the sound sources (e.g., on their directional characteristics; Giron 1994).*

The central controller has the following functions. It collects information about incoming "events" produced by the listeners when they move their heads, or events that are created by the world model itself. It evaluates these events, decides the system's reactions to them, and initiates the steps necessary to implement the events. Also, the central controller may be in charge of monitoring the listeners' performance or of adapting the virtual world using rules defining the virtual tasks of the system. Furthermore, the central controller sychronizes the

---

*It should be mentioned in passing that the collection of directional characteristics of natural sound sources such as talkers or musical instruments is not an easy task (Meyer, 1980, Giron 1996).

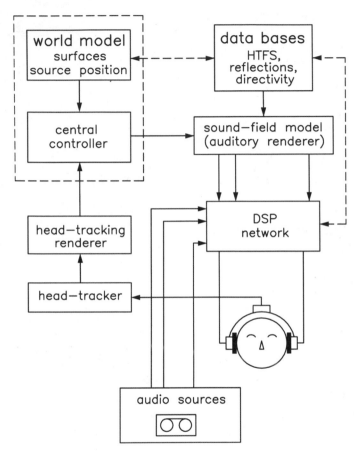

Figure 5.8
Block diagram of the auditory component of the system in figure 5.7, including auditory rendering, head-position tracking and interactive control of the auditory representation. HTFS, head-related transfer functions; DSP, digital signal processor.

various components of the system by managing the information exchange between them.

There are two (modal) pathways linking virtual world and listener. The head-position pathway transmits information on the actual coordinates of the head (six degrees of freedom) onto the central controller, whereby the head tracker measures head position and orientation and feeds position data into the head-tracking renderer, which analyzes these and renders results compatible with the coordinate system of the world model. The auditory pathway, which is in charge of creating the acoustic signals sent to the listener, also consists of two main modules, the auditory renderer and the auralization unit.

The auditory renderer is, essentially, the sound-field model, that is, the set of programs and databases which compute the effective cloud of visible, spectrally weighted direct and mirror-sound sources at discrete moments in time. The databases contain the necessary data of the acoustical environment (e.g., linear dimensions, positions, orientations, reflectances of reflecting or absorbing surfaces) and of the listeners (catalogs of HRTFs or the corresponding impulse responses).

The stream of parameters, as determined by the sound-field model, are then forwarded to the auralization unit, a dedicated cluster of programmable digital-signal processors, or DSPs, which process anechoic audio signals, for example, speech or music, in real time so as to create the desired auditory perceptual scenario when played to listeners through headphones.

There are, as a matter of fact, three separable steps of signal processing to be performed in the auralization module for each direct source and for each reflection: a temporal, spectral and spatial step (Lehnert 1995, Lehnert and Richter 1995, Shinn-Cunningham et al. 1996). The temporal step adds an initial delay to the signal component that is proportional to its traveling time. The spectral step performs a spectral weighting taking account of the spectral modifications due to one or multiple reflections and directional source characteristics. The spatial step, finally, performs a convolution of the signal components with the external-ear impulse responses specific to their direction of incidence relative to the actual position of the listener's head.

In an interactive system, obviously, most processes have to run in real time. This poses a severe challenge to today's technology. From a perceptual point of view, there are two characteristics of a virtual-reality system which have to be considered in this context, namely its "responsiveness" and its "smoothness" (Appino et al. 1992).

Responsiveness is correlated with the delay with which the system responds to an action of the subject. If this delay is too long, the listener may lose the sense of synchrony of action and reaction, and therefore the sense of being present in the virtual scenario. Smoothness is correlated with the refresh rate with which the auralization unit takes account of a changing auditory scenario, for example, when the listener is moving. Too slow a refresh rate will cause unnatural, nonuniform movement to be perceived (auditory flicker), and, again, cause a lack of the sense of presence.

It goes without saying that a design goal for virtual-reality systems must be that the initial delay be small enough and the refresh rate be high enough not to cause any disturbing perceptual effects. Single-number design criteria, though, cannot be specified, as the perceptual thresholds depend on the individual sensitivities of the subjects and on the specific situation to be mimicked, such as the kind of signals the sources emit, the speed of moving objects, and the question of whether important direct or mirror sources are obstructed by particular changes of positions.

Designers of the auditory component of virtual-reality systems will encounter the problem of real-time performance especially when building the central controller and the auditory renderer. Modern concepts imply a reasonable degree of parallelization and incrementation of the corresponding algorithms. It is worth mentioning at this point that minimum system delay and a high refresh rate may even lead to contradictory demands in the light of implementation, for example, nonsequential processing may increase the refresh rate but also the system delay (see Shinn-Cunningham et al. 1996).

If the time between two frames of computation is too short to take account of all parameter changes, the system can make a decision on what to do first. A reasonable tactic would be to take account of those changes that are perceptually most salient, for example, changes in the direct sound and the strongest early reflections, and to apply further necessary changes "incrementally" during the following frames. Careful individual analysis of each variation in the scenario may also reveal that only some of the parameters are affected and need reconsideration. The following list, as developed by Lehnert (see Shinn-Cunningham et al. 1996), serves as an illustration of this idea.

Examples of variations in the scenario that demand complete recalculation of the sound field are translatory movements of either subjects or sound sources; and modification of the geometry of the environment, such as repositioning of reflecting and absorbing surfaces. Examples of variation in the scenario which only demand a parameter update of the auralization unit are rotational movement of subjects and sound sources and variations in the directional characteristics of sound sources or of absorption characteristics.

The auralization unit can be driven efficiently by making the number of available filter coefficients flexible. For a direct-sound signal, most filtering resources are needed for precise spatial representation. Spectral modification has also to be taken care of additionally in the case of early reflections, but the spatial precision can be less accurate (Lehnert and Richter 1995). The later the reflections, the less important the spatial cues become, and reflections may even be bundled before being sent through the same spatial filter. Last but not least, reverberance can be handled by a specialized algorithm.

From the discussion above it becomes clear that a major difference between binaural room simulation and the auditory representation in virtual reality is that virtual reality, in contrast to binaural room simulation, necessarily requires real-time processing because of to its interactive character. Some relief may come from the fact that, while in binaural room simulation perceptual authenticity is often a prominent design goal, virtual reality mainly aims at creating a sense of presence for the listener. Consequently, perceptual plausibility of the auditory representation is more important than authenticity. On the other hand, interactivity introduces a number of further complications. Two of them, arising from the non-stationarity of the scenario and the perceptual involvement of the listener, are discussed below.

Since binaural room simulation is static, the transmission paths of the signals as emitted by the sound source to the auditory system of the listeners can be considered linear time-invariant systems and consequently they can be described mathematically by transfer functions or impulse responses. In a spatially nonstationary scenario, the situation is more complicated. Consider, for example, a moving sound source in

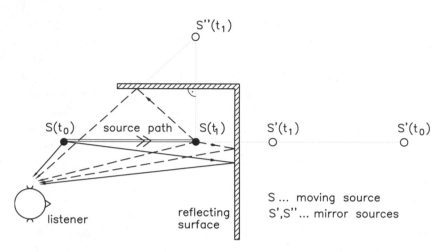

Figure 5.9
Sketch to illustrate the time variance and nonlinearity of an acoustical situation with moving sound sources. Mirror sources may appear or disappear as a function of their position and the path lengths to different sources may vary individually. Doppler shifts may occur.

front of a reflecting wall and another wall to the side, as depicted in figure 5.9. While the source is moving toward the wall in front, the direct sound path to the listener becomes longer and the (frontal) reflective path becomes shorter at the same time. The sideways reflection is ineffective until the source has reached a point where the mirror source suddenly becomes "visible" to the listener.

From a mathematical point of view, the system is now time-variant. A representation of its components by transfer functions or impulse responses can only be attempted piecewise, if at all. The determination of the pieces is nontrivial as the position of a listener is not known at the time the sound components that will reach the listener later are sent out, possibly after multiple reflections. Further, the fact that the sound-path lengths vary as a function of time, even differently for different direct and mirror sources, leads to a specific kind of non-linearity known as Doppler shifts. Doppler shifts cannot be accounted for by transfer functions or impulse responses. Their simulation, which becomes perceptually indispensable when the speed of movements in the scenario is sufficiently high, requires specific modules that perform spectral transformation.

Particular problems arising from the perceptional involvement of the listener arise when listeners are given the possibility of vocalization, as, for instance, in a virtual teleconference scenario where all the listeners are also potential talkers. The issue is that the voice of each talker must be represented so as to sound reasonably natural to the talker himself as well as to the other participants. Some issues which Lehnert and Giron (1995) have identified in this context are considered in the following paragraphs.

As far as the self-perception of the talker is concerned, we have a unique situation in that the source positions and the receiver positions coincide spatially. The voice of the talker will normally be picked up by a close-talk microphone. A first step is to correct the microphone signals as if they stemmed from a far-field pick-up point. Starting from these far-field speech signals, both the direct sound and the reflected sounds can be derived.

The reflected sounds present less of a problem because they are derived in a way that is usual for any sound source. The only complication is that the directional characteristics of the talker must be included. A parametric six-monopole representation of speaker directivity (Giron 1994, Lehnert and Giron 1995) has proved to be a reasonable solution. As to the direct sound, the self-perception of a talker is composed of two components, an airborne and a bone-conducted component (figure 5.10). Only the airborne component has to be provided by the virtual-reality system. It is delivered through the headphones that the listener is wearing. Assuming that the headphones are the supra-aural (open) type, the bone-conducted component will not be affected. The "real" airborne component, however, must be compensated by adequate filtering of the virtual one. Active noise cancellation may help at this point and may also reduce other unwanted signals from the real environment.

If more than one participant of a virtual teleconference scenario is simultaneously present in the same real room, the real-sound signals may interfere with the virtual ones. If the real signals are not sufficiently shielded from concurrent participants, they may govern their process of auditory localization so that the participants localize the speaker at its real and not at its virtual position. A solution is offered by the precedence effect (see section 3.1.2), where the first incoming wavefronts determine the directions at which the auditory events are

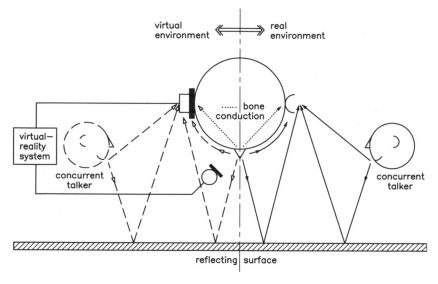

Figure 5.10
Active talker in real vs. virtual environment: airborne and bone-conducted
components involved in self-perception and effect of concurrent talker in the same
real room.

formed. Consequently, the initial delay of the virtual-reality system
has to be adjusted so that the first virtual sounds arrive before the first
real ones.

In conclusion, the following can be said. Applications based on the
physics of the external ear have established themselves as an important
basis for a novel enabling technology, binaural technology. Spatially
static acoustic scenarios can be represented with sufficient authenticity, even very complex ones such as the acoustics of a concert hall.
Nonstatic, interactive scenarios are more difficult to cope with and
cannot be tackled in a straightforward manner. The necessity of real-
time processing, as well as the fact that these scenarios require time-
variant, nonlinear systems to be represented, create a special challenge
to binaural technology. Nevertheless, situation-specific systems have
already been demonstrated that provide sufficient auditory plausibility
and hence a sense of presence and immersion to the listeners (e.g.,
Wenzel 1992, Blauert and Lehnert 1993, 1995b, McKinley et al. 1994,
Begault 1994).

5.3 Binaural Signal Processing and Speech Enhancement

In binaural hearing, that is, hearing with two functional ears, the auditory system is provided with differences in the input signals to the two ears that would not be available if only one ear were functioning (monaural hearing). As a consequence, binaural hearing offers a number of advantages over monaural hearing. The most obvious ones are the following:

• Spatial hearing. The formation of an auditory space is improved with regard to the positions (azimuth, elevation, distance) and the spatial extents of the auditory events. Localization blur is reduced.
• Separation of sound signals from concurrent sound sources. Signals stemming from concurrent sources become more distinguishable, at least when the sources are spatially separated. This improves the listeners' ability to concentrate on one and disregard the others. See the cocktail-party effect (see sections 3.2.2 and 4.4.3) in the case of concurrent talkers.
• Suppression of the perceptual effects of reflected sounds. Coloration and reverberance as induced by reflected sounds are reduced. The dominant role of the first wavefront in the formation of the direction of the auditory event (precedence effect; see sections 3.1.2, 4.4.2, and 5.3) is supported.

These features of binaural hearing make it attractive from a technological point of view. As a matter of fact, binaural technology efforts are aiming at modeling the processes of binaural signal processing as a means of building applications such as improved source-position finders and cocktail-party processors (see Blauert, 1996, for a list of further application ideas).

An overview of the state of the art of modeling of binaural signal processing up to 1983 has been given in sections 3.2.1 and 4.4.4. In the following, recent progress is reported, the focus being on work performed at our laboratory at Bochum, Germany. This work is part of a developmental stream that has led to technological applications. General coverage of recent binaural modeling is not intended (see Stern and Trahiotis, 1996, for a broader survey of the field).

A starting point for many modeling efforts in binaural hearing is the model of Jeffress (1948), the essence of which is depicted in figures 3.32

to 3.34 and 4.30. Observed from a signal-processing point of view, the Jeffress model produces estimates of cross-correlation functions of its two inputs, in other words, a running interaural cross-correlation function.

Cross-correlation is an adequate means of analyzing interaural differences in arrival time. Consequently, analyses of binaural running cross-correlation patterns, such as those shown in figure 4.32, can be used to support tasks, such as the following:

• Detection, identification, and separation of incoherent sound sources
• Determination of the azimuth of these sound sources
• Detection and identification of echoes
• Estimation of the amount of auditory spaciousness (see section 4.5.1)

The human auditory system takes interaural level differences into account, as well as interaural arrival time differences. Among various approaches to incorporating the evaluation of both kinds of interaural cues into one consolidated model, an algorithm designed by Lindeman, known as the Lindemann extension to the Jeffress model, will now be described. This algorithm also deals with the fact that humans can still hear in the absence of interaural cues (monaural hearing), for instance, with one ear occluded.

Lindemann's algorithm has the advantage of computational simplicity and covers a broad range of binaural psychophysical phenomena, at least qualitatively (Lindemann 1985, 1986a,b, Lindemann and Blauert 1982, Blauert and Lindemann 1982, Gaik and Wolf 1988, Blauert 1983, 1991). It has further proved to be a basis for technological applications such as position finders and cocktail-party processors. The algorithm is physiologically driven, as its elements are physiologically feasible. In fact, various researchers have found elements with time-delay, inhibitory, excitatory, and coincidence-detection features in the auditory system. (e.g., Wagner et al. 1981, Pickles 1982, Caird and Klinke 1983, Yin et al., 1987, Popper and Fay 1992, Yin 1994). More, isomorphy with physiology has not (yet?) been verified (see Sujaku et al., 1981, for a closely related model based on physiologic evidence). However, one has to be aware that the auditory system most likely performs different processes simultaneously or intercurrently

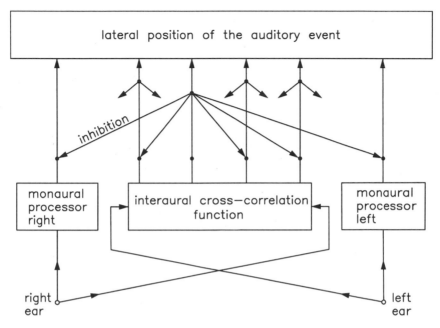

Figure 5.11
A mechanism of inhibition, superimposed on a Jeffress type of interaural cross-correlation model. Note that monaural pathways are added in such a way that monaural activity can be inhibited by a binaural one, but not vice versa.

because of massive parallel processing (see also section 4.4.4). Certainly, a single algorithm cannot cover all of the complex auditory functions.

The special feature of Lindemann's algorithm is the way in which it integrates inhibitory elements into the purely excitatory structure of the Jeffress model. The basic idea of adding inhibition is illustrated in figure 5.11, while figure 5.12 depicts its specific implementation by Lindemann.

Figure 5.11 shows that whenever the cross-correlation line generates an output at a certain position, which corresponds to a certain correlation delay, this output may trigger a mechanism that inhibits activity at other positions. Furthermore, there are two monaural pathways (left and right), which can also be inhibited by binaural activity. Since interaural cross-correlation equals zero in the case of

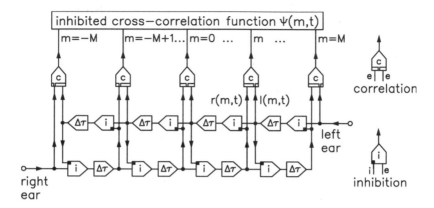

Figure 5.12
A specific implementation of the functions of the structure of figure 5.11: the
Lindemann extension to the Jeffress model.

no interaural cues, all activity will then be restricted to the monaural
pathways.*

Lindemann's specific implementation (see figure 5.12) makes use of
a mechanism called contralateral inhibition, which works as follows.
Any activity running down one of the two tapped delay lines of the
cross-correlation processor can inhibit the activity at the corresponding
positions on the opposite delay line. Consider, as an example, the
situation after the ears have been hit by a single sound impulse from a
lateral direction. Both delay lines receive a bandpass impulse as an
input, though at different arrival times. The respective neural activities
travel along both delay lines in opposite directions. On their way they
cause inhibition at the respective positions in the opposite delay lines.
Finally, the activities from both sides meet somewhere on the line
and stimulate the coincidence detector ("multiplier") connected to this
position. Owing to the contralateral inhibition described, activities
originating from positions along the delay lines other than the one
where the coincidence occurred are suppressed. In other words, the
circuit creates an output pattern that could similarly be generated by
the circuit shown in figure 5.11.

---

*There is no contralateral inhibition if there are no interaural cues. This happens, for
instance, when only one ear receives a sound signal, or when the sound signals to the
two ears are incoherent.

Several parameters of the Lindemann extension can be set to demand, for example, the amount and persistence with which the inhibition is applied. The amount can be adjusted between full and zero inhibition. The persistence can be set such that only simultaneous inhibition takes place or that any triggered inhibition persists for a while, according to a specified memory function. Further, the "multipliers" can be modified to perform a "weighted multiplication" adjusted between the following two extremes: (1) the output depends on both input activities in the same way; or (2) the output depends on the input activities from only one of the delay lines. The first setting is adequate for a position on the delay line that corresponds to diotic presentation (zero interaural arrival-time difference); the second creates a monaural detector. For a mathematical formulation of the Lindemann extension, see Lindemann (1986a,b). In the following, some interesting functional features of the algorithm have been summarized.

Lindemann's extension produces a sharpening of the peaks of the cross-correlation function when compared with those rendered by a pure Jeffress model. It further suppresses secondary peaks which otherwise would rise owing to the periodic nature of the cross-correlation function for bandpass signals. Both interaural arrival-time differences and interaural level differences are accounted for in that both result in a plausible shift of the peak of the inhibited cross-correlation function (figure 5.13). Spatially separate incoherent sources create separate peaks, the width of which depends on the amount of interaural correlation, thus indicating more or less auditory spaciousness.*

With contralateral inhibition set to persist for a while after its initial triggering, the Lindemann algorithm is able to create a kind of a precedence effect, at least for some simple scenarios. Figure 5.14 shows the output for an impulsive sound from a frontal direction, followed by a lateral reflection. The right panel gives the output rendered by a pure Jeffress-type model, the left one the output of the Lindemann extension. The delay of the reflections is varied. The memory function for the inhibition is exponential with a time constant of 10 ms. It is

---

*Auditory spaciousness is an important quality issue of spaces for musical performance (see section 4.5.1, and, for example, Blauert 1986a,b, 1987, Blauert et al. 1985, 1986, Blauert and Lindemann 1985, 1986a,b, Lindemann et al. 1985).

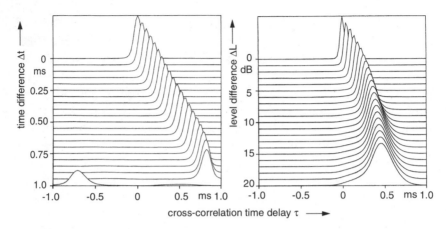

Figure 5.13
Lateral shift of the peak of the inhibited cross-correlation function as a function of
interaural arrival-time differences (left panel) and of interaural level differences (right
panel) for 500-Hz pure tones. Note the sharpness of the peak and the absence of
secondary peaks.

obvious from the Lindemann results that the reflection is suppressed
for short delays.

Lindemann's extension, though very useful for modeling the basic
effects of binaural hearing in the laboratory, needs to be further refined
to be able to cope with "natural" binaural signals, such as the output
signals of a dummy head. Since the interaural level difference occurring in such signals varies considerably between frequency bands
(from almost zero at low frequencies to more than 30 dB at the higher
ones), the Lindemann algorithm tends to generate output that is inconsistent across frequency bands. For instance, it may produce solely
monaural output at high frequencies, although interaural cues are
actually present, namely, in the case of high interaural level differences.

Gaik (1990, 1993) has proposed amending Lindemann's algorithm
to avoid these undesirable effects. The amendment begins with the
understanding that any binaural model must adapt to the transfer
function of the specific external ears that it is bound to listen through.
To this end, Gaik adds weighting elements that do not affect the
activity in the opposite delay line, but rather control the activity traveling along each (tapped) delay line. These weighting elements may
be placed equidistantly, for example, one at each tap (figure 5.15). The

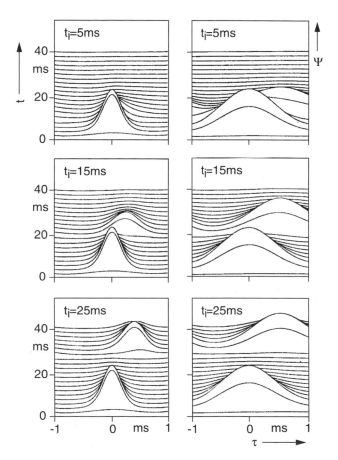

Figure 5.14
Output of a pure Jeffress model (right panel) compared with that of the Lindemann extension (left panel). Signals are critical-band-wide impulses at 500 Hz, one frontal direct sound plus one lateral reflection with three different delays, $t_i = 5$, 15, and 25 ms. The upper left plot indicates that the reflection has been suppressed. (Data from Lindemann 1985.)

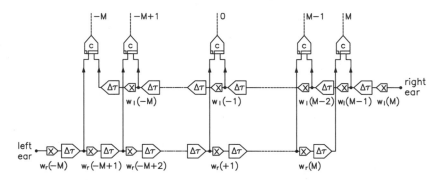

Figure 5.15
Gaik's amendment to the Lindemann extension of the Jeffress model. When
compared with Lindemann's, there are additional weighting elements along each
delay line which can be adjusted according to external-ear transfer functions. The
inhibitory elements of Lindemann have been omitted for clarity (cf. figure 5.12).

amount of inhibition in each is adjustable (normally between 0% and
100%, but negative values are also admitted: excitation).

The idea is to adjust the additional elements to compensate for the
excessive effects of interaural level differences in such a way that,
for any "natural" combination of interaural arrival-time and level
differences, the remaining level difference of the activities at the "correct" point of coincidence is simply zero. This would have the effect
of natural binaural signals leading to coincidence positions at corresponding positions along the delay lines across frequency bands.
"Natural," in this context, means occurring with a distinct sound
source anywhere around the listener in an anechoic space.

In order to be able to set the inhibition values reasonably, Gaik has
analyzed a catalog of measured external-ear impulse responses provided by Pösselt from the projects reported in Schröter et al. (1986)
and Pösselt (1987). A most interesting finding was that, by and large,
any natural interaural level difference comes with a specific interaural
arrival-time difference, yet some ambiguities may occur for extreme
lateral source positions. Figure 5.16 shows, as an example, the combinations of interaural arrival-time and level differences in two critical
bands.

The adjustment of Gaik's inhibition elements is performed using
an iterative, recursive algorithm based on measured sets of external-
ear transfer functions. As a matter of fact, it is not far from the mark

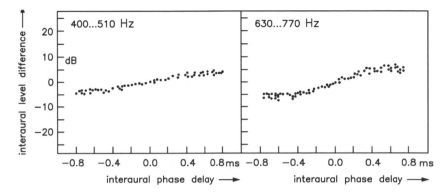

Figure 5.16
"Natural" combinations of interaural arrival-time differences and interaural level differences in two critical bands.

to state that the Jeffress-Lindemann-Gaik model represents, on the whole, a special artificial time-delay neural network adaptable to specific ears by means of a supervised learning procedure.

Figure 5.17 gives examples of binaural activities in adjacent bands for impulsive sounds from different angles of incidence in the horizontal plane resulting from Gaik's algorithm. Note the increasing spread of positions with increasing azimuth in accordance with the perceptual findings (increasing localization blur; see figure 2.2). The different heights of the peaks in different bands are due to the external ears.

Essentially, the Jeffress-Lindemann-Gaik algorithm provides a means of mapping the sounds impinging on a listener's head in terms of their temporal and spatial structure (with the spatial dimensions currently restricted to one: laterality). There are many possible applications for such a tool. As an example, figure 5.18 gives the plot of a binaural impulse response recorded in a concert hall. The pattern indicates the direct sound plus a dense series of early reflections from different directions. Plots of this kind can, for instance, aid architectural acoustics experts to evaluate the quality of spaces for musical performances.

For signals like ongoing speech or music under reverberant conditions, that is, in the presence of reflected sounds, the Jeffress-Lindemann-Gaik model may have problems discriminating the direct sound from the reflections and thus may sometimes miss the source position. These problems become even greater when multiple sound

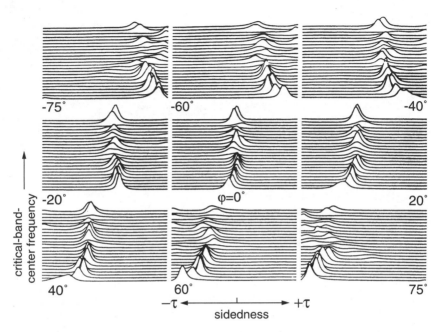

Figure 5.17
Output patterns of the Jeffress-Lindemann-Gaik model for white noise (20 Hz...
15.5 kHz) from various directions in the horizontal plane. Each curve represents the
output of one of 24 adjacent critical bands.

sources are simultaneously or intercurrently active. Wolf (1990, 1991)
has shown how to deal with these complications. Instead of performing the interaural cross-correlation on the binaural signals as they
come from the cochlea modules, an additional module is inserted into
each of the two signal pathways. This additional module recognizes
prominent onset slopes in the signals and, since these onset slopes most
likely stem from direct sounds rather than from reflections, enhances
them over the other portions of the signal. Cross-correlation is then
performed on the processed signals and, additionally, the resulting
running cross-correlation pattern is subject to a specific two-dimen-
sional filtering across correlation delays and critical bands. As a result,
mapping of sound sources becomes possible, even in reverberant
conditions (see Hartung et al. 1994, Grabke 1994, for further improvement of the algorithm).

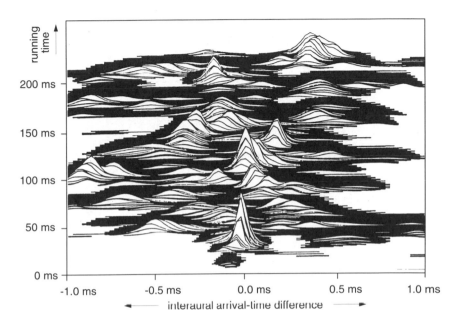

Figure 5.18
Pattern generated by the Jeffress-Lindemann-Gaik model from a binaural impulse response recorded in the Grosser Musikvereinsaal in Vienna (critical band 630...770 Hz).

Models of binaural signal processing have yet another important field of application, namely as a kernel of systems for separating sound signals from different sources – in perceptual terms, auditory-stream segregation (Bregman 1990, 1992). If the sources to be separated are concurrent talkers or talkers under otherwise adverse acoustical conditions, these systems are often called cocktail-party processors, in reference to the so-called cocktail-party effect (see sections 3.2.2 and 3.3).

In the following, an outline of a specific, successful implementation of a cocktail-party processor is given (Bodden and Gaik, 1989, Bodden, 1992a,b, 1993, Bodden and Blauert, 1992). There have been further attempts to tackle the problem in Germany (e.g., Gaik and Lindemann 1986, Peissig and Kollmeier 1990, Koch 1990, 1992, Peissig 1993, Slatky 1994, Kollmeier and Koch 1994.

The cocktail-party processor of Bodden is based on the Jeffress-Lindemann-Gaik model with some of Wolf's ideas incorporated. The

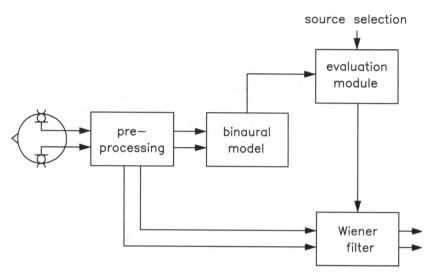

Figure 5.19
Architecture of the cocktail-party processor by Bodden.

basic concept behind it is to use information supplied by the binaural model to enhance the sound energy stemming from a specified sound source and to blend out all the other sound energy. Figure 5.19 shows the architecture of the system.

Binaural two-channel signals as, for example, recorded via a dummy head, provide the input signals to the system. A preprocessing stage decomposes these signals into critical-band−wide components. The preprocessed multichannel signals go two different ways. On the one hand, they are fed into a binaural model of the Jeffress-Lindemann-Gaik type with an extra evaluation module on top of it. On the other hand, they go to controllable filters, whose coefficients can be adjusted in a time-variant way. The information to control the filters is rendered by the evaluation module. The aim is to drive the time-variant filters in such a way as to optimally estimate the signal of the desired talker from the corrupted signal, that is, from the mixture of the signals of multiple talkers and noise.

For the limiting case of stationary signals, the optimal transfer function for the filters, $H(f)$, a purely real function, would result from

$$H(f) = C_{ss}(f)/C_{xx}(f)$$

where $C_{ss}(f)$ and $C_{xx}(f)$ are the power-density spectra of the desired signal, $s(t)$, and the corrupted signal, $x(t)$. Filters of this kind are known as Wiener filters. As, in fact, both the signals from the desired talker and the concurrent talkers plus eventual noise are nonstationary, the optimal transfer function, here, becomes a running transfer function, $H(f, t)$.

Since both channels of the binaural signal have been decomposed into sets of critical-band–wide bandpass signals in the preprocessing stage, $H(f, t)$ can be implemented approximately by multiplying each critical-band component with a time-variant coefficient. The coefficients reflect the running power relation of the desired and corrupted signals as determined by the evaluation module on top of the binaural model. To put it simply, what the filters actually do is the following. Whenever the evaluation stage signals that the power in a specific critical band most probably stems from the desired talker, the signal in this channel is put through. Whenever it is less probable that the band stemmed from the desired talker, it is gradually faded out. In this way, signal components from the desired talker are enhanced compared with the rest of the signals. Of course, the algorithm cannot influence the (simultaneous) proportion of desired and undesired components inside bands.

Analyzing the filtering process with two spatially separated talkers whose speech signals are known reveals a theoretical increase of the signal-to-noise ratio (SNR) of up to 18 dB. The corresponding suppression of the undesired talker is even higher (up to 26 dB), and the increase in intelligibility for the desired talker can be dramatic: The data predict recovery of a nonunderstandable talker (SNR $= -15$ dB) to almost 80% word intelligibility (1000-word corpus).

It is obvious that the practical effectiveness of the filtering process depends on the reliability and precision of the binaural model and evaluation stage in discriminating any signal components stemming from the desired talker. The binaural model, as described here, works on the basis of interaural arrival-time and level differences. Consequently, it can only separate signals from sources at different lateral positions.*

---

*To include further signal attributes, the model would have to be amended by additional signal-processing steps; for possibilities, see, for example, Lim 1983).

In the case of multiple talkers the model needs information on the actual position of the desired talker. The position data can either be given continuously to the model, or the model can track the desired talker, once his or her initial position has been identified. Position tracking is actually comparatively easy for a small number of concurrent sound sources in anechoic spaces. Complications may arise when reflections or reverberations are present. The method of Wolf (1991), as mentioned above, cannot readily be used to overcome these problems, as Wolf enhances the onset slopes and suppresses the ongoing parts of the signals in a way that would distort speech to an unacceptable degree. Nevertheless, Bodden has incorporated the basic idea of weighting different parts of the signals with respect to their relevance in the process of identifying the source position. In figure 5.20, two exemplary results of his source tracking algorithm are given.

The necessary estimation of the running power of the desired signal is performed with the help of "space" windows which allow those signal components to pass through that show up close to predicted positions on the cross-correlation axis. In contrast, the power of the complete signal is obtained by estimating from the cross-correlation function as a whole, after some adequate transformation. The cocktail-party processor definitely has a considerable number of free parameters: bandwidth of filters, integration times for the running cross correlation, "space" windows for the pattern evaluation, and compression functions for the filter coefficients, among others. The parameter settings that were finally used by Bodden represent the result of a tedious experimental optimization phase with the goal of a maximum source separation but continuing to have only tolerable distortion of the desired speech. Audible distortions appear particularly for negative SNRs due to the time-variant filtering process.

Auditory tests of Bodden's system with different speech materials, selected on phonetic principles, have proved to be a remarkable enhancement with respect to consonant-cluster discrimination and word and sentence intelligibility. It is especially remarkable that a significant enhancement of consonant clusters could be shown, which is difficult to achieve by more conventional methods. As a typical example, a hearing-impaired subject experienced an increase in sentence intelligibility from 55% to 85% in a two-talker scenario and from 35% to 65% in a three-talker scenario.

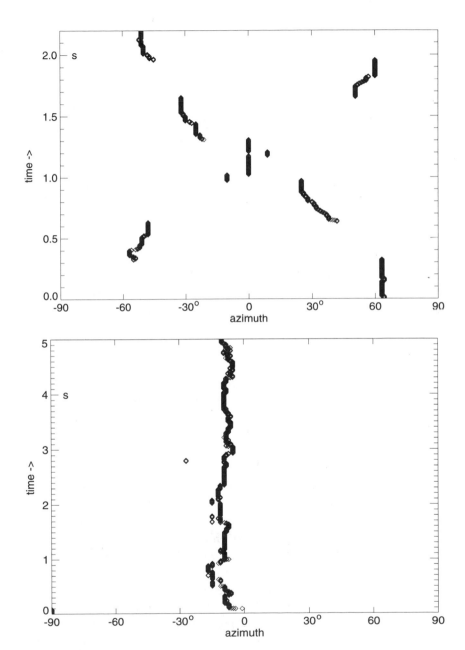

Figure 5.20
Results of the source-tracking method implemented by Bodden. (Top) Two moving talkers in an anechoic room. (Bottom) Circular saw in a reverberant factory hall.

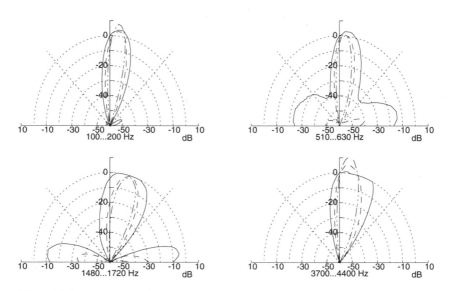

Figure 5.21
Polar plots of the sensitivity of Bodden's cocktail-party processor (horizontal plane, critical bands of different center frequency, F_0). Solid, broken, and solid-dotted lines reflect different parameter settings.

In an application study where the system was used as a front end for a automatic speech recognizer under acoustically adverse conditions, an increase in the rate of correct recognition could be shown equivalent to a 21-dB improvement of the SNR ratio (Bodden and Anderson, 1995).

A binaural cocktail-party processor is a device that enhances sound signals from one direction of incidence and suppresses those from other directions. The spatial selectivity of the system can be illustrated as polar plots of the system's sensitivity. Figure 5.21 gives examples of a specific parameter setting, as chosen in one experiment under anechoic conditions.

Although there is some variation in the actual form of the polar plots of sensitivity, depending on the system parameters chosen and on the sound field encountered, profound spatial selectivity is generally observed, even at low frequencies. This is surprising insofar as the system's performance only rests on the two signals picked up by the microphones of a dummy head, that is, of two sensors spaced roughly 13 cm apart. Multisensor linear arrays, which have also been proposed as a front ends for cocktail-party processors (e.g., Mitchell et al. 1971, Zelinski 1988), would require linear dimensions on the order of 3.4 m at 100 Hz to achieve a comparable effect.

In summary, it is believed that cocktail-party processors based on the principles of binaural signal processing will soon find their way into many applications and, as such, will contribute considerably to binaural technology. The next step along this road will be to develop computer-friendly algorithms for real-time processing (e.g., Peissig and Kollmeier 1990, Kollmeier et al. 1990, Grabke and Blauert, 1995). Furthermore, the evaluation of additional information in the binaural signals, for example, the profile of the internal spectrum at the coincidence position, will have to be considered.

5.4 The Precedence Effect: A Case of Cognition

In sections 3.2.1 and 4.4.4 a functional diagram of binaural hearing was proposed. In the diagram the signals arriving at a listener's two ears are assumed to have been processed monaurally first and then to have been combined binaurally. The combination results in a kind of a sophisticated "running representation of binaural activity" somewhere in the auditory system (see figures 3.34 and 4.29). It was understood that the signal processing, as depicted in the diagram, is basically "signal-driven", that is, the input signals to the two ears essentially determine the resulting representation of binaural activity. In terms of information flow, the system has a so-called bottom-up architecture.

Yet the ultimate and relevant output of the auditory systems is not any hypothetical internal representation of binaural activity, but rather auditory perceptual scenes, that is to say, arrays of auditory events arranged in time and space. Consequently, the question has to be tackled as to how the positions and spatial extents of the auditory events are linked to the assumed internal representation of binaural activity. In figures 3.34 and 4.29 it is suggested that more central stages of the auditory system perform some kind of a pattern-recognition process in the course of evaluating and interpreting the binaural-activity representation.

The idea behind pattern recognition is that patterns of characteristic attributes of the binaural-activity representation are known to the system, such as corresponding to specific sound-source positions. The system then evaluates the representation of binaural activity with the aim of identifying any patterns that might be contained in it. Once a pattern or a set of patterns has been identified, auditory events are formed accordingly.

Pattern recognition is a "hypothesis-driven" process. At a given moment in time the system typically sets up the hypothesis that a certain pattern of attributes is contained in the data. This hypothesis is then checked and subsequently accepted or rejected. In terms of information flow, such a system shows a so-called top-down architecture.

In figure 5.1, which is an extension of figures 3.34 and 4.29, bottom-up (signal-driven) and top-down (hypothesis-driven) divisions are explicitly marked. Note that a specific feature of the top-down division is the following. The system is assumed to have prior knowledge of what can be expected in the data and sets up hypotheses on the basis of this knowledge. Such an architecture is certainly in line with conventional understanding of sensory perception. We think of conciously perceiving organisms as more or less autonomous systems which, among other things, are able to actively collect information from the environment by paying selective attention to some sensory input while disregarding others, depending on the specific situation.

It is a widely accepted concept in this context that the central nervous system of an organism develops an internal model of the world, and that this model forms the basis of the perceptual world of this organism. The model and, consequently, the perceptual world are maintained and updated using information from different sources, such as input from the different sensory modalities and prior knowledge, or both. Note at this point that the central nervous system is a powerful biological computer with massive parallel, distributed processing and a huge amount of memory!

As far as auditory signal processing with respect to spatial hearing is concerned, it obviously has to be considered that the formation of the positions and spatial extents of auditory events is not only dependent on the actual acoustic input to the system but also on information from other senses (e.g., vision) as well as on cognitive (knowledge-based) processes. As an example to support this point, recent results obtained for the precedence effect will be put forward and discussed in the following paragraphs.

When signals from two or multiple coherent sources, for example, a direct sound and successive reflections, reach a listener from different directions, the auditory event will, nevertheless, often appear in a single direction only. Given that this "perceived" direction corresponds to the direction of the first wavefront, the directional information of this wavefront has obviously gained "precedence" over the directional information contained in successive wavefronts, and distinct echoes are thus not perceived, a case of the "law of the first wavefront" (see sections 3.1.2 and 4.4.2).*

The question, now, is whether precedence of the first wavefront in forming the direction of the auditory event is an effect that is necessarily driven by the auditory input signals, or whether this precedence is subject to modification in the sense that the central auditory system may interpret the auditory input differently in different situations, eventually also using information from other modalities or cognition, or both.

The precedence effect has recently been an issue of intense discussion in the field of auditory research. For comprehensive reviews, see Gaskell (1983), Zurek (1987), Berkley 1987, Clifton and Freyman (1996), and Hartman (1996). As a matter of fact, it appears that it has been known for quite some time that nonacoustic "cross-modal" information may influence the direction of the auditory event. See section 2.5, for the influence of visual, tactile and proprioceptive cues, and Thurlow and Jack (1973) and Thurlow and Rosenthal (1976) for the "ventriloquism" effect. Incidentally, precedence of the first wavefront does not necessarily presuppose that the successive sounds are coherent with the primary sound (Zurek 1987, Blauert and Divenyi 1988, Divenyi and Blauert 1986, 1987). In addition, precedence can also be observed for spatial features other than direction, for example, for the acoustical cues that are correlated with the spatial extents of the auditory events (Aoki and Houtgast, 1992, 1994, Houtgast and Aoki, 1994). Furthermore, it has been shown that precedence does not

*The use of the term "law of the first wavefront" (from the German *Gesetz der ersten Wellenfront*) is no longer recommended in Germany. The relevant standard on acoustic terminology (DIN 1320, 1991) advises use of the term *Präzedenzeffekt* ("precedence effect") instead.

necessarily mean that all spatial information is suppressed for those sounds that have not gained precedence (e.g., Perrott 1984, Yost and Sonderquist 1984, Perrott et al. 1987, 1988, Saberi and Perrott 1990; see also figure 2.101 for a bimodal paradigm on this subject).

The most interesting observations pertaining to this section, however, reveal that the probability of a reflection inducing an audible echo depends not only on the temporal, spectral, and spatial characteristic of a sound field but also on the context in which it is presented. (Note that the occurence of echoes means that precedence of the first wavefront over reflections is not effective!) Furthermore, there is evidence that the occurence of echoes can to a certain degree be controlled mentally, for example, by experience and selective attention.*

Both the influence of the context and of the listeners' mental states provide an indication of the involvement of top-down processes in spatial hearing. In the following, a case for cognition in spatial hearing is given as an example on the basis of results from our laboratory in Bochum with special reference to results from R.K. Clifton and her associates but also with reference to relevant suggestions from other authors (e.g., Thurlow and Parks 1961, Theile 1980, Hartman 1983, 1988, Rakert and Hartman 1985, 1986, 1992, Hafter et al. 1988, Budzynski 1985, Berkley 1987, Santon 1989, Hartmann and Rakert 1989, Wagenaars 1990, Bech 1989, Divenyi 1992).

The first experiment to be discussed is illustrated by figure 5.22, which shows two loudspeakers in a standard stereo arrangement (see figure 3.1) with a delay line connected to enable "classic" precedence-effect observations (see figure 3.12) to be made. In addition, a switch allows one of the two loudspeakers to be selected to radiate the leading signal.

Clifton (1987) has excited this equipment with an equidistant series of impulses (clicks) with a rate of $1/s$ and an interloudspeaker delay of $\tau_e = 5$ ms. In the course of an impulse train, the listeners experience precedence as expected, that is, the auditory events appear in the direction of the leading loudspeaker. Yet, at the moment in time when the switch is operated, the auditory event does not switch, and the listeners hear clicks at both loudspeakers for a few impulses. Then

*See the discussion of the so-called Franssen effect (first published by Kietz 1959) in section 3.3, for an interesting aspect of selective attention in spatial hearing.

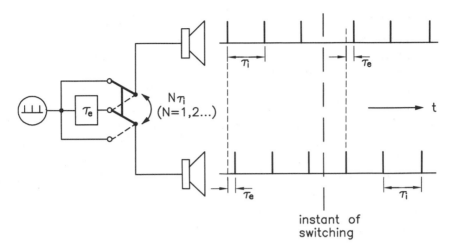

Figure 5.22
Experimental setup to produce the precedence effect and its eventual breakdown.
(From Clifton 1987.)

precedence resumes and the clicks are heard at the loudspeaker that is now leading.

The precedence effect, in other words, breaks down for a while, following an instance of a refiguration in the set of stimuli, and is only reasserted after some time delay. Clifton and her associates have analyzed this breakdown (the "Clifton effect") over a wide range of parameters (Clifton and Freyman 1989, 1996, Freyman et al. 1991a,b). Among other things, it appears that rebuilding precedence after the switching depends mainly on the number of impulses rather than on the presentation time or impulse rate.*

In addition to broadband impulses, broadband noise bursts or bandpass-filtered impulses or noise bursts produce the Clifton effect as well (Blauert and Col 1989, 1992, Freyman et al. 1991a,b). A time span, or rather a number of conditioning impulses during which the precedence effect becomes fully effective, has also been observed following the initial start of the impulse train and not only after reconfiguring the stimuli. This has been confirmed by Blauert and Col

---

* See, for example, Hafter and Dye (1983), Hafter et al. (1988), or the review by Hafter (1996) for related findings with regard to the effect of "binaural adaptation," whose relation to the precedence effect has not yet been conclusively established.

(1989, 1992) and Clifton and Freyman (1989) following a suggestion by Thurlow and Parks (1961). It has been argued that in ongoing "natural" signals like speech and music, signal features like pronounced onset slopes take on the role of the conditioners for the buildup of precedence. It should also be remembered at this point that buildup times for auditory spatial scenarios have been reported in various contexts. For example, Plenge (1972, 1974; see end of section 2.3.2) argues that the externalization of auditory events must allow some time for the subject to become accustomed to the sound field, and Platte (1979; see figure 4.11) found that, in a specific experiment, it took a few seconds for binaural fusion to occur.

In order to allow for a more detailed evaluation of the buildup and breakdown of precedence, Wolf (1988, 1990, 1991) designed an experimental paradigm in which these effects can be quantified via threshold measurements. This paradigm was later adopted by the Clifton group. Figure 5.23 explains the idea.

A main loudspeaker in an anechoic space radiates a (conditioning) train of impulses with an equally spaced interimpulse delay, τ_i. At the end of the train a test impulse is emitted by one of two adjacent speakers, positioned to the left and right of the main speaker. The test impulse will give rise to a spatially distinct echo unless the precedence effect is operative. The listeners respond by giving the echo direction

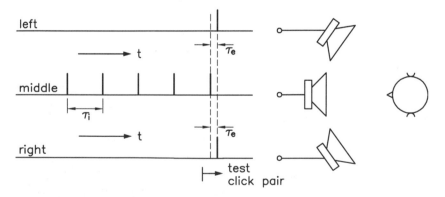

Figure 5.23
Experimental setup to quantitatively evaluate the echo-threshold level following presentation of a conditioning stimulus train. (From Wolf, 1988.)

(left or right of the main loudspeaker). More than 75% "right" answers or more than 75% "left" answers indicate echo perception.

The following results have been reported by Wolf (1988, 1990, 1991) from experiments using the setup shown in figure 5.23. The echo threshold in terms of the level of the test impulse, L_e, clearly increases with the number of impulses in the conditioning impulse train ($N = 1$ $\dots 8, \tau_i = \tau_e$), that is, the precedence effect becomes more effective. Variation of the interimpulse interval, $\tau_i = 250$ or 500 ms, does not make a difference. With increasing test-impulse delay, τ_e, the echothreshold level decreases again, that is, the precedence effect fades away.

With a slightly modified setup (figure 5.24), Wolf extended his experiments. Two loudspeakers were used (left and right). A conditioning impulse train was sent out by one of them. The last impulse in the train formed a test-impulse pair together with an additional impulse sent out by the second loudspeaker. The interimpulse interval in the train was $\tau_i = 250$ ms. The delay within the test-impulse pair was

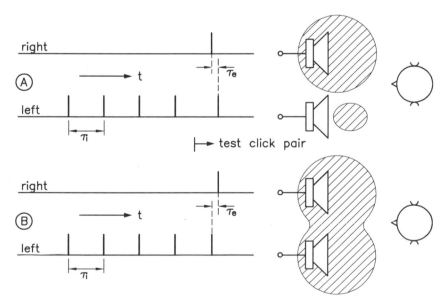

Figure 5.24
Stimulus scheme and plot of results by Wolf (1988, 1991) concerning echo loudness following a conditioning stimulus train.

$\tau_e = +2$ ms or $\tau_e = -2$ ms, that is, the impulse in the second speaker appeared either before or after the last impulse in the train. Listeners had three alternatives to choose from when responding to the test-impulse pair: (1) the clicks in both loudspeakers are of equal loudness, (2) the click in the left loudspeaker is clearly louder, or (3) the click in the right loudspeaker is clearly louder.

As a matter of fact, the question of loudness adds a new dimension to the precedence effect as it implies that suppressing the spatial information from the test impulse goes hand in hand with reducing echo loudness, that is, partial masking. This issue may be debatable*, but Wolf's results are, nevertheless, extremely interesting. As the results are symmetrical, the discussion can be restricted to the case where the left loudspeaker sends out the impulse train (see figure 5.24, upper panel). If the second member of the test-impulse pair (sent out by the right speaker) is leading, it produces the click with the greater loudness (right). If it is lagging, both clicks (left and right) are judged to be of about equal loudness (see Freyman et al. 1991a,b, for confirmation in principle).

Wolf offers the following explanation for his results. If the second member of the test-impulse pair is leading, it stands out as a new event to the auditory system. Consequently, it is regarded as important, while the other member of the test-click pair is just a continuation of the known conditioning impulse train and can thus be neglected. In the opposite case, where the second member is lagging, there is a conflict of interpretation. On the one hand, the second impulse could be a new event; on the other hand, it could just be a delayed version (a reflection) of the last impulse in the train. The auditory system reacts by not disregarding either of the two impulses, but forms two clicks of equal loudness.

The important implication of Wolf's explanation is the postulate that the auditory system evaluates sounds with respect to their "information content" and hence their amount of possible significance to the listener. Less important sounds are disregarded while important cues are processed or even enhanced.

---

*The precedence effect is usually understood as being the effect whereby spatial information carried by sound components is suppressed, but not that these components are generally suppressed (see section 4.4.2).

The ideas of Wolf have prompted Blauert and Col (1989, 1991, Col 1990, Blauert 1993) to conduct a series of experiments closer to the original Clifton paradigms. As a first step the setup of figure 5.22 was used, although the switching program was different from Clifton's (1987). Instead of a single switching, multiple switching was performed at regular or random intervals, each the length of one or multiple interimpulse intervals, τ_i. The impulse train was equidistant (typically $\tau_i = 500$ ms); the delay between impulse pairs was typically $\tau_e = 3$ ms for broadband impulses.

In the first experiment switching was performed regularly, for example, after a series of 20 impulse pairs each. The Clifton effect was observed as expected, that is, directly after each switching, echo became audible in the lag loudspeaker for a number of impulses. Yet, in addition to the Clifton effect, the following was observed. When the directional switching was performed more than once at regular intervals in such a way that the subjects could anticipate it, the echoes became increasingly fainter with repetitive switching. They finally vanished completely for some subjects.

In the next experiment the switching was performed after each single impulse pair. According to the expected breakdown of the precedence effect after each switching, one would expect that the listener heard a primary click in one and an echo in the other loudspeaker continuously. This was indeed the case, but the listeners were also able to indicate which was the primary click and which was the echo for each impulse pair. Again, similar to the experiment, the following interesting effect was observed. Once the subjects had definitely "picked up" the spatial movement, that is to say, the to-and-fro jumping of the primary click between the two loudspeakers, the echoes faded away. One subject coined the term "picking up the spatial melody" as a prerequisite of echo suppression. The perceptual situation is delineated in figure 5.25.

There are two conclusions to be drawn from these experiments: Firstly, the precedence effect does not require the source of primary sound to be fixed in space. If the movement of the source is reasonably slow (more than 250 ms for a full jump between left and right loudspeakers; cf. Aschoff 1963, Blauert 1968a, 1970a), the central nervous system is capable of collecting the information relevant to the formation of an appropriately moving auditory event and of suppressing

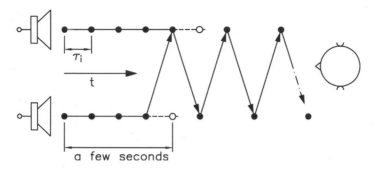

Figure 5.25
Schematic plot of primary auditory events and echoes in the case of a "jumping"
sound source with one opposite reflection. (From Blauert and Col, 1989, 1991.)

echoes. As a prerequisite, the central nervous system must "pick up
the spatial melody", that is, understand the spatial trajectory of the
source. If the trajectory of the sound source is not understood by the
listener, the reflections give rise to the formation of audible echoes. In
other words — and this is the second thing to conclude — if reflections
are unexpected and thus a possible carrier of significant information to
the listener, the precedence effect breaks down. This interpretation is,
in fact, congruent with Wolf's explanation of his results, as reported
above.

   To further elaborate on the hypothesis that the precedence effect is
codetermined by top-down processes where the information content
of the delayed sounds is an important criterion for triggering a breakdown of echo suppression, additional experiments were carried out by
Blauert and Col (1989, 1992). They started with the idea that any
sudden change in a reflection series that cannot be readily understood
by a source movement in a space with reflecting walls would be unexpected to the listener, would catch his or her selective attention, and
would consequently (or intercurrently?) cause the precedence effect to
break down.

   Two different kinds of sudden changes in the reflections were applied, namely, temporal and spatial ones. The temporal changes were
as follows. In a periodic presentation of primary sounds and reflections, the primary source being either fixed or jumping, reflections
were sometimes left out either on a regular or on a random basis. The
spatial changes were such that, with a fixed direction of the primary

source, the direction of reflections was switched either regularily or randomly between two alternatives. Both manipulations of the reflection pattern, which were unexpected to the listeners and could not be understood on the grounds of "normal" variations in reflective sound fields, led to a release from the precedence effect. Echoes that were not heard without the manipulation stood out clearly. In some cases subjects even reported that they could "concentrate" on the echoes to such an extent that they could almost completely disregard the primary clicks — a case of "backward inhibition" (see section 3.1.3).

In related studies along a similar line of thinking, Clifton et al. (1994) and Freyman et al. (1994) basically confirmed the findings reported above, but explored the observed effects for a wider range of parameters. After a train of conditioning stimulus pairs (short noise bursts), a test pair followed whose parameters were varied. The delayed component of the test pair was sent out alternatively in random order from one of two loudspeakers, at different directions. The subjects indicated echo detection by correctly identifying the lag loudspeaker.

Release of the precedence effect was observed when the delayed component of the test pair was suddenly changed with respect to delay, intensity, or spectral contents. Yet release was not observed when both components of the test pair were suddenly modified in the same way with respect to either intensity or spectral contents. Note that the first class of changes would normally not occur in the environment, as they imply sudden changes of positions or absorption characterics of the reflecting surfaces. In contrast to this, the second class of changes are perfectly normal, as they occur with any source emitting everyday sounds, with a running short-term spectrum changing from moment to moment, for example, speech, music, traffic noise (see also Blauert et. al. 1987, in this context).

All in all, the following picture of the breakdown of the precedence effect emerges. Whenever a sudden change of the reflection pattern occurs that is "implausible" to the listeners on the grounds of their conception of the trajectories of the sound sources or possible variations of the room acoustics of the space they are in, echo suppression is halted and the incoming signals to the two ears are rescanned (see Rakert and Hartman, 1985, Hartman 1996, for the concept of "plausibility" in sound localization in rooms). During the rescanning phase, localization performance may temporarily break down. This may affect, by the way, apart from echo suppression, for example, externalization (Plenge, 1972, 1974) and binaural fusion (Platte, 1979).

The ability to develop a conception of the sound field in enclosed spaces (a "spatial impression"; see section 3.3) and, consequently, to make sense of the reflection patterns received, seems to be an ability that evolves rather early in life. Newborn babies may react to sound sources by directing their heads toward the source, but they do not do so in cases where a direct-sound–reflection series is presented. The ability to discriminate the direct-sound direction from the direction of a successive reflection is only observed at an age of more than 16 weeks in newborn humans and more than 6 weeks in dogs (Clifton et al. 1981, 1984, Clifton 1985, Ashmead et al. 1986; see also Muir 1982). Obviously the precedence effect, although codetermined by higher stages of the nervous system, does not necessarily require profound intellectual effort to become effective, but rather can be set into force "intuitively" as well.

In view of the results and ideas reported above, one may arrive at the following general conclusion with regard to the precedence effect (Blauert and Col 1989, 1991), a conclusion that in principle is shared by a number of authors (e.g., Hafter et al. 1988, Hafter 1996, Clifton and Freyman 1996, Hartman 1996).

The precedence effect is the result of evaluation and decision processes in higher stages of the nervous system during which, in addition to auditory cues, cues from other sensory modalities and prior knowledge are taken into consideration. As a result, cues are identified which provide less important spatial information than do others. Less important are, for example, cues that are redundant or irrelevant from the listener's point of view. These cues are, subsequently, more or less disregarded in the course of forming the spatial attributes of the auditory events (directions, distances, spatial extents).

In the process of providing sensory cues for the higher stages of the nervous system, adequate preprocessing takes place. In the auditory pathway, spectral decomposition, masking, coincidence detection, lateral and contralateral inhibition, adaptation, and enhancement of onset slopes are known features, among others. In this sense, peripheral auditory processing must certainly be seen as a major part of the precedence effect as well. There is some indication that feedback

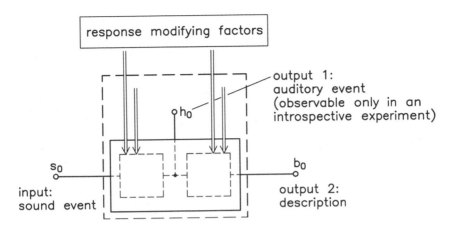

Figure 5.26
Schematic representation of the subject of an auditory experiment modified to take
account of top-down influences on perception and judgment and measurement (cf. to
figure 1.1).

from the central nervous system back to the peripheral nervous system
has to be anticipated in such a way that the nervous system, when it
has decided to suppress or enhance a certain cue, can control peripheral functions to this end (see figure 5.1). Consider the retriggering of
binaural adaption (Hafter and Buell, 1990) or the efferent control of
cochlea filters by selective attention (Scharf et al. 1987, Scharf 1995) as
examples in this context.

    The evaluation and decision as to whether certain cues are to be
suppressed are not necessarily experienced as a conscious or deliberate
processes. It may take quite some training for listeners to "recover" an
echo in a situation where it is normally suppressed "automatically"
(Blauert and Col 1989). In comparison to visual perception, the following analogies may be appropriate. Deliberate head-and-eye orientation in vision may be compared to direction-finder movements of the
head in audition, which, as is known (see section 2.5.1), may provide
crucial cues to spatial hearing and, hence, to the precedence effect. The
precedence effect itself, however, may be more reasonably compared
to the perception of stereoscopic images via a binaural visor, where,
once the 3-D image has popped up, it is hard to decompose it at will.

    In summing up, it must be stated that the precedence effect is still
not understood in such detail as to allow its effective modeling for

technological purposes. This is regrettable as the upcoming implementation of cognitive (knowledge-based) components in binaural technology products has created urgent demand for the relevant knowledge (Blauert 1996). Earlier models of the precedence effect are either too vague for technogical implementation (e.g., the association model of Theile 1980), or too specific for broad application (e.g., the evaluation-and-decision model of Wolf 1988).

Among builders of cocktail-party processors (see section 5.3), there seems to be some consensus that the incorporation of precedence-effect modules into these processors is an indispensable feature if they are to work effectively under reverberant conditions. The onset-slope models of Wolf (1987, 1988, 1991), the feature catalog of Bodden (1992b), and the recent work of Grabke (Grabke 1994, Grabke and Blauert 1995) must be regarded in this context. Grabke's work starts from the Jeffress-Lindemann-Gaik model, incorporating the onset-slope module of Wolf as well as a dedicated analysis unit for binaural-activity representations. As an output, it renders hypotheses concerning azimuths of auditory events, which certainly need further evaluation.

As a conclusion to this section it should be mentioned that the schematic of a subject in an auditory experiment, as put forward in section 1.2 (see figures 1.1 and 1.3), needs some modification in the light of the current discussion on the precedence effect. It has to be respected that auditory perception and judgment are more or less influenced by cross-modal information and cognitive processes. The least that can be done with regard to the schematic is to include a concept of the response-modifying factor as depicted in figure 5.26.

Bibliography

Asterisks (*) indicate surveys of spatial hearing or of branches of the subject.

Abel, J. S., and S. Foster (1994): Measuring HRTFs in a reflective environment. In: Proc. 2nd Int. Conf. Auditory Display ICAD 94, Santa Fe, p. 267.

Ahnert, W., and W. Reichardt (1981): Grundlagen der Beschallungstechnik [Fundamentals of public address technology]. VEB-Verlag Technik, Berlin.

Allen, J. B., D. A. Berkley, and J. Blauert (1977): Multimicrophone signal processing technique to remove room reverberation from speech signals. J. Acoust. Soc. Amer. 62, 912–915.

Allers, R., and O. Bénésy (1922): Zur Frage nach der Wahrnehmung der Schallrichtung [On the question of the perception of the direction of sound]. Z. ges. Neurol. u. Psychiatrie 67, 18–41.

Alrutz, H., and D. Gottlob (1978): Der Einfluss der frühen seitlichen Reflexionen auf die Räumlichkeit [The effect of early lateral reflections on spaciousness]. Fortschritte der Akustik, DAGA '78, VDE-Verlag, Berlin, pp. 579–582.

*Altman, J. A. (1972/78): Sound localization – neurophysiological mechanism. Beltone Institute of Hearing Research, Chicago (original Russian edition: Nauka, Leningrad, 1972).

Altman, J. A., and O. V. Viskov (1977): Discrimination of perceived movement velocity for fused auditory image in dichotic stimulation. J. Acoust. Soc. Amer. 61, 816–819.

Ando, Y. (1977): Subjective preference in relation to objective parameters of music sound fields with a single echo. J. Acoust. Soc. Amer. 62, 1436–1441.

Ando, Y. (1981): Preferred delay and level of early reflections in concert halls. In: Fortschritte der Akustik, DAGA '81, VDE-Verlag, Berlin, pp. 157–160.

Angell, J. R., and W. Fite (1901a): The monaural localization of sound. Psychol. Rev. 8, 225–243.

Angell, J. R., and W. Fite (1901b): Further observations on the monaural localization of sound. Psychol. Rev. 8, 449–458.

Aoki, S., and T. Houtgast (1992): A precedence effect in the perception of interaural cross correlation. Hearing Res. 59, 25–30.

Aoki, S., and T. Houtgast (1994): Onset dominance in the precedence effect with loudspeaker reproduction in a free field. J. Acoust. Soc. Jpn. (E) 15, 197–199.

Appino, P. A., J. B. Lewis, L. Koved, D. T. Ling, D. A. Rabenhorst, and C. F. Codella (1992): An architecture for virtual worlds. Presence 1, 1–17.

Arnheim, F. (1887): Beiträge zur Theorie der Lokalisation von Schallempfindungen mittels der Bogengänge [Contributions to the theory of the localization of sensations of sound by means of the semicircular canals]. Dissertation, University of Jena, cited in Bloch (1892).

Arnoult, M. D. (1950): Post-rotatory localization of sound. Amer. J. Psychol. 63, 229–235.

Arps, G. F., and O. Klemm (1913): Untersuchungen über die Lokalisation von Schall-reizen I: Der Einfluss der Intensität auf die Tiefenlokalisation [Investigations of the localization of sound stimuli I: The influence of intensity on the localization of depth]. Psychol. Stud. Wundt **8**, 226–270.

Aschoff, V. (1958): Probleme der akustischen Einkanalübertragung [Problems of single-channel acoustic transmission]. Arbeitsgem. f. Forschung Nordrhein-Westfalen **33**, 7–38, Westdeutscher Verlag, Köln.

Aschoff, V. (1960): Zur Frage der Rauminformation [On the question of spatial infor-mation]. Proceedings, 5th Conference of Sound Engineers, Detmold.

*Aschoff, V. (1963): Über das räumliche Hören [On spatial hearing]. Arbeitsgem. f. Forschung Nordrhein-Westfalen **138**, 7–38, Westdeutscher Verlag, Köln.

Aschoff, V. (1968): Nachrichtenübertragungstechnik [Information transmission tech-nology]. Springer-Verlag, Berlin.

Ashmead, D., R. Clifton, and E. Reese (1986): Development of auditory localization in dogs: Single source and precedence-effect sounds. Develop. Psychobiol. **19**, 91–104.

Atal, B. S., M. R. Schroeder, and K. H. Kuttruff (1962): Perception of coloration in filtered gaussian noise; short-time spectral analysis by the ear. Proceedings, 4th Int. Congr. on Acoustics, Copenhagen, H 31.

Atal, B. S., and M. R. Schroeder (1966): Nachahmung der Raumakustik durch Elek-tronenrechner [Simulation of room acoustics using electronic computers]. Gravesaner Blätter **27/28**, 124–137.

Babkoff, H., and S. Sutton (1966): End point of lateralization of dichotic clicks. J. Acoust. Soc. Amer. **39**, 87–102.

Babkoff, H., and S. Sutton (1969): Binaural interaction of transients: Interaural inten-sity asymmetry. J. Acoust. Soc. Amer. **46**, 887–892.

Babkoff, H., S. Sutton, and M. Barris (1973): Binaural interaction of transients: Inter-aural time and intensity asymmetry. J. Acoust. Soc. Amer. **53**, 1028–1036.

Ballantine, S. (1928): Effect of diffraction around the microphone in sound measure-ments. Phys. Rev. **32**, 988–992.

Banister, H. (1924): A further note on the phase effect in the localization of sound. Brit. J. Psychol. **15**, 80–81.

Banister, H. (1925): The effect of binaural phase differences on the localization of tones at various frequencies. Brit. J. Psychol. **15**, 280–307.

Banister, H. (1926): Three experiments on the localization of tones. Brit. J. Psychol. **16**, 226–279. See also Amer. J. Psychol. **38**, 436–440.

Banks, S. M., and D. M. Green (1973): Localization of high- and low-frequency transients. J. Acoust. Soc. Amer. **53**, 1432–1433.

Barron, M. (1971): The subjective effects of first reflections in concert halls – the need for lateral reflections. J. Sound and Vibration **15**, 475–494.

Barron, M. (1974a): Early lateral reflections and cross-section ratio in concert halls. Proceedings, 8th Int. Congr. on Acoustics, London, vol. 2, p. 602.

Barron, M. (1974b): The effects of early reflections on subjective acoustical quality in concert halls. Dissertation, University of Southhampton.

Barron, M., and A. H. Marshall (1981): Spatial impression due to early lateral reflec-tions in concert halls: The derivation of a physical measure. J. Sound and Vibration **77**, 211–232.

Batteau, D. W. (1967): The role of the pinna in human localization. Proc. Roy. Soc. London **B168**, 158–180.

Batteau, D. W. (1968): Listening with the naked ear. In: S. J. Freedman (Ed.), The neuropsychology of spatially oriented behavior, Dorsey Press, Homewood, IL, pp. 109–133.

Bauer, B. B. (1960): Broadening the area of stereophonic perception. J. Audio Eng. Soc. **8**, 91–94.

Bauer, B. B. (1961a): Phasor analysis of some stereophonic phenomena. J. Acoust. Soc. Amer. **33**, 1536–1539.

Bauer, B. B. (1961b): Stereophonic earphones and binaural loudspeakers. J. Audio Eng. Soc. **9**, 148–151.

Bauer, B. B., and E. L. Torick (1966): Experimental studies in underwater directional communication. J. Acoust. Soc. Amer. **39**, 25–34.

Bauer, R. W., J. L. Matuzsa, R. F. Blackmer, and S. Glucksberg (1966): Noise localization after unilateral attenuation. J. Acoust. Soc. Amer. **40**, 441–444.

Bech, S. (1989): Audibility of single reflections with short delay times. In: Proc. 13th Int. Congr. Acoust. ICA '89, 447–450, Belgrade, pp. 447–450.

Becker, R. (1971): Zur Psychobiologie des Sehorgans [On the psychobiology of the organ of vision]. Psychobiol. **19**, 1–5.

*Begault, D. R. (1994): 3-D sound for virtual reality and multimedia. AP Professional, Cambridge MA.

Belendiuk, K., and A. R. Butler (1975): Monaural localization of low-pass noise bands in the horizontal plane. J. Acoust. Soc. Amer. **58**, 701–705.

Bense, M. (1961): Bewusstseinstheorie [Theory of consciousness]. Grundlagenstud. aus Kybern. u. Geisteswiss. **2**, 65–73.

Beranek, L. L. (1949): Acoustic measurements. John Wiley, New York.

Berger, R. (1952): Das Menschenohr [The human ear]. Verlag E. Jaster, Berlin.

Bergmann, M. (1957): Binaural hearing. Arch. Otolaryngol. **66**, 572–578.

Berkley, D. A. (1987): Hearing in rooms. In: W. A. Yost and G. Gourevitch (Eds.): Directional hearing, Springer, New York, pp. 249–260.

Bielek, K. H. (1975): Spektrale Dominanz bei der interauralen Signalanalyse [Spectral dominance in interaural signal analysis]. Unpubl. thesis, Ruhr-Universität Bochum.

Bilsen, F. A., and J. Raatgever (1973): Spectral dominance in lateralization. Acustica **28**, 131–132.

Bilsen, F. A. (1977): Pitch of noise signals: Evidence for a "central spectrum." J. Acoust. Soc. Amer. **61**, 150–161.

Bischof, N. (1966): Stellungs-, Spannungs- und Lagewahrnehmung [Perception of posture, tension, and position]. In: Handbuch der Psychologie [Handbook of psychology], vol. 1, part 1, Verlag für Psychologie, Dr. C. J. Hogrefe, Göttingen, pp. 409–497.

Blauert, J. (1966): Zur Methode der Nachrichtentechnik bei der Erforschung und Beschreibung der menschlichen Wahrnehmung [On the method used in communications technology in researching and describing human perceptions]. Psychobiol. **14**, 49–55.

Blauert, J. (1967): Bemerkungen zur Theorie bewusst wahrnehmender Systeme [Remarks on the theory of consciously perceiving systems]. Grundlagenstud. aus Kybern. u. Geisteswiss. **8**, 45–56.

Blauert, J. (1968a): Ein Beitrag zur Trägheit des Richtungshörens in der Horizontalebene [A contribution to the study of the persistence of directional hearing in the horizontal plane]. Acustica **20**, 200–206.

Blauert, J. (1968b): Ein Beitrag zur Theorie des Vorwärts-Rückwärts-Eindruckes beim Hören [A contribution to the theory of the front–back impression in hearing]. Proceedings, 6th Int. Congr. on Acoustics, Tokyo, A-3-10.

Blauert, J. (1969a): Untersuchungen zum Richtungshören in der Medianebene bei fixiertem Kopf [Investigations of directional hearing in the median plane with the head immobilized]. Dissertation, Technische Hochschule, Aachen.

Blauert, J. (1969b): Die Beschreibung von Hörversuchen anhand eines einfachen, systemtheoretischen Modells [The description of auditory experiments according to a simple, system-theoretical model]. Kybernetik **5**, 45–49.

Blauert, J. (1969/70): Sound localization in the median plane. Acustica **22**, 205–213.

Blauert, J. (1970a): Zur Trägheit des Richtungshörens bei Laufzeit- und Intensitätsstereophonie [On the persistence of directional hearing in connection with time- and intensity-difference stereophonic sound]. Acustica **23**, 287–293; also Int. Audiol. (1972) **11**, 265–270.

Blauert, J. (1970b): Ein Versuch zum Richtungshören bei gleichzeitiger optischer Stimulation [An experiment in directional hearing with simultaneous optical stimulation]. Acustica **23**, 118–119.

Blauert, J. (1971): Localization and the law of the first wavefront in the median plane. J. Acoust. Soc. Amer. **50**, 466–470.

Blauert, J., and R. Hartmann (1971): Verlustfaktoren und Schallkennimpedanzen von Schädelknochen unterschiedlichen Pneumatisationsgrades [Loss factors and characteristic acoustic impedances of cranial bone of varying degrees of air-filled porosity]. Acustica **24**, 226–229.

Blauert, J., R. Hartmann, and P. Laws (1971): Entfernungs- und Richtungsabhängigkeit des Übertragungsfaktors des äusseren Ohres [Distance and direction dependence of the transfer factor of the external ear]. Proceedings, 7th Int. Congr. on Acoustics, Budapest, 25 H 5.

Blauert, J. (1972a): Die Schallausbreitung im äusseren Ohr und Konsequenzen für das räumliche Hören [Sound propagation in the external ear and its consequences for spatial hearing]. Convention '72, Audio Eng. Soc., München.

Blauert, J. (1972b): Zur Auswertung interauraler Signalunterschiede beim räumlichen Hören [On the evaluation of interaural signal differences in spatial hearing]. HNO **20**, 313–316.

Blauert, J. (1973): Bemerkungen zur binauralen Signalanalyse durch Kreuzkorrelation [Notes on binaural signal analysis by means of cross-correlation]. In: Fortschritte der Akustik, DAGA '73, VDI-Verlag, Düsseldorf, pp. 443–446.

Blauert, J., and P. Laws (1973): Verfahren zur orts- und klanggetreuen Simulation von Lautsprecherbeschallungen mit Hilfe von Kopfhörern. [Process for positionally and tonally accurate simulation of sound presentation over loudspeakers using headphones]. Acustica **29**, 273–277.

Blauert, J. (1974a): Impulse measurements of eardrum impedance. Proceedings, 8th Int. Congr. on Acoustics, London, vol. 1, p. 172.

Blauert, J. (1974b): Vergleich unterschiedlicher Systeme zur originalgetreuen elektroakustischen Übertragung [Comparison of various systems for accurate electroacoustical transmission]. Rundfunktech. Mitt. **18**, 222–227.

Blauert, J., P. Laws, and H.-J. Platte (1974): Impulsverfahren zur Messung von Aussenohrübertragungsfunktionen [Impulse procedure for measurement of the transfer function of the external ear]. Acustica **31**, 35–41.

Blauert, J., and H.-J. Platte (1976): Impulse measurement of human eardrum impedance. J. Audiol. Tech. **15**, 34–44.

Blauert, J. (1978): Some aspects of three-dimensional hearing in rooms. Proceedings, Meeting of the Federated Acoustical Societies of Europe, Warsaw, vol. 3, pp. 65–68.

Blauert, J., and W. Cobben (1978): Some consideration of binaural crosscorrelation analysis. Acustica **39**, 96–104.

Blauert, J., and P. Laws (1978): Group delay distortions in electroacoustical systems. J. Acoust. Soc. Amer. **63**, 1478–1483.

*Blauert, J., V. Mellert, H.-J. Platte, P. Laws, H. Hudde, P. Scherer, T. Poulsen, D. Gottlob, and G. Plenge (1978): Wissenschaftliche Grundlagen der kopfbezogenen Stereophonie [Scientific fundamentals of head-related stereophony]. Rundfunktech. Mitt. **22**, 195–218.

Blauert, J., and G. Tüttemann (1978/80): Primärschallunterdrückung in Konzertsälen [Auditory backward inhibition in concert halls]. Acustica **40**, 132–133; English translation: J. Audio Eng. Soc. **28**, 718–719.

*Blauert, J. (1980a): Neuere Ergebnisse zum räumlichen Hören [Recent results in the area of spatial hearing]. Rheinisch-Westfälische Akademie der Wissenschaften, Vorträge **N292**, Westdeutscher Verlag, Opladen.

Blauert, J. (1980b): Modelling of interaural time and intensity difference discrimination. In: G. van den Brink and F. A. Bilsen (Eds.), Psychophysical physiological, and behavioural studies in hearing, Delft University Press, Delft, pp. 421–424.

Blauert, J. (1980c): Interaural arrival time difference: Envelope vs. fine structure. Proceedings, 10th Int. Congr. on Acoustics, Sydney, vol. 2, B-10.7.

Blauert, J., H. Els, and J. Schröter (1980): A review of progress in external ear physics regarding the objective performance evaluation of personal ear protectors. Proceedings, INTER-NOISE '80, Miami, pp. 653–658.

Blauert, J. (1981): Lateralization of jittered tones. J. Acoust. Soc. Amer. **70**, 694–697.

Blauert, J. (1982a): Binaural localization: Multiple images and applications in room- and electroacoustics. In: R. W. Gatehouse (Ed.), Localization of sound: Theory and application, The Amphora Press, Groton, CT, pp. 65–84.

Blauert, J. (1982b): Binaural localization. In: O. J. Pedersen and T. Poulsen (Eds.), Binaural effects in normal and impaired hearing, Scandinavian Audiol. Suppl. **15**.

Blauert, J., and W. Lindemann (1982): Zur Entwicklung von Modellen der binauralen Signalverarbeitung [Study regarding the development of models of binaural signal processing]. In: Fortschr. Akustik, FASE/DAGA '82, Göttingen, pp. 1161–1164.

*Blauert, J. (1983): Psychoacoustic binaural phenomena. In: R. Klinke and R. Hartmann (Eds.), Hearing – psychological bases and psychophysics, Springer-Verlag, New York, pp. 182–199.

Blauert, J. (1984a): Akustische Untersuchungen mit verkleinerten Modellen [Acoustical investigations with scaled-down models]. Bundesbaubl. 1984, 601–604.

Blauert, J. (1984b): Psychoakustik des binauralen Hörens [Psychoacoustics of binaural hearing]. In: Fortschr. Akustik, DAGA '84, DPG-GmbH, Bad Honnef, pp. 117–128.

Blauert, J., K. Gruber, and W. Lindemann (1985): Zur Psychoakustik der auditiven Räumlichkeit [Study regarding the psychoacoustics of auditory spaciousness]. In: Fortschr. Akustik, DAGA '85, DPG-GmbH, Bad Honnef, pp. 495–498.

Blauert, J., and W. Lindemann (1985): Auditory spaciousness in concert halls – New aspects. In: Proc. 5th FASE Symp., Thessaloniki, pp. 179–182.

Blauert, J. (1986a): Further explorative studies of auditory spaciousness. 12th Int. Congr. Acoust., In: Proc. Vancouver Symp. Acoust. and Theatre Planning for the Performing Arts, Toronto, pp. 39–44.

Blauert, J. (1986b): Neuere Aspekte zum Entwurf von Aufführungsstätten für Musik [Recent aspects regarding the design of spaces for musical performances]. Bundesbaubl. 1986, 170–173.

Blauert, J., and W. Lindemann (1986a): Auditory spaciousness: Some further psychoacoustic analyses. J. Acoust. Soc. Amer. **80**, 533–541.

Blauert, J., and W. Lindemann (1986b): Spatial mapping of intracranial auditory events for various degrees of interaural coherence. J. Acoust. Soc. Amer. **79**, 806–813.

Blauert, J., U. Möbius, and W. Lindemann (1986): Supplementary psychoacoustical results on auditory spaciousness. Acustica **59**, 292–293.

Blauert, J. (1987): Some fundamentals of auditory spaciousness. In: S. Bech, and O. J. Pedersen (Eds.), Perception of reproduced sound, Ingenørhøskolen, Aarhus, pp. 33–40.

Blauert, J., G. Canévet, and T. Voinier (1987): The precedence effect: No evidence for an active release process found. J. Acoust. Soc. Am. **85**, 2581–2586.

Blauert, J., and P. Divenyi (1988): Spectral selectivity in binaural contralateral inhibition. Acustica **66**, 267–274.

Blauert, J., and J.-P. Col (1989): Etude de quelques aspects temporels de l'audition spatiale [A study of certain temporal effects of spatial hearing]. Note-laboratoire LMA, No. 118, CNRS, Marseille.

Blauert, J., and Ch. Pösselt (1989): Application of modeling tools in the process of planning electronic room acoustics. In: T. Tuzzle (Ed.), Sound reinforcement. Audio Engr. Soc., New York, pp. 510–517.

Blauert, J. (1991): Application-oriented modelling of binaural interaction. Nederlands-akoestisch-genootschap (NAG)-Journ. **104**, 51–57.

Blauert, J., M. Bodden, and H. Lehnert (1991a): La technologie binaurale appliquée à l'acoustique des salles [Binaural technologie as applied to room acoustics and sound perception]. In: Genese et perception des sons, Publ. L.M.A. No. 128, CNRS, Marseille, pp. 249–255.

Blauert, J., H. Lehnert, W. Pompetzki, and N. Xiang (1991b): Binaural room simulation. Acustica **72**, 295–296.

*Blauert, J. (Ed.), (1992): Auditory virtual environment and telepresence, J. Appl. Acoust. **36** (special issue).

Blauert, J., and J.-P. Col, (1992): A study of temporal effects in spatial hearing. In: Y. Cazals, L. Demany and K. Horner (Eds.), Auditory psychology, and perception. Pergamon Press, Oxford, pp. 531–538.

Blauert, J., and H. Lehnert (1992): Aspects of auralization in binaural room simulation. 93rd AES Conv., Audio Engr. Soc., New York, preprint 3390-G-6.

Blauert, J., and W. Pompetzki (1992): Auditory virtual environment. In: Proc. 6th FASE Congr., Zurich, pp. 23–29.

Blauert, J. (1993): Anomalien des Gesetzes der ersten Wellenfront [Anomalities of the law of the first wavefront]: In: Fortschr. Akust. DAGA '93, DPG-GmbH, Bad Honnef, pp. 788–791.

Blauert, J., M. Bodden, and H. Lehnert (1993): Binaural signal processing and room acoustics, IEICE Transact. Fundamentals E75 (Japan), 1454–1458.

Blauert, J., and H. Lehnert (1993): Zur Erzeugung interaktiver auditiv-taktiler Schein-welten für die psychophysikalische Forschung [Generation of interactive auditory virtual environments for psychophysical research]. In: Fortschr. Akust. DAGA '93, DPG-GmbH, Bad Honnef, pp. 546–549.

Blauert, J. (1994): La technologie binaurale: bases scientifiques et domaines d'applica-tion génériques [Binaural technology: scientific bases and generic application areas]. J. Phys. IV, Coll. C5, Les Editions des Physiques, Les Ulis, pp. 11–50.

Blauert, J., and H. Lehnert (1995a): Binaural technology and virtual reality. In: Proc. 2nd. Int. Conf. Acoust. Music. Res. CIARM 95, Ferrara, pp. 3–10.

Blauert, J., and H. Lehnert (1995b): The auditory representation in virtual reality. In: Proc. Int. Conf. Acoustics ICA 95, TAPIR, Trondheim, pp. 207–210.

*Blauert, J. (1996): An introduction to binaural technology. In: R. Gilkey and T. Anderson (Eds.), Binaural and spatial hearing, Lawrence Erlbaum, Hilldale NJ, (in press).

*Bloch, E. (1893): Das binaurale Hören [Binaural hearing]. Z. Ohren-Nasen-Kehl-kopfheilk. 24, 25–83.

Blodgett, H. C., W. A. Wilbanks, and L. A. Jeffress (1956): Effect of large interaural time differences upon the judgement of sidedness. J. Acoust. Soc. Amer. 28, 639–643.

Bloom, P. J. (1977a): Determination of monaural sensitivity changes due to the pinna by use of minimum-audible-field measurements in the lateral vertical plane. J. Acoust. Soc. Amer. 61, 820–828.

Bloom, P. J. (1977b): Creating source elevation illusions by spectral manipulation. J. Aud. Eng. Soc. 25, 560–565.

Bloom, P. J., and P. J. Jones (1978): Lateralization thresholds based on interaural time differences for middle- and high-frequency three-tone harmonic complexes. Acustica 39, 284–291.

Blumlein, A. D. (1931): Improvements in and relating to sound-transmission, sound-recording and sound-reproducing systems. British Patent No. 394325.

Bodden, M., and W. Gaik (1989): Untersuchungen zur Störsprecherunterdrückung mit einer gesteuerten Bandpassfilterbank [Studies in suppression of undesired talkers with a controlled bandpass filter bank]. In: Fortschr. Akust. DAGA '89, DPG-GmbH, Bad Honnef, pp. 195–198.

Bodden, M. (1992a): Cocktail-party processing: Concept and results. In: Proc. 14th Int. Conf. Acoustics ICA, vol. 4, Beijing, L3–2.

*Bodden, M. (1992b): Binaurale Signalverarbeitung: Modellierung der Richtungser-kennung und des Cocktail-Party-Effektes [Binaural signal processing: Modeling of direction finding and of the cocktail-party effect], vol. 85, series 17: Biotechnik, VDI-Verlag, Düsseldorf.

Bodden, M., and J. Blauert (1992): Separation of concurrent speech signals: A cocktail-party processor for speech enhancement. In: Proc. ESCA Worksh. Speech processing in adverse conditions, Europ. Speech Comm. Ass., Grenoble, pp. 147–150.

Bodden, M. (1993): Modeling human sound-source localization and the cocktail-party effect. Acta Acustica 1, 43–55.

Bodden, M., and T. R. Anderson (1995): A binaural-selectivity model of speech recognition. Proc. Eurospeech, Europ. Speech Comm. Ass., Grenoble, pp. 127–130.

*Boerger, G. (1965a): Die Lokalisation von Gausstönen [The localization of Gaussian tones]. Dissertation, Technische Universität, Berlin.

Boerger, G. (1965b): Über die Trägheit des Gehörs bei der Richtungsempfindung [On the persistence of the directional sensation in hearing]. Proceedings, 5th Int. Congr. on Acoustics, Liège, B 27

Boerger, G., and U. Kaps (1973): Kopfhörerstereophonie; Steuerung von Übertragungsparametern durch Kopfdrehung [Headphone stereophony, variation of transmission parameters by means of rotation of the head]. In: Fortschritte der Akustik, DAGA '73, VDI-Verlag, Düsseldorf, pp. 398–401.

Boerger, G., P. Laws, and J. Blauert (1977): Stereophone Kopfhörerwiedergabe mit Steuerung bestimmter Übertragungsfaktoren durch Kopfdrehbewegungen [Stereophonic headphone reproduction with variation of various transfer factors by means of rotational head movements]. Acustica 39, 22–26.

Bolt, R. H., and P. E. Doak (1950): A tentative criterion for the short-term transient response of auditoriums. J. Acoust. Soc. Amer. 22, 507–509.

*Boring, E. G. (1926): Auditory theory with special reference to intensity, volume and localization. Amer. J. Psychol. 37, 157–188.

Boring, E. G. (1942): Sensation and perception in the history of experimental psychology. Appleton-Century-Crofts, New York.

Bothe, S. J., and L. F. Elfner (1972): Monaural vs. binaural auditory localization for noise bursts in the median vertical plane. J. Aud. Res. 12, 291–296.

Bowlker, T. J. (1908): On the factors serving to determine the direction of sound. Phil. Mag. 15, 318–331.

*Bregman, A. S. (1990): Auditory scene analysis: The perceptual organization of sounds. MIT-Press, Cambridge MA.

Bregman, A. S. (1992): Auditory scene analysis: Hearing in complex environments. In: S. McAdams and E. Bigand (Eds.), Thinking in sound: the cognitive psychology of human audition, Clarendon Press, Cambridge, pp. 10–36.

Briggs, R. M., and D. R. Perrott (1972): Auditory apparent movement under dichotic listening conditions. J. Exp. Psychol. 92, 83–91.

Brittain, F. H., and D. M. Leakley (1956): Two-channel stereophonic sound systems. Wireless World 206–210.

Brunzlow, D. (1925): Über die Fähigkeit der Schallokalisation in ihrer Bedingtheit durch die Schallqualitäten und die Gestalt der Ohrmuschel [On the ability to localize sound as determined by the qualities of sound and the shape of the pinna]. Z. Sinnesphysiol. 56, 326–363.

Brunzlow, D. (1939): Über das räumliche Hörvermögen und die Fähigkeit zur Schallokalisation [On the faculty of spatial hearing and the ability to localize sound]. Hals-Nasen-Ohrenarzt 30, 1–6.

Budzynski, G. (1985): Theory of reflective localization of sound sources, In: Proc. 5th Symp. Fed. Acoust. Soc. Europe, FASE '85, Thessaloniki, pp. 151–155.

Burger, J. F. (1958): Front–back discrimination of the hearing system. Acustica 8, 301–302.

Burgtorf, W. (1961): Untersuchungen zur Wahrnehmbarkeit verzögerter Schallsignale [Investigations of the perceptibility of delayed sound signals]. Acustica 11, 97–111.

Burgtorf, W. (1963): Zur subjektiven Wirkung von Schallfeldern in Räumen (Rückverdeckung, Phantomschallquellen) [On the subjective effect of sound fields in rooms (backwards masking, phantom sound sources)]. Acustica 13, 86–91.

Burgtorf, W., and H. K. Oehlschlägel (1964): Untersuchungen über die richtungsabhängige Wahrnehmbarkeit verzögerter Schallsignale [Investigations of the direction dependence of the perceptibility of delayed sound signals]. Acustica 14, 254–265.

Burgtorf, W., and B. Wagener (1967/68): Verdeckung durch subjektiv diffuse Schallfelder [Masking by means of subjectively diffuse sound fields]. Acustica 19, 72–79.

Burkhardt, M. D., and R. M. Sachs (1975): Anthropometric manikin for acoustic research. J. Acoust. Soc. Amer. 58, 214–222.

Butler, R. A., and R. F. Naunton (1964): Role of stimulus frequency and duration in the phenomenon of localization shifts. J. Acoust. Soc. Amer. 36, 917–922.

Butler, R. A., and K. Belendiuk (1977): Spectral cues utilized in the localization of sound in the median sagittal plane. J. Acoust. Soc. Amer. 61, 1264–1269.

Caird, D., and R. Klinke (1983): Processing of binaural stimuli by cat superior olivary complex neurons. Exp. Brain. Res. 52, 385–399.

Campbell, N. R. (1938): Symposium: Measurement and its importance for philosophy. Aristotelian Soc. Suppl. 17.

Campbell, P. A. (1959): Just noticeable differences of changes of interaural time differences as a function of interaural time differences. J. Acoust. Soc. Amer. 31, 123.

Canévet, G., R. Germain, and B. Scharf (1980): Localisation d'une information sonore en présence de bruit masquant [Sound localization in the presence of a masking noise]. Acustica 46, 96–99.

Carhart, R., T. W. Tillman, and K. R. Johnson (1966): Binaural masking of speech by periodically modulated noise. J. Acoust. Soc. Amer. 39, 1037–1050.

Carhart, R., T. W. Tillman, and K. R. Johnson (1968): Effects of interaural time delays on masking by two competing signals. J. Acoust. Soc. Amer. 43, 1223–1230.

Carhart, R., T. W. Tillman, and E. S. Greetis (1969a): Release from multiple maskers: Effect of interaural time disparities. J. Acoust. Soc. Amer. 45, 411–418.

Carhart, R., T. W. Tillman, and E. S. Greetis (1969b): Perceptual masking in multiple sound backgrounds. J. Acoust. Soc. Amer. 45, 694–703.

Carsten, H., and H. Salinger (1922): Zur Frage der Lokalisation von Schallreizen [On the question of the localization of sound stimuli]. Naturwiss. 14, 329–330.

Chaudière, H. T. (1980): Ambiophonie: Has its time finally arrived? J. Audio Eng. Soc. 28, 500–509.

Chernyak, R. I., and N. A. Dubrovsky (1968): Pattern of the noise images and the binaural summation of loudness for the different interaural correlation of noise. Proceedings, 6th Int. Congr. on Acoustics, vol. 1, Tokyo, A-3-12.

Cherry, E. C. (1953): Some experiments on the recognition of speech with one and with two ears. J. Acoust. Soc. Amer. 25, 975–979.

Cherry, E. C., and W. K. Taylor (1954): Some further experiments upon recognition of speech with one and with two ears. J. Acoust. Soc. Amer. 26, 554–559.

Cherry, E. C., and B. McA. Sayers (1956): "Human crosscorrelator" — A technique for measuring certain parameters of speech perception. J. Acoust. Soc. Amer. 28, 889–895.

Chistovich, L. A., and V. A. Ivanova (1959): Mutual masking of short sound pulses. Biophys. **4**, 46–57.

Chocholle, R. (1957): La sensibilité auditive differentielle d'intensité en présence d'un son contralatéral de même fréquence [The differential auditory sensitivity to intensity in the presence of a contralateral sound at the same frequency]. Acustica **7**, 75–83.

Christian, W., and D. Röser (1957): Ein Beitrag zum Richtungshören [A contribution to the study of directional hearing]. Z. Laryngol. u. Rhinol. **36**, 431–445.

Clark, B., and A. Graybiel (1949): The effect of angular acceleration on sound localization: The auditory illusion. J. Psychol. **28**, 235–244.

Clark, H. A. M., G. F. Dutton, and P. B. Vanderlyn (1957): The "stereosonic" recording and reproducing system. Proc. IEE **104B**, 417–432.

Clifton, R. K., B. A. Morrongiello, J. W. Kulig, J. W., and J. M. Dowd, (1981): Newborns' orientation towards sound: Possible implications for cortical development, Child Develop. **52**, 833–838.

Clifton, R. K., B. A. Morrongiello, and J. M. Dowd (1984): A developmental look at an auditory illusion: The precedence effect. Develop. Psychobiol. **17**, 519–536.

Clifton, R. K. (1985): The precedence effect: Its implications for developmental questions. In: S. Trebhub and B. Schneider (Eds.), Auditory development in infancy, Plenum, New York, pp. 85–90.

Clifton, R. K. (1987): Breakdown of echo suppression in the precedence effect, J. Acoust. Soc. Am. **82**, 1834–1835.

Clifton, R. K., and R. L. Freyman (1989): Effect of click rate and delay on breakdown of the precedence effect. Percept. Psychophys. **46**, 139–145.

Clifton, R. K., R. L. Freyman, R. Y. Litovski, and D. D. McCall, (1994): Listeners' expectations about echoes can raise and lower echo threshold. J. Acoust. Soc. Am. **95**, 1525–1533.

Clifton, R. K., and R. L. Freyman (1996): The precedence effect: Beyond echo suppression. In: R. Gilkey, and T. Anderson (Eds.), Binaural and spatial hearing, Lawrence Erlbaum, Hilldale NJ, (in press).

Cochran, P., J. Throop, and W. E. Simpson (1968): Estimation of distance of a sound source. Amer. J. Psychol. **81**, 198–206.

Cohen, M. F. (1978): Lateralization performance in the presence of background noise. J. Acoust. Soc. Am. **64**, S35.

Cohen, M. F. (1981): Interaural time discrimination in noise. J. Acoust. Soc. Amer. **70**, 1289–1293.

Col, J.-P. (1990): Localisation auditiv d'un signal et aspects temporels de l'audition spatiale [Auditory localization of a signal and temporal aspects of spatial hearing]. Dissertation, Marseille.

Colburn, H. S. (1969): Some physiological limitations on binaural performance. Dissertation, MIT, Cambridge, MA.

Colburn, H. S. (1973): Theory of binaural interaction based on auditory-nerve data, I. General strategy and preliminary results on interaural discrimination. J. Acoust. Soc. Amer. **54**, 1458–1470.

Colburn, H. S. (1977a): Theory of binaural interaction based on auditory-nerve data, II. Detection of tones in noise. J. Acoust. Soc. Amer. **61**, 525–533; **62**, 1315.

Colburn, H. S. (1977b): Some properties of narrow-band, high-frequency waveforms. J. Acoust. Soc. Amer. **61**, S62(A).

*Colburn, H. S., and N. I. Durlach (1978): Models of binaural interaction. In: E. C. Carterette and M. P. Friedman (Eds.), Handbook of perception, Academic Press, New York, vol. 4, pp. 467–518.

Colburn, H. S., and J. S. Latimer (1978): Theory of binaural interaction based on auditory-nerve data, III. Joint dependence on interaural time and amplitude differences in discrimination and detection. J. Acoust. Soc. Amer. **64**, 95–106.

Colburn, H. S., and R. Hausler (1980): Note on the modelling of binaural interaction in impaired auditory systems. In: G. van den Brink and F. A. Bilsen (Eds.), Psychophysical, physiological and behavioural studies in hearing, Delft University Press, Delft, pp. 412–420.

Colburn, H. S., and P. J. Moss (1981): Binaural interaction models and mechanism. In: J. Syka and L. Aitkin (Eds.), Neural mechanisms of hearing, Plenum, New York.

Coleman, P. D. (1962): Failure to localize the source distance of an unfamiliar sound. J. Acoust. Soc. Amer. **34**, 345–346.

*Coleman, P. D. (1963): An analysis of cues to auditory depth perception in free space. Psychol. Bull. **60**, 302–315.

Coleman, P. D. (1968): Dual role of frequency spectrum in determination of auditory distance. J. Acoust. Soc. Amer. **44**, 631–632.

Conant, D. A. (1976): Physical correlates to the spatial impression in concert halls through binaural simulation. J. Acoust. Soc. Amer. **59**, S11.

*Cremer, L. (1948): Die wissenschaftlichen Grundlagen der Raumakustik [The scientific foundations of architectural acoustics], vol. 1. S. Hirzel Verlag, Stuttgart.

Cremer, L. (1971): Vorlesungen über technische Akustik [Lectures on technical acoustics]. Springer-Verlag, Berlin.

Cremer, L. (1976): Zur Verwendung der Worte "Korrelationsgrad" und "Kohärenzgrad" [On the use of the terms "degree of correlation" and "degree of coherence"]. Acustica **35**, 215–218.

*Cremer, L., and H. A. Müller (1978/82): Die wissenschaftlichen Grundlagen der Raumakustik, vol. 1, pt. 3: Psychologische Raumakustik [The scientific fundamentals of architectural acoustics, vol. 1, pt. 3: Psychological architectural acoustics]. S. Hirzel Verlag, Stuttgart. English translation by T. J. Schultz: Principles and applications of room acoustics, vol. 1, Applied Science Publishers, Essex, England, 1982.

Curthoys, I. S. (1969): Auditory location during binaural masking. J. Acoust. Soc. Amer. **46**, 125.

Damaske, P. (1967/68): Subjektive Untersuchungen von Schallfeldern [Subjective investigations of sound fields]. Acustica **19**, 198–213.

Damaske, P., and B. Wagener (1969): Richtungshörversuche über einen nachgebildeten Kopf [Investigations of directional hearing using a dummy head]. Acustica **21**, 30–35.

Damaske, P. (1969/70): Richtungsabhängigkeit von Spektrum und Korrelationsfunktionen der an den Ohren empfangenen Signale [Direction dependence of the spectrum and the correlation function of the signals received at the ears.] Acustica **22**, 191–204.

Damaske, P., and V. Mellert (1969/70): Ein Verfahren zur richtungstreuen Schallabbildung des oberen Halbraumes über zwei Lautsprecher [A procedure for generating directionally accurate sound images in the upper half-space using two loudspeakers]. Acustica **22**, 154–162.

*Damaske, P. (1971a): Die psychologische Auswertung akustischer Phänomene [The psychological interpretation of acoustical phenomena]. Proceedings, 7th Int. Congr. on Acoustics, Budapest, 21 G 2.

Damaske, P. (1971b): Head-related two-channel stereophony with loudspeaker reproduction. J. Acoust. Soc. Amer. 50, 1109–1115.

Damaske, P. (1971c): Richtungstreue Schallabbildung über zwei Lautsprecher [Directionally accurate sound images generated using two loudspeakers]. In: Gemeinschaftstagung für Akustik und Schwingungstechnik, Berlin, VDI-Verlag, Düsseldorf, pp. 403–406.

Damaske, P., and V. Mellert (1971): Zur richtungstreuen stereophonen Zweikanalübertragung [On directionally accurate two-channel stereophonic transmission]. Acustica 24, 222–225.

Damaske, P., and Y. Ando (1972): Interaural crosscorrelation for multichannel loudspeaker reproduction. Acustica 27, 231–238.

Damper, R. I. (1976): Tracking of complex binaural images. Audiology 15, 488–500.

Danilenko, L. (1967): Binaurales Hören im nichtstationären, diffusen Schallfeld [Binaural hearing in a nonstationary, diffuse sound field]. Dissertation, Technische Hochschule, Aachen.

Danilenko, L. (1969): Binaurales Hören im nichtstationären, diffusen Schallfeld [Binaural hearing in a nonstationary, diffuse sound field]. Kybernetik 6, 50–57.

David, E. E., N. Guttman, and W. A. van Bergeijk (1958): On the mechanism of binaural fusion. J. Acoust. Soc. Amer. 30, 801–802.

David, E. E. (1959): Comment on the precedence effect. Proceedings, 3d Int. Congr. on Acoustics, Stuttgart, vol. 1, pp. 144–146.

*David, E. E., N. Guttman, and W. A. van Bergeijk (1959): Binaural interaction of high-frequency complex stimuli. J. Acoust. Soc. Amer. 31, 774–782.

David, E. E., and R. L. Hanson (1962): Binaural hearing and free field effects. Proceedings, 4th Int. Congr. on Acoustics, Copenhagen, H 24.

Davis, J. R., and S. D. G. Stephens (1974): The effect of intensity on the localization of different acoustical stimuli in the vertical plane. J. Sound and Vibration 35, 223–229.

Deatherage, B. H., and I. J. Hirsh (1959): Auditory localization of clicks. J. Acoust. Soc. Amer. 31, 486–492.

Deatherage, B. H., (1961): Binaural interactions of clicks of different frequency content. J. Acoust. Soc. Amer. 33, 139–145.

*Deatherage, B. H. (1966): Examination of binaural interaction. J. Acoust. Soc. Amer. 39, 232–249.

Deatherage, B. H., and T. R. Evans (1969): Binaural masking: Backward, forward and simultaneous effects. J. Acoust. Soc. Amer. 46, 362–371.

de Boer, K., and R. Vermeulen (1939): On improving defective hearing. Philips Tech. Rev. 4, 316–319.

*de Boer, K (1940a): Stereofonische Geluidsweergave [Stereophonic sound reproduction]. Dissertation, Institute of Technology, Delft.

de Boer, K (1940b): Plastische Klangwiedergabe [Three-dimensional sound reproduction]. Philips Tech. Rev. 5, 107–115.

de Boer, K., and A. T. van Urk (1941): Some particulars of directional hearing. Philips Tech. Rev. 6, 359–364.

de Boer, K (1946): The formation of stereophonic images. Philips Tech. Rev. **8**, 51–56.

de Boer, K (1947): A remarkable phenomenon with stereophonic sound reproduction. Philips Tech. Rev. **9**, 8–13; also Frequenz **3** (1949), 24–25.

de Burlet, H. M. (1934): Vergleichende Anatomie des stato-akustischen Organs [Comparative anatomy of the stato-acoustical organ]. In: E. Bolk, E. Goppert, W. Kallius, and W. Lubosch (Eds.), Handbuch der vergleichenden Anatomie der Wirbeltiere [Handbook of comparative vertebrate anatomy], Berlin, part 2, vol. 2, pp. 1293–1432.

Delany, M. E. (1964): The acoustical impedance of human ears. J. Sound and Vibration **1**, 455–467.

Deutsch, D. (1978): Lateralization by frequency for repeating sequences of dichotic 400 and 800 Hz tones. J. Acoust. Soc. Amer. **63**, 184–186.

Diamant, H. (1946): Sound localization and its determination in connection with some cases of severely impaired function of vestibular labyrinth, but with normal hearing. Acta Oto-laryngol. **34**, 576–586.

Diercks, K. J., and L. A. Jeffress (1962): Interaural phase and the absolute threshold for tone. J. Acoust. Soc. Amer. **34**, 981–984.

DIN 1318 (1970): Lautstärkepegel [Loudness levels]. Beuth-Vertrieb, Berlin.

DIN 1320 (1959): Allgemeine Benennungen in der Akustik [Common terms used in acoustics]. Beuth-Vertrieb, Berlin.

DIN 1320 (1991): Akustik Begriffe [Acoustics terminology], Beuth-Vertrieb, Berlin.

DIN 45590 (1974): Mikrophone: Begriffe, Formelzeichen, Einheiten [Microphones: Concepts, formulas, units of measurement]. Beuth-Vertrieb, Berlin.

DIN 45591 (1974): Mikrophon–Prüfverfahren: Messbedingungen und Messverfahren fur Typprüfungen [Microphone test procedures: Measurement conditions and procedures for testing types]. Beuth-Vertrieb, Berlin.

DIN 45630 (1966): Grundlagen der Schallbewertung, Blatt 2: Normalkurven gleicher Lautstärke von Sinustönen [Fundamentals of sound evaluation, sheet 2: Standard curves of equal loudness for sinusoidal tones]. Beuth-Vertrieb, Berlin.

Divenyi, P. L., and J. Blauert (1986): The precedence effect revisited: Echo suppression within and across frequency bands. In: Proc. 12th Int. Congr. Acoust. vol. 1, Toronto, B2–9.

Divenyi, P. L., and J. Blauert (1987): On creating a precedent for binaural pattern. In: W. A. Yost and C. S. Watson, (Eds.), Auditory processing of complex sounds, Lawrence Erlbaum, Hillsdale NJ, pp. 147–156.

Divenyi, P. L. (1988): Echo suppression or lateral masking?, J. Acoust. Soc. Am. **84**, S79.

Divenyi, P. L. (1992): Binaural suppression of non-echoes. J. Acoust. Soc. Am. **91**, 1078 1084.

Dolan, T. R., and D. E. Robinson (1967): An explanation of masking-level differences that result from interaural intensity disparities of noise. J. Acoust. Soc. Amer. **42**, 977–981.

Dolan, T. R. (1968): Effects of masker spectrum level on MLD at low frequencies. J. Acoust. Soc. Amer. **44**, 1507–1512.

Dolan, R., and C. Trahiotis (1970): Binaural interaction in backward masking. J. Acoust. Soc. Amer. **47**, 131.

Domnitz, R. H. (1973): The interaural time JND as a simultaneous function of interaural time and interaural amplitude. J. Acoust. Soc. Amer. **53**, 1549–1552.

Domnitz, R. H., and H. S. Colburn (1977): Lateral position and interaural discrimination. J. Acoust. Soc. Amer. **61**, 1586–1598.

Dubrovsky, N. A., and R. 1. Chernyak (1971): The size and the localization of noise images at different durations of noise. Proceedings, 7th Int. Congr. on Acoustics, Budapest, 25H4.

Duifhuis, H. (1972): Perceptual analysis of sound. Dissertation, Technische Hochschule, Eindhoven.

Durlach, N. I. (1963): Equalization and cancellation theory of binaural masking level differences. J. Acoust. Soc. Amer. **35**, 1206–1218.

*Durlach, N. I. (1972): Binaural signal detection: Equalization and cancellation theory. In: J. V. Tobias (Ed.), Foundations of modern auditory theory, vol. 2, Academic Press, New York, pp. 369–462.

*Durlach, N. I., and H. S. Colburn (1978): Binaural phenomena. In: E. C. Carterette and M. P. Friedman (Eds.), Handbook of perception, vol. 4, Academic Press, New York, pp. 365–466.

Eargle, J. M. (1960): Stereophonic localization – An analysis of listener reactions to current techniques. Transactions IRE, AU8, 174–178.

Ebata, M., and T. Sone (1968): Binaural fusion of tone bursts different in frequency. Proceedings, 6th Int. Congr. on Acoustics, Tokyo, A-3-7.

Ebata, M., T. Sone, and T. Nimura (1968a): On the perception of direction of echo. J. Acoust. Soc. Amer. **44**, 542–547.

Ebata, M., T. Sone, and T. Nimura (1968b): Improvement of hearing ability by directional information. J. Acoust. Soc. Amer. **43**, 289–297.

Ebata, M., T. Nimura, and T. Sone (1971): Effects of preceding sound on time-intensity trading ratio. Proceedings, 7th Int. Congr. on Acoustics, Budapest, 19 H 2.

Edwards, A. S. (1955): Accuracy of auditory depth perception. J. Gen. Psychol. **52**, 327–329.

Egan, J. P., and W. Benson (1966): Lateralization of a weak signal presented with correlated and with uncorrelated noise. J. Acoust. Soc. Amer. **40**, 20–26.

Eichhorst, O. (1959): Zur Frühgeschichte der stereophonischen Übertragung [On the early history of stereophonic transmission]. Frequenz **13**, 273–277.

Elfner, L., and D. Perrott (1966): Effect of prolonged exposure to a binaural intensity mismatch on the locus of a dichotically produced tonal image. J. Acoust. Soc. Amer. **39**, 716–719.

Elfner, L. F., and D. R. Perrott (1967): Lateralization and intensity discrimination. J. Acoust. Soc. Amer. **42**, 441–445.

Elfner, L. F., and R. T. Tomsic (1968): Temporal and intensive factors in binaural lateralization of auditory transients. J. Acoust. Soc. Amer. **43**, 746–751.

Elliott, L. L (1962): Backward masking: Monotic and dichotic conditions. J. Acoust. Soc. Amer. **34**, 1108–1115.

Elphern, B. S., and R. F. Naunton (1964): Lateralizing effects of interaural phase differences. J. Acoust. Soc. Amer. **36**, 1392–1393.

Els, H. (1985): Ein Miniaturkunstkopf für die akustische Modelltechnik [A minature dummy head for acoustic scale modeling]. In: Fortschr. Akust. DAGA '85, DPG-GmbH, Bad Honnef, pp. 423–426.

Els, H., and J. Blauert (1985): Measuring techniques for acoustic models – upgraded. In: Proc. Internoise '85, Schriftenr. Bundesanst. Arbeitsschutz Unfallforsch., vol. Ib 39/II, Dortmund, pp. 1359–1362.

Els, H. (1986): Ein Messystem für die akustische Modelltechnik [A measurement system for acoustic scale models]. Schriftenr. Bundesanst. Arbeitsschutz, vol. Fb 477, Dortmund.

Els, H., and J. Blauert (1986): A measuring system for acoustic scale models. 12th Int. Congr. Acoust. In: Proc. Vancouver Symp. Acoustics and theatre planning for the performing arts, Toronto, pp. 65–70.

Enkl, F. (1958): Die Übertragung räumlicher Schallfeldstrukturen über einen Kanal mit Hilfe unterschwelliger Pilotfrequenzen [The transmission of spatial sound field structures over one channel aided by pilot tones below the threshold]. Elektron. Rdsch. 12, 347–349.

*Erulkar, S. D. (1972): Comparative aspects of spatial localization of sound. Physiol. Rev. 52, 237–360.

Ewert, P. H. (1930): A study of the effect of inverted retinal stimulation upon spatially coordinated behaviour. Genetic Psychol. Monog. 7, 242–244.

Eyshold, U., D. Gottlob, K. F. Siebrasse, and M. R. Schroeder (1975): Räumlichkeit und Halligkeit, Untersuchung zur Auffindung korrespondierender objektiver Parameter [Spatiousness and reverberance: Investigation to evolve corresponding objective parameters]. In: Fortschritte der Akustik, DAGA '75, Physik-Verlag, Weinheim, pp. 471–474.

Eyshold, U. (1976): Subjektive Untersuchungen an digitalen Nachbildungen von Schallfeldern aus Konzertsälen [Subjective investigations of the digital imitation of concert-hall sound fields]. Dissertation, Universität Göttingen.

Fasbender, A. (1981): Messungen früher seitlicher Schallreflexionen in Sälen [Measurements of early lateral reflections in concert halls]. In: Fortschritte der Akustik, DAGA '81, VDE-Verlag, Berlin, pp. 145–148.

Fechner, G. T. (1860): Elemente der Psychophysik [Elements of psychophysics]. Breitkopf und Härtel, Leipzig.

Feddersen, W. E., T. T. Sandel, D. C. Teas, and L. A. Jeffress (1957): Localization of high-frequency tones. J. Acoust. Soc. Amer. 29, 988–991.

Feinstein, S. H. (1966): Human hearing under water: Are things as bad as they seem? J. Acoust. Soc. Amer. 40, 1561–1562.

Feldman, A. S., and J. Zwislocki (1965): Effect of the acoustic reflex on the impedance at the eardrum. J. Speech and Hearing Res. 8, 213–222.

Feldmann, H. (1963): Untersuchungen über binaurales Hören unter Einwirkung von Störgeräusch [Investigations of binaural hearing in conjunction with noise interference]. Arch. Ohren-, Nasen- und Kehlkopfheilk. 181, 337–374.

Feldmann, H., and G. Steimann (1968): Die Bedeutung des äusseren Ohres für das Hören im Wind [The importance of the external ear to hearing under windy conditions]. Arch. klin. u. exp. Ohren-Nasen-Kehlkopfheilk. 190, 69–85.

Feldmann, H. (1972): Paper presented to the annual conference of the professional association of German audiologists, Heidelberg.

Ferree, C. E., and R. Collins (1911): An experimental demonstration of the binaural ratio as a factor in auditory localization. Amer. J. Psychol. 250–292.

Fettweis, A. (1977): On the significance of group delay in communication engineering. Arch. Elektronik Übertragungstech. 31, 342–348.

Firestone, F. A. (1930): The phase difference and amplitude ratio at the ears due to a source of pure tones. J. Acoust. Soc. Amer. **2**, 260–270.

Fischer, F. A. (1969): Einführung in die statistische Übertragungstheorie [Introduction to statistical communications theory]. Bibliographisches Institut, Mannheim.

Fischler, H., M. Hohenberger, E. H. Frei, M. Rubinstein, and D. Kretzer (1966): Acoustic input impedance of the human ear. Acta Oto-laryngol. **62**, 373–383.

Fisher, H., and S. J. Freedman (1968): The role of the pinna in auditory localization. J. Auditory Res. **8**, 15–26.

Flanagan, J. L., E. E. David, and B. J. Watson (1962): Physiological correlates of binaural lateralization. Proceedings, 4th Int. Congr. on Acoustics, Copenhagen, H 27.

Flanagan, J. L., E. E. David, and B. J. Watson (1964): Binaural lateralization of cophasic and antiphasic clicks. J. Acoust. Soc. Amer. **36**, 2184–2193.

Flanagan, J. L., and B. J. Watson (1966): Binaural unmasking of complex signals. J. Acoust. Soc. Amer. **40**, 456–468.

Fletcher, H. (1934): Auditory perspective – Basic requirements. Elec. Eng. **53**, 9–11.

Ford, A. (1942): The binaural intensity disparity limen. J. Acoust. Soc. Amer. **13**, 367–372.

Franssen, N. V. (1959): Eigenschaften des natürlichen Richtungshörens und ihre Anwendung auf die Stereophonie [The properties of natural directional hearing and their application to stereophony]. Proceedings, 3rd Int. Congr. on Acoustics, Stuttgart, vol. 1, pp. 787–790.

Franssen, N. V. (1960): Some considerations of the mechanism of directional hearing. Dissertation, Institute of Technology, Delft.

*Franssen, N. V. (1963): Stereophony. Philips Tech. Bibl., Eindhoven.

Frei, E. H., M. Hohenberger, S. Shtrikman, and A. Szöle (1966): Methods of measuring the vibrations of the middle ear. Med. Biol. Eng. **4**, 507–508.

Frey, H. (1912): Über die Beeinflussung der Schallokalisation durch Erregungen des Vestibularapparates [On the influence of stimulation of the vestibular apparatus on sound localization]. Monatsschr. Ohrenheilk. **46**, 16–21.

Freyman, R. L., R. K. Clifton, and R. Y. Litovsky (1991a): Changing echo thresholds. J. Acoust. Soc. Am. **89**, 1995–1996.

Freyman, R. L., R. K. Clifton, and R. Y. Litovsky (1991b): Dynamic processes in the precedence effect. J. Acoust. Soc. Am. **90**, 874–884.

Freyman, R. L., R. K. Clifton, and D. D. McCall (1994): Sudden changes in simulated room acoustics influence echo suppression. J. Acoust. Soc. Am **95**, 2898.

Fukudome, K. (1980a): Equalization for the dummy-head–headphone system capable of reproducing true directional information. J. Acoust. Soc. Japan (E) **1**, 59–67.

Fukudome, K. (1980b): The Thevenin acoustic impedance and pressure of dummy heads. Proceedings, 10th Int. Congr. on Acoustics, Sydney, L-13.2.

Gabor, D. (1946): Theory of communication. JIEE **93**, 429–457.

Gage, F. H. (1935): The variation of the uniaural differential threshold with simultaneous stimulation of the other ear by tones of the same frequency. Brit. J. Psychol. **25**, 458–464.

Gaik W., and W. Lindemann (1986): Ein digitales Richtungsfilter, basierend auf der Auswertung interauraler Parameter von Kunstkopfsignalen [A digital directional filter, based on the evaluation of interaural parameters of dummy-head signals]. In: Fortschr. Akust. DAGA '86, DPG-GmbH, Bad Honnef, pp. 721–724.

Gaik, W., and S. Wolf (1988): Multiple images: Psychological data and model predictions. In: H. Duifhius, J. W. Horst and H. P. Wit (Eds.), Basic issues of hearing, Academic Press, London, pp. 386–393.

*Gaik, W. (1990): Untersuchungen zur binauralen Verarbeitung kopfbezogener Signale [Investigations into binaural signal processing of head-related signals]. vol. 63, series 17: Biotechnik, VDI-Verlag, Düsseldorf.

Gaik, W. (1993): Combined evaluation of interaural time and intensity differences: Psychoacoustic results and computer modeling. J. Acoust. Soc. Am. **94**, 98–110.

Galginaitis, S. V. (1956): Dependence of localization on azimuth. J. Acoust. Soc. Amer. **28**, 153–154.

Gardner, M. B. (1967): Comparison of lateral localization and distance estimation for single- and multiple-source speech signals. J. Acoust. Soc. Amer. **41**, 1592.

Gardner, M. B. (1968a): Lateral localization of 0° or near-0°-oriented speech signals in anechoic space. J. Acoust. Soc. Amer. **44**, 797–803.

Gardner, M. B. (1968b): Proximity image effect in sound localization. J. Acoust. Soc. Amer. **43**, 163.

Gardner, M. B. (1968c): Historical background of the Haas and/or precedence effect. J. Acoust. Soc. Amer. **43**, 1243–1248.

Gardner, M. B. (1969a): Distance estimation of 0° or apparent 0°-oriented speech signals in anechoic space. J. Acoust. Soc. Amer. **45**, 47–53.

Gardner, M. B. (1969b): Image fusion, broadening and displacement in sound localization. J. Acoust. Soc. Amer. **46**, 339–349.

Gardner, M. B. (1973): Some monaural and binaural facets of median plane localization. J. Acoust. Soc. Amer. **54**, 1489–1495.

Gardner, M. B., and R. S. Gardner (1973): Problem of localization in the median plane: Effect of pinnae cavity occlusion. J. Acoust. Soc. Amer. **53**, 400–408.

Gaskell, H. (1976): Anomalous lateralization in the precedence effect. J. Acoust. Soc. Amer. **60**, S102 (A).

Gaskell, H. (1978): Some aspects of the localization of transient sounds in man. Dissertation, Oxford University.

Gaskell, H., and G. B. Henning (1979): The effect of noise on time/intensity trading in lateralization. J. Acoust. Soc. Amer. **65**, S121.

Gaskell, H., and G. B. Henning (1981): The effect of noise on time-intensity trading in lateralization. Hearing Res. **4**, 161–174.

*Gaskell, H. (1983): The precedence effect. Hearing Res. **11**, 277–303.

*Gatehouse, R. W. (Ed.) (1982): Localization of sound: Theory and application. The Amphora Press, Groton, CT.

Geffcken, W. (1934): Untersuchungen über akustische Schwellenwerte. Über die Bestimmung der Reizschwelle der Hörempfindung aus Schwellendruck und Trommelfellimpedanz [Investigations of acoustical thresholds. On determining the threshold of stimulus to produce an audible sensation from sound pressure and the impedance of the eardrum]. Ann. Phys. Lpz., 5th series, **19**, 829–848.

Genuit, K., and J. Blauert (1992): Evaluation of sound environment from the viewpoint of binaural technology. In: Proc. ASJ Intern. Symp. on: Contribution of acoustics to the creation of comfortable sound environment, Osaka, pp. 27–38.

Gilad, P., S. Shtrikman, and P. Hillman (1967): Application of the Mössbauer method to ear vibrations J. Acoust. Soc. Amer. **41**, 1231–1236.

Gierlich, H. W., (1992): The application of binaural technology, J. Appl. Acoust. **36**, 219–258.

*Gilkey, R., and T. Anderson. (Eds.) (1996): Binaural and spatial hearing, Lawrence Erlbaum, Hilldale NJ.

Giron, F. (1994): Modellierung der Richtcharakteristik eines Sprechers mittels der Monopolsynthese [Modeling of the spatial characteristics of a talker with monopole synthesis]. In: Fortschr. Akust. DAGA '94, DPG-GmbH, Bad Honnef, pp. 841–844.

Giron, F. (1996): Binaural room simulation as applied to a grand piano in a medium sized room, In: Proc. Perugia Classico, Perugia (in press).

Goeters, K.-M. (1972): Personal correspondence.

Goldstein, K., and O. Rosenthal-Veit (1926): Über akustische Lokalisation und deren Beeinflussbarkeit durch andere Sinnesreize [On acoustical localization and the ability of other sensory stimuli to influence it]. Psychol. Forsch. **8**, 318–335.

Gotoh, T., Y. Kimura, A. Yamada, and K. Watanabe (1980): A new sound localization control system for stereophonic recording. 67th Convention, Audio Eng. Soc., New York, preprint 1700 (B-3).

Gotoh, T., Y. Kimura, and N. Sakamoto (1981): A proposal of normalization for binaural recording. 70th Convention, Audio Eng. Soc., New York, preprint 1811 (B-2).

Gottlob, D. (1973): Vergleich objektiver akustischer Parameter mit Ergebnissen subjektiver Untersuchungen an Konzertsälen [Comparison of objective acoustical parameters with the results of subjective investigations in concert halls]. Dissertation, Universität Göttingen.

Gottlob, D., K. F. Siebrasse, and M. R. Schroeder (1975): Neuere Ergebnisse zur Akustik von Konzertsälen [Recent results on the acoustics of concert halls]. In: Fortschritte der Akustik, DAGA '75, Physik-Verlag, Weinheim, pp. 467–470.

Gottlob, D. (1978): Anwendung der kopfbezogenen Stereophonie in der akustischen Forschung [Application of head-related stereophony in acoustical research]. Rundfunktech. Mitt. **22**, 214–216.

Grabke, J. W. (1994): Modellierung des Präzedenz-Effektes [Modeling the precedence effect]. In: Fortschr. Akust., DAGA '94, DPG-GmbH, Bad Honnef, pp. 1145–1148.

Grabke, J. W., and J. Blauert (1997): Cocktail-party processors based on binaural models. In: H. Okuno and D. Rosenthal (Eds.), Readings in Computational Auditory Scene Analysis, Erlbaum, Hilldale NJ (in press).

Graf, U., H.-J. Henning, and K. Stange (1966): Formeln und Tabellen der mathematischen Statistik [Formulas and tables of mathematical statistics]. Springer-Verlag, Berlin.

Gran, S. (1966): Transformation der Frequenzcharakteristiken des Gehörganges [The transform of the frequency characteristics of the auditory canal]. Acustica **20**, 76–81.

Grantham, D. W., and F. L. Wightman (1978): Detectability of varying interaural temporal differences. J. Acoust. Soc. Amer. **63**, 511–523.

Grantham, D. W., and F. L. Wightman (1979): Detectability of a pulsed tone in the presence of a masker with time-varying interaural correlation. J. Acoust. Soc. Amer. **65**, 1509–1517.

Green, D. M. (1966): Interaural phase effects in the masking of signals of different durations. J. Acoust. Soc. Amer. **39**, 720–724.

*Green, D. M., and G. B. Henning (1969): Audition. Ann. Rev. Psychol. **20**, 105–128.

Green, D. M. (1973): Minimum integration time. In: A. R. Møller (Ed.), Basic mechanisms in hearing, Academic Press, New York, pp. 829–846.

*Green, D. M. (1976): An introduction to hearing. Lawrence Erlbaum, Hillsdale, NJ.

Groen (1972): Physik und Physiologie der Otolithen und Bogengänge [Physics and physiology of the otoliths and semicircular canals]. In: O. H. Gauer, K. Kramer, and R. Jung (Eds.), Lehrbuch der Physiologie des Menschen [Textbook of human physiology], Urban & Schwarzenberg, München.

Gruber, J. (1967): Hörversuche mit moduliertem Rauschen unterschiedlicher interauraler Korrelation [Auditory experiments using modulated noise of different degrees of interaural correlation]. Dissertation, Technische Universität, Berlin.

Gruber, J., and G. Boerger (1971): Binaurale Verdeckungspegeldifferenzen (BMLD) und Vor- und Rückwärtsverdeckung [Binaural masking level differences and forward and backward masking]. Proceedings, 7th Int. Congr. on Acoustics, Budapest, 23 H 5.

Guilford, J. P. (1950): Fundamental statistics in psychology and education, 2d ed. McGraw-Hill, New York.

Guilford, J. P. (1954): Psychometric methods, 2d ed. McGraw-Hill, New York.

Güttich, A. (1937): Schallrichtungsbestimmung und Vestibularapparat [Determination of the direction of sound and the vestibular apparatus]. Arch. Ohren-Nasen-Kehlkopfheilk. **142**, 139–149.

Güttich, A. (1939): Zur Schallrichtungsbestimmung bei doppelseitigem Vestibularisausfall [On determination of the direction of sound with bilateral vestibular dysfunction]. Arch. Ohren-Nasen-Kehlkopfheilk. **146**, 298–301.

Güttich, A. (1940): Zur Klinik der Tumoren des IV. Ventrikels, zugleich ein Beitrag zur Schallrichtungsbestimmung bei intaktem Cochlearis und fehlendem Vestibularis [On clinical practice in cases of tumors of the fourth ventricle, and also a contribution to the study of the determination of the direction of sound with an intact cochlea and absent vestibule]. Arch. Ohren-Nasen-Kehlkopfheilk. **147**, 5–7.

Guttman, N., W. A. van Bergeijk, and E. E. David (1960): Monaural temporal masking investigated by binaural interaction. J. Acoust. Soc. Amer. **32**, 1329–1336.

Guttman, N. (1962): A mapping of binaural click lateralization. J. Acoust. Soc. Amer. **34**, 87–92.

Guttman, N. (1965): Binaural interaction of three clicks. J. Acoust. Soc. Amer. **37**, 145–150.

Haas, H. (1951): Über den Einfluss eines Einfachechos auf die Hörsamkeit von Sprache [On the influence of a single echo on the intelligibility of speech]. Acustica **1**, 49–58.

Hafter, E. R., and L. A. Jeffress (1968): Two image lateralization of tones and clicks. J. Acoust. Soc. Amer. **44**, 563–569.

Hafter, E. R., W. T. Bourbon, A. S. Blocker, and A. Tucker (1969): A direct comparison between lateralization and detection under conditions of antiphasic masking. J. Acoust. Soc. Amer. **46**, 1452–1456.

Hafter, E. R., and S. C. Carrier (1969): Inability of listeners to trade completely interaural time for interaural intensity in a detection task. J. Acoust. Soc. Amer. **46**, 125.

Hafter, E. R., and S. C. Carrier (1970): Masking-level differences obtained with a pulsed tonal masker. J. Acoust. Soc. Amer. **47**, 1041–1047.

Hafter, E. R. (1971): Quantitative evaluation of a lateralization model of masking level differences. J. Acoust. Soc. Amer. **50**, 1116–1122.

Hafter, E. R., and S. C. Carrier (1972): Binaural interaction in low-frequency stimuli: The inability to trade time and intensity completely. J. Acoust. Soc. Amer. **51**, 1852–1862.

Hafter, E. R., and J. de Maio (1975): Difference threshold for interaural delay. J. Acoust. Soc. Amer. **57**, 181–187.

Hafter, E. R. (1977): Lateralization model and the role of time-intensity tradings in binaural masking: Can the data be explained by a time-only hypothesis? J. Acoust. Soc. Amer. **62**, 633–635.

Hafter, E. R., R. H. Dye, J. M. Nuetzel, and H. Aronow (1977): Difference threshold for interaural intensity. J. Acoust. Soc. Amer. **61**, 829–833.

Hafter, E. R., R. H. Dye, and R. H. Gilkey (1979): Lateralization of tonal signals which have neither onsets nor offsets. J. Acoust. Soc. Amer. **65**, 471–477.

Hafter, E. R., and P. Kimball (1980): The threshold of binaural interaction. J. Acoust. Soc. Amer. **67**, 1823–1825.

Hafter, E. R., R. H. Dye, and J. M. Nuetzel (1981): Lateralization of high-frequency stimuli on the basis of time and intensity. In: G. van den Brink and F. A. Bilsen (Eds.), Psychophysical, physiological and behavioural studies in hearing, Delft University Press, Delft, pp. 393–400.

Hafter, E. R., and R. H. Dye, Jr. (1983): Detection of interaural differences in time in trains of high-frequency clicks as a function of interclick interval and number. J. Acoust. Soc. Am. **73**, 644–651.

Hafter, E. R., T. N. Buell, and V. Richards (1988): Onset coding in lateralization: Its form, site and function. In: G. M. Edelmann, W. E. Gall and W. M. Cowan (Eds.), Function of the auditory system, Wiley, New York, pp. 647–676.

Hafter, E. R., and T. N. Buell (1990): Restarting the adapted binaural system. J. Acoust. Soc. Am. **88**, 806–812.

Hafter, E. R. (1996): Binaural adaption and the effectiveness of a stimulus beyond its onset. In: R. Gilkey, and T. Anderson (Eds.), Binaural and spatial hearing, Lawrence Erlbaum, Hilldale NJ, (in press).

Hall, J. L. (1964): Minimum detectable change in interaural time or intensity difference for brief impulsive stimuli. J. Acoust. Soc. Amer. **36**, 2411–2413.

Hall, J. L. (1965): Binaural interaction in the accessory superior olivary nucleus of the cat. J. Acoust. Soc. Amer. **37**, 814–824.

Halverson, H. M. (1922): Binaural localization of tones as dependent upon differences of phase and intensity. Amer. J. Psychol. **33**, 178–212.

Hammershøi, D., H. Møller, M. F. Sørensen, and K. A. Larsen (1992): Head-related transfer functions: Measurements on 40 human subjects. 92nd AES Conv., Audio Engr. Soc., New York, preprint 3289.

Hanson, R. L., and W. E. Kock (1957): Interesting effect produced by two loud-speakers under free space conditions. J. Acoust. Soc. Amer. **29**, 145.

Hanson, R. L. (1959): Sound localization. J. Acoust. Soc. Amer. **31**, 830.

Harkness, E. L. (1974): Localization of strong and weak sounds. J. Acoust. Soc. Amer. **55**, 1352.

Harris, G. G. (1960): Binaural interaction of impulsive stimuli and pure tones. J. Acoust. Soc. Amer. **32**, 685–692.

Harris, G. G., J. L. Flanagan, and B. J. Watson (1963): Binaural interaction of a click with a click pair. J. Acoust. Soc. Amer. **35**, 672–678.

Harris, J. D. (1964): Sound shadow, cast by head and ears. J. Acoust. Soc. Amer. **36**, 1049.

Harrison, J. M., and P. Downey (1970): Intensity changes at the ear as a function of the azimuth of a tone source: A comparative study. J. Acoust. Soc. Amer. **47**, 1509–1518.

Hartley, R. V. L., and T. C. Fry (1921): The binaural location of pure tones. Phys. Rev. **18**, 431–442.

*Hartman, W. M. (1983): Localization of sounds in rooms. J. Acoust. Soc. Am. **74**, 1380–1391.

Hartman, W. M. (1988): Listening to sound in rooms. J. Acoust. Soc. Am. **83**, S74.

Hartman, W. M., and B. Rakert (1989): Localization of sound in rooms, IV: The Franssen effect. J. Acoust. Soc. Am. **86**, 1366–1373.

Hartman, W. M. (1996): Listening in a room and the precedence effect. In: R. Gilkey and T. Anderson (Eds.), Binaural and spatial hearing, Lawrence Erlbaum, Hilldale NJ, (in press).

Hartung, K., J. Grabke, K. Rateitschek, and M. Bodden (1994): Eine physiologienahe Strategie zur Modellierung des binauralen Hörens [A physiology-related strategy for modeling binaural hearing]. In: Fortschr. Akust., DAGA '94, DPG-GmbH, Bad Honnef, pp. 1141–1144.

Hartung, K. (1995): Messung, Verifikation und Analyse von Aussenohrübertragungsfunktionen [Measurement, verification and analysis of HRTFs]. In: Fortschr. Akust., DAGA '95, Deutsch. Ges. Akust., Oldenburg, pp. 755–758.

Harvey, F. K., and M. R. Schroeder (1961): Subjective evaluation of factors affecting two-channel stereophony. J. Audio Eng. Soc. **9**, 19–28.

Haustein, B. G. (1969): Hypothesen über die einohrige Entfernungswahrnehmung des menschlichen Gehörs [Hypotheses about the perception of distance in human hearing with one ear]. Hochfrequenztech. u. Elektroakustik **78**, 46–57.

Haustein, B. G., and W. Schirmer (1970): Messeinrichtung zur Untersuchung des Richtungslokalisationsvermögens [A measuring apparatus for the investigation of the faculty of directional localization]. Hochfrequenztech. u. Elektroakustik **79**, 96–101.

Hawkins, J. E., and S. S. Stevens (1950): The masking of pure tones and of speech by white noise. J. Acoust. Soc. Amer. **22**, 6–13.

Hebrank, J., and D. Wright (1974a): Are two ears necessary for localization of sound sources on the median plane? J. Acoust. Soc. Amer. **56**, 935–938.

Hebrank, J., and D. Wright (1974b): Spectral cues used in the localization of sound sources on the median plane. J. Acoust. Soc. Amer. **56**, 1829–1834.

Hebrank, J., and D. Wright (1975): The effect of stimulus intensity upon the localization of sound sources on the median plane. J. Sound and Vibration **38**, 498–500.

Hebrank, J. H. (1976): Pinna disparity processing: A case of mistaken identity? J. Acoust. Soc. Amer. **59**, 220–221.

Hecht, H. (1922a): Über die Lokalisation von Schallquellen [On the localization of sound sources]. Naturwiss. **10**, 107–112.

Hecht, H. (1922b): Zur Frage der Lokalisation von Schallquellen [On the question of the localization of sound sources]. Naturwiss. **14**, 329–330.

Heinz, R. (1993): Binaurale Raumsimulation mit Hilfe eines kombinierten Verfahrens
– Getrennte Simulation der geometrischen und der diffusen Schallanteile [Binaural
spatial simulation using a combined method: Separate simulation of the geometrical
and diffuse sound components]. Acustica **79**, 207–220.

Held, R. (1955): Shifts in binaural localization after prolonged exposures to atypical
combinations of stimuli. Amer. J. Psychol. **68**, 526–548.

Henneberg, B. (1941): Über die Bedeutung der Ohrmuschel – Die Ohrmuschel als
Schliessapparat für den äusseren Gehörgang [On the significance of the pinna: The
pinna as termination of the exterior auditory canal]. Z. Anat. Entwicklungsgesch. **111**,
307–310.

Henning, G. B. (1974a): Detectability of interaural delay in high-frequency complex
waveforms. J. Acoust. Soc. Amer. **55**, 84–90.

Henning, G. B. (1974b): Lateralization and the binaural masking-level difference. J.
Acoust. Soc. Amer. **55**, 1259–1262.

Henning, G. B. (1980): Some observations on the lateralization of complex waveforms.
J. Acoust. Soc. Amer. **68**, 446–454.

Henning, G. B. (1981): Lateralization of complex waveforms. In: G. van den Brink and
F. A. Bilsen (Eds.), Psychophysical, physiological and behavioural studies in hearing,
Delft University Press, Delft, pp. 386–392.

Henning, G. B., and J. Ashton (1981): The effect of carrier and modulation frequency
on lateralization based on interaural phase and interaural group delay. Hearing Res. **4**,
185–194.

Henry, J. (1849): Presentation before the American Association for the Advancement
of Science on the 21st of August. Cited in: Scientific writings of Joseph Henry, part II,
pp. 295–296, Smithsonian Institution, Washington, DC (1851).

Hershkowitz, R. M., and N. I. Durlach (1969a): Interaural time and amplitude JNDs
for a 500-Hz tone. J. Acoust. Soc. Amer. **46**, 1464–1467.

Hershkowitz, R. M., and N. I. Durlach (1969b): An unsuccessful attempt to determine
the tradability of interaural time and interaural intensity. J. Acoust. Soc. Amer. **46**,
1583–1584.

Hirsch, H. R. (1968): Perception of the range of a sound source of unknown strength.
J. Acoust. Soc. Amer. **43**, 373–374.

Hirsch I. J. (1948): The influence of interaural phase on interaural summation and
inhibition. J. Acoust. Soc. Amer. **20**, 536–544.

Hirsch, I. J., and F. A. Webster (1949): Some determinants of interaural phase effects.
J. Acoust. Soc. Amer. **21**, 468–469.

Hirsch, I. J., and M. Burgeat (1958): Binaural effects in remote masking. J. Acoust.
Soc. Amer. **30**, 827–832.

HNO-Handbuch (1965): Hals-Nasen-Ohrenheilkunde – Ein kurzgefasstes Handbuch
in drei Bänden [Ear, nose, and throat medicine – A brief handbook in three volumes].
Georg Thieme Verlag, Stuttgart, vol. 3, part I.

Holt, E. B. (1909): On ocular nystagmus and the localization of sensory data during
dizziness. Psychol. Rev. **16**, 377–398.

Holt, R. E., and W. R. Thurlow (1969): Subject orientation and judgment of distance
of a sound source. J. Acoust. Soc. Amer. **46**, 1584–1585.

Houtgast, T., and R. Plomp (1968): Lateralization threshold of a signal in noise.
J. Acoust. Soc. Amer. **44**, 807–812.

Houtgast, T. (1977): Phase effects in the two-tone suppression investigated with a binaural lateralization paradigm. In: E. F. Evans and J. P. Wilson (Eds.), Psychophysics and physiology of hearing, Academic Press, London, pp. 165–170.

Houtgast, T., and S. Aoki (1994): Stimulus-onset dominance in the perception of binaural information. Hearing Res. **72**, 29–36.

Hudde, H. (1976): Zur Ungenauigkeit der Trommelfellimpedanzbestimmung nach der Impulsmethode [On the inaccuracy of the eardrum impedance determined by the impulse method]. In: Fortschritte der Akustik, DAGA '76, VDI-Verlag, Düsseldorf, pp. 629–632.

Hudde, H. (1978a): Methoden zur Bestimmung der menschlichen Trommelfellimpedanz unter Berücksichtigung der Querschnittsfunktion des Ohrkanals. Rundfunktech. Mitt. **22**, 206–208.

Hudde, H. (1978b): Ein neues System zur Erfassung breitbandiger akustischer Signale [A new system for picking up broadband acoustical signals]. In: Fortschritte der Akustik, DAGA '78, VDE-Verlag, Berlin, pp. 593–596.

Hudde, H. (1980a): Messung der Trommelfellimpedanz des menschlichen Ohres bis 19 kHz [Measurement of the human eardrum impedance up to 19 kHz]. Dissertation, Ruhr-Universität Bochum.

Hudde, H. (1980b): Messung der menschlichen Trommelfellimpedanz bis 19 kHz [Measurement of human eardrum impedance up to 19 kHz]. In: Fortschritte der Akustik, DAGA '80, VDE-Verlag, Berlin, pp. 579–582.

Hudde, H., and J. Schröter (1980): The equalization of artificial heads without exact replication of the eardrum impedance. Acustica **44**, 302–307.

Hudde, H., and R. Lackmann (1981): Systematische Fehler bei Messungen mit Sondenmikrofonen [Systematic errors in measurements using probe microphones]. Acustica **47**, 27–33.

Hudde, H., and J. Schröter (1981): Verbesserungen am Neumann-Kunstkopfsystem [Improvements to the Neumann dummy-head system]. Rundfunktech. Mitt. **25**, 1–6.

Huggins, A. W. F. (1974): On perceptual integration of dichotically alternating pulse trains. J. Acoust. Soc. Amer. **56**, 939–943.

Huizing, E. H. (1970): Lateralization of bone conduction into the better ear in conductive deafness. Acta Oto-laryngol. **69**, 395–401.

Ikenberry, L. D., and C. E. Shutt (1898): Experiments in judging the distance of sound. Kansas Univ. Quart **7**, series A, 9–16.

Ingård, U. (1953): A review of the influence of meteorological conditions on sound propagation. J. Acoust. Soc. Amer. **25**, 405–411.

Ito, Y., C. L. Thompson, and H. S. Colburn (1979): Interaural time discrimination in noise. J. Acoust. Soc. Amer. **65**, S121.

Jacobsen, T. (1976): Localization in noise. Tech. Rep. 10, Acoustics Lab, Technical University, Lynby, Denmark.

Jahn, G. (1958): Über die Beziehung zwischen der Lautstärke und dem Schalldruck am Trommelfell [On the relationship between loudness and sound pressure at the eardrum]. Hochfrequenztech. u. Elektroakustik **67**, 69–81.

Jahn, G., and S. Vogelsang (1959): Die einohrige Richtcharakteristik des menschlichen Gehörs [The directional characteristics of human hearing with one ear]. Hochfrequenztech. u. Elektroakustik **68**, 50–56.

Jahn, G. (1960): Über den Unterschied zwischen den Kurven gleicher Lautstärke in der ebenen Welle und im diffusen Schallfeld [On the differences between the curves of equal loudness for plane waves and for a diffuse sound field]. Hochfrequenztech. u. Elektroakustik 69, 75–81.

Janovsky, W. H. (1948): Einrichtung zur plastischen Wiedergabe elektroakustischer Darbietungen [An apparatus for 3-dimensional reproduction in electroacoustical presentations]. German Federal Republic Patent No. 973570.

Jeffress, L. A. (1948): A place theory of sound localization. J. Comp. Physiol. Psych. 61, 468–486.

Jeffress, L. A., H. C. Blodgett, and B. H. Deatherage (1952): The masking of tones by white noise as a function of the interaural phases of both components. J. Acoust. Soc. Amer. 24, 523–527.

Jeffress, L. A., H. C. Blodgett, T. T. Sandel, and C. L. Wood (1956): Masking of tone signals. J. Acoust. Soc. Amer. 28, 416–426.

Jeffress, L. A. (1957): Note on the "Interesting effect produced by two loudspeakers under free space conditions" by L. R. Hanson and W. E. Kock. J. Acoust. Soc. Amer. 29, 655.

Jeffress, L. A., and R. W. Taylor (1961): Lateralisation versus localization. J. Acoust. Soc. Amer. 33, 482–483.

Jeffress, L. A., H. C. Blodgett, and B. H. Deatherage (1962): Effect of interaural correlation on the precision of centering a noise. J. Acoust. Soc. Amer. 34, 1122–1123.

Jeffress, L. A., and D. E. Robinson (1962): Formulas for the coefficient of interaural correlation of noise. J. Acoust. Soc. Amer. 34, 1658.

Jeffress, L. A., and D. McFadden (1970): Detection, lateralization and the phase angle α. J. Acoust. Soc. Amer. 47, 130.

Jeffress, L. A., and D. McFadden (1971): Differences of interaural phase and level in detection and lateralization. J. Acoust. Soc. Amer. 49, 1169–1179.

Jeffress, L. A. (1972): Binaural signal detection: Vector theory. In: J. V. Tobias (Ed.), Foundations of modern auditory theory, vol.2, Academic Press, New York, pp. 349–368.

Johansen, P. A. (1975): Measurement of the human ear canal. Acustica 33, 349–351.

Jones, P. J., and R. P. Williams (1981): An experiment to determine whether the interaural time difference used in lateralizing middle- and high-frequency complex tones is dependent in any way on fine-structure information. Acustica 47, 164–169.

Jongkees, L. B. W., and J. J. Groen (1946): On directional hearing. J. Laryngol. Otol. 61, 494–504.

Jongkees, L. B. W. (1953): Über die Untersuchungsmethoden des Gleichgewichtsorgans [On techniques for investigating the organ of balance]. Fortschr. Hals-Nasen-Ohrenheilk. 1, 1–147.

Jongkees, L. B. W., and R. A. van de Veer (1958): On directional sound localization in unilateral deafness and its explanation. Acta Oto-laryngol. 49, 119–131.

Jordan, V. L. (1954): A system for stereophonic reproduction. Acustica 4, 36–38.

Jordan, V. L. (1980): Acoustical design of concert halls and theaters. Applied Science Publishers, London.

Joswig, M., and H. Hudde (1978): Eine Messrohrmethode zur Bestimmung der Querschnittsfunktion von Rohren [A measuring-tube method for determining the function of cross-sectional area of tubes]. In: Fortschritte der Akustik, DAGA '78, VDE-Verlag, Berlin, pp. 597–600.

Joswig, M. (1981): Messung der Trommelfellimpedanz des Menschen mit einer Messrohrmethode [Measurement of the human eardrum impedance using a measuring-tube method]. In: Fortschritte der Akustik, DAGA '81, VDE-Verlag, Berlin, pp. 709–712.

Kaiser, J. F., and E. E. David (1960): Reproducing the cocktail party effect. J. Acoust. Soc. Amer. **32**, 918.

Kasynski, G., and W. Ortmeyer (1961): Die Zweikanal-Stereophonie und ihre Aufnahmeverfahren [Two-channel stereophony and sound-collecting procedures applicable to it]. Bild und Ton **14**, 107–111, 155–157.

Katzvey, W., and F. K. Schröder (1958): Die Grundlagen des stereophonen Hörens [The fundamentals of stereophonic hearing]. Radio Mentor **6**, 377–380.

Keet, W. deV. (1968): The influence of early reflections on the spatial impression. Proceedings, 6th Int. Congr. on Acoustics, Tokyo, E-2-4.

Keibs, L. (1936): Methode zur Messung von Schwellendrucken und Trommelfellimpedanzen in fortschreitenden Wellen [Techniques for the measurement of threshold pressures and impedances of the eardrum using propagating waves]. Dissertation, Technische Hochschule, Breslau; also Ann. Phys. Lpz., 5th series, **26**, 585–608.

Keibs, L. (1965): Kompatible stereo-ambifone Schallübertragung auf zwei Kanälen [Compatible stereophonic-ambiphonic sound transmission using two channels]. Nachrichtentechnik **15**, 246–253.

Keibs, L. (1966): Universelles System zur stereo-ambiphonen Aufnahme und Wiedergabe [A universal system for stereophonic-ambiphonic sound collection and reproduction]. Reports of the 7th Conference of Audio Engineers, Cologne, WDR Köln, pp. 10–14.

Keidel, W. D., M. E. Wigand, and U. O. Keidel (1960): Lautheitseinfluss auf die Informationsverarbeitung beim binauralen Hören des Menschen [The influence of loudness on the processing of information in human binaural hearing]. Pflügers Arch. **270**, 370–389.

*Keidel, W. D. (1966): Das räumliche Hören [Spatial hearing]. In: Handbuch der Psychologie, vol. 1, part 1, Verlag für Psychologie, Dr. C. J. Hogrefe, Göttingen, pp. 518–555.

Kessel, J. (1882): Über die Funktion der Ohrmuschel bei den Raumwahrnehmungen [On the function of the pinna in connection with spatial perceptions]. Arch. Ohrenheilk. **18**, 120–129.

Kiang, N. Y. S., T. Watanabe, E. C. Thomas, and L. F. Clark (1965): Discharge patterns of single fibers in the cat's auditory nerve. The MIT Press, Cambridge, MA.

Kietz, H. (1952): Das Problem des räumlichen Richtungshörens [The problem of spatial directional hearing]. Arch. Hals-Nasen-Ohrenheilk., 91–94.

*Kietz, H. (1953): Das räumliche Hören [Spatial hearing]. Acustica **3**, 73–86.

Kietz, H. (1957): Die physikalischen Vorgänge bei der Schallbildübertragung vom Stapes bis zum Zentralorgan [The physical processes of sound conduction from the stapes to the central organ]. Lärmbekämpfung **1**, 109–116, 131–136.

Kietz H. (1959): Der echte und ein falscher Haas-Effekt [The genuine and a false Haas effect]. Proceedings, 3rd. Int. Congr. on Acoustics, Stuttgart, vol. 1, pp. 147–149.

Kikuchi, Y. (1957): Objective allocation of sound image from binaural stimulation. J. Acoust. Soc. Amer. **29**, 124–128.

Killion, M. C. (1979): Equalization filter for eardrum-pressure recording using a KEMAR manikin. J. Audio Eng. Soc. **27**, 13–16.

King, W. G., and D. A. Laird (1930): The effect of noise intensity and pattern on locating sounds. J. Acoust. Soc. Amer. **2**, 99–102.

Kirikae, I., K. Nakamura, T. Sato, and T. Shitara (1970): A study of binaural interaction. Ann. Bull. No. 5, Res. Inst. of Logopedics-Phoniatrics, University of Tokyo.

Kleiner, M. (1978): Problems in the design and use of "dummy heads." Acustica **41**, 183–193.

Kleis, D. (1955): Experimente zur Verbesserung der Raumwirkung von Schall [Experiments in improving the spatial quality of sound]. Elektron. Rdsch. **9**, 64–68.

Klemm, O. (1909): Lokalisation von Sinneseindrücken bei disparaten Nebenreizen [Localization of sensory impressions in connection with disparate additional stimuli]. Psychol. Stud. **5**, 73–162.

Klemm, O. (1913): Untersuchungen über die Lokalisation von Schallreizen II: Versuche mit einem monotischen Beobachter [Investigations of the localization of sound stimuli II: Experiments with a monotic observer]. Psychol. Stud. **8**, 497–505.

Klemm, O. (1914): Über die Lokalisation von Schallreizen [On the localization of sound stimuli]. Report on the 4th Congress of Experimental Psychology, vol. 2, Leipzig, pp. 169–258.

Klemm, O. (1918): Untersuchungen über die Lokalisation von Schallreizen III: Über den Anteil des beidohrigen Hörens [Investigations of the localization of sound stimuli III: On what is contributed by two-eared hearing]. Arch. ges. Psychol. **38**, 71–114.

Klemm, O. (1920): Untersuchungen über die Lokalisation von Schallreizen IV: Über den Einfluss des binauralen Zeitunterschiedes auf die Lokalisation [Investigations of the localization of sound stimuli IV: On the influence of binaural time difference on localization]. Arch. ges. Psychol. **40**, 117–145.

Klensch, H. (1948): Beitrag zur Frage der Lokalisation des Schalles im Raum [A contribution to the study of the localization of sound in space]. Pflügers Arch. **250**, 492–500.

Klensch, H. (1949): Die Lokalisation des Schalles im Raum [The localization of sound in space]. Naturwiss. **36**, 145–149.

Klinke R. (1972): Physiologie des Hörens I: Das mittlere und das innere Ohr [The physiology of hearing I: The middle and inner ear]. In: O. H. Gauer, K. Kramer, and R. Jung (Eds.), Lehrbuch der Physiologie des Menschen, vol. 12, Urban & Schwarzenberg, München.

Klumpp, R. G. (1953): Discriminability of interaural time difference. J. Acoust. Soc. Amer. **25**, 823.

Klumpp, R. G., and H. R. Eady (1956): Some measurements of interaural time difference thresholds. J. Acoust. Soc. Amer. **28**, 859–860.

Knowles, H. S. (1954): Artificial acoustical environment control. Acustica **4**, 80–82.

Koch, R. (1990): Störgeräuschunterdrückung für Hörhilfen – ein adaptiver "Cocktail-Party-Prozessor" [Noise suppression for hearing aids – an adaptive cocktail-party processor]. In: Fortschr. Akust. DAGA '90, DPG-GmbH, Bad Honnef, pp. 1019–1021.

Koch, R. (1992): Gehörgerechte Schallanalyse zur Vorhersage und Verbesserung der Sprachverständlichkeit [Hearing-adequate sound analysis for the prediction and enhancement of speech intelligibility]. Dissertation, Gîttingen.

Kock, W. E. (1950): Binaural localization and masking. J. Acoust. Soc. Amcr. 22, 801–804.

Koenig, A. H., J. B. Allen, D. A. Berkley, and T. H. Curtis (1977): Determination of masking-level differences in a reverberant environment. J. Acoust. Soc. Amer. 61, 1374–1376.

Koenig, W. (1950): Subjective effects in binaural hearing. J. Acoust. Soc. Amer. 22, 61–62.

Kollmeier, B., V. Hohmann, and J. Peissig (1992): Digital processing for binaural hearing. In: Proc. 14th Int. Congr. Acoust. ICA, Beijing, H 3–4.

Kollmeier, B., and R. Koch (1994): Speech enhancement based on physiological and psychological models of modulation perception and binaural interaction. J. Acoust. Soc. Am. 95, 1593–1602.

König, G., and W. Sussmann (1955): Zum Richtungshören in der Mediansagittalebene [On directional hearing in the median-sagittal plane]. Arch. Ohren-Nasen-Kehlkopfheilk. 167, 303–307.

Kraus, M. (1953): Probleme der Ohrphysiologie und neue Lösungsversuche [Problems of the physiology of the ear, and new attempts to solve them]. Springer-Verlag, Vienna.

Kreidl, A., and S. Gatscher (1923): Über die Lokalisation von Schallquellen [On the localization of sound sources]. Naturwiss. 11, 337–338.

Kreyszig, E. (1967): Statistische Methoden und ihre Anwendungen [Statistical techniques and their applications]. Vandenhoek und Ruprecht, Göttingen.

Kronberg, H. (1975): Eigenschaften der dichotischen Pulsationsschwelle [Properties of the threshold of perceptibility for dichotic (binaural) beats]. In: Fortschritte der Akustik, DAGA '75, Physik-Verlag, Weinheim, pp. 343–346.

Kronberg, H. (1976): Ermittlung dichotischer Pulsationsschwellen als psychoakustische Messmethode neuronaler Wechselwirkungen [Applying dichotic (binaural) beat thresholds as a psychoacoustical measuring method relative to neuronal mutual effects]. In: Fortschritte der Akustik, DAGA '76, VDI-Verlag, Düsseldorf, pp. 573–576.

Krückel, A. (1972): Bestimmung von akustischen Rohrabschlussmpedanzen mit Hilfe einer Doppelrohrmethode [Determining the acoustical impedance of the terminations of tubes by means of a double-tube technique]. Dissertation, Technische Hochschule, Aachen.

Krumbacher, G. (1969): Über die Leistungsfähigkeit kopfbezüglicher Stereophonie [On the capabilities of head-related stereophony]. Acustica 21, 288–293.

Kuhl, W. (1939): Über die Abhängigkeit der Lautstärke des subjektiven Differenztones von der Frequenz der Primärtöne [On the dependence of the loudness of the subjective difference tone on the frequency of the primary tone]. Akust. Z. 4, 43–50.

Kuhl, W., and J. M. Zosel (1956): Untersuchungen zur Stereophonie [Investigations of stereophony]. Acustica 6, 474–481.

Kuhl, W. (1969): Unterschiedliche Bedingungen beim Hören in einem Raum und bei elektroakustischen Übertragungen [Differences between hearing in a room and electroacoustic transmissions]. Rundfunktech. Mitt. 13, 205–208.

Kuhl, W., and R. Plantz (1972): Die Lokalisierung einer vorderen und einer hinteren Schallquelle bei frei beweglichem Kopf [The localization of a front and a rear sound source with the head free to move]. Acustica 27, 108–112.

Kuhl, W., and R. Plantz (1975): Kopfbezogene Stereophonie und andere Arten der Schallübertragung im Vergleich mit dem natürlichen Hören [Head-related stereophony and other types of sound transmission in comparison with natural hearing]. Rundfunktech. Mitt. 19, 120–132.

Kuhl, W., and R. Plantz (1976): Die Kombination eines Verzögerungsgerätes mit einem Nachhallgerät zur Erzeugung eines Raumeindruckes bei mehrkanaligen Schallübertragungen [The combination of a delay unit with a reverberation unit in generating a spatial impression in multiple-channel sound transmissions]. Rundfunktech. Mitt. 20, 39–43.

Kuhl, W. (1977): In der Raumakustik benutzte, hörakustische Termini [Acoustical terms related to hearing and used in architectural acoustics]. Acustica 39, 57–58.

Kuhl, W. (1978): Räumlichkeit als eine Komponente des Höreindruckes [Spatiousness as a component of the auditory impression]. Acustica 40, 167–181.

Kuhn, G. F. (1977): Model for the interaural time difference in the azimuthal plane. J. Acoust. Soc. Amer. 62, 157–167.

Kunov, H., and S. M. Abel (1981): Effect of rise/decay time on the lateralization of interaurally delayed 1-kHz tones. J. Acoust. Soc. Amer. 69, 769–773.

Küpfmüller, K. (1968): Die Systemtheorie der elektrischen Nachrichtentechnik [The systems theory of electrical communications technology], 3d ed. S. Hirzel Verlag, Stuttgart.

Kürer, R., G. Plenge, and H. Wilkens (1969): Correct spatial sound perception rendered by a special 2-channel recording method. Proceedings, 37th Convention of the Audio Eng. Soc., New York, vol. 3.

Kuttruff, H. (1963): Raumakustische Korrelationsmessungen mit einfachen Mitteln [Measurements of correlation in room acoustics using simple means]. Acustica 13, 120–122.

Lange, F. H. (1962): Korrelationselektronik [Correlation electronics]. VEB Verlag Technik, Berlin.

Langenbeck, B. (1958): Die Lateralisation des Knochenleitungshörens beim Weber'schen Versuch [The lateralization of bone conduction hearing in Weber's experiment]. Arch. Ohren-Nasen-Kehlkopfheilk. 172, 451–456.

Langford, T. L., and L. A. Jeffress (1964): Effect of noise crosscorrelation on binaural signal detection. J. Acoust. Soc. Amer. 36, 1455–1458.

Lauridsen, H. (1954): Nogle Forsog med Forskellige Former Rumakustik Gengivelske. Ingenioren 47, 906 (cited in Schroeder 1961).

Lauridsen, H., and F. Schlegel (1956): Stereofonie und richtungsdiffuse Klangwiedergabe [Stereophony and directionally diffuse reproduction of sound]. Gravesaner Blätter 5, 28–50.

Laws, P. (1971): Entfernung des Hörereignisses bei Simulation des Nahfeldes eines Kugelstrahlers nullter Ordnung [The distance of the auditory event in connection with the simulation of the near field of a spherical radiator of the zeroth order]. In: Gemeinschaftstagung für Akustik und Schwingungstechnik, Berlin 1970, VDI-Verlag, Düsseldorf, pp. 397–401.

*Laws, P. (1972): Zum Problem des Entfernungshörens und der Im-Kopf-Lokalisiertheit von Hörereignissen [On the problem of distance hearing and the localization of auditory events inside the head]. Dissertation, Technische Hochschule, Aachen; also personal correspondence.

Laws, P., and H.-J. Platte (1975): Spezielle Experimente zur kopfbezogenen Stereo-phonie [Some experiments in head-related stereophony]. In: Fortschritte der Akustik. DAGA '75, Physik-Verlag, Weinheim, pp. 365–368.

Laws, P., J. Blauert, and H.-J. Platte (1976/77): Anmerkungen zur stereophonen, kopf-bezogenen Übertragungstechnik [Observations on the technique of stereophonic, head-related reproduction]. Acustica 36, 45–47.

Laws, P. (1978): Messung und Nachbildung von Trommelfellimpedanzen [Measure-ment and simulation of eardrum impedances]. Rundfunktech. Mitt. 22, 201–205.

Laws, P., and H.-J. Platte (1978): Ein spezielles Konzept zur Realisierung eines Kunst-kopfes für die kopfbezogene stereophone Aufnahmetechnik [A specific concept related to the construction of a dummy head for head-related stereophonic sound pickup]. Rundfunktech. Mitt. 22, 28–31.

Lazarus-Mainka, G., and H. Lazarus (1976): Monaurale und binaurale Wahrnehmung maskierter Sprache. Ein Beitrag zum Problem der BILD [Monaural and binaural perception of masked speech. A contribution on the problem of the BILD]. In: Fort-schritte der Akustik, DAGA '76, VDI-Verlag, Düsseldorf, pp. 585–588.

Leakey, D. M. (1957): Further effects produced by two loudspeakers in echo-free conditions. J. Acoust. Soc. Amer. 29, 966.

Leakey, D. M., and E. C. Cherry (1957): Influence of noise upon the equivalence of intensity differences and small time delays in two-loudspeakers systems. J. Acoust. Soc. Amer. 29, 284–286.

Leakey, D. M., B. M. Sayers, and C. Cherry (1958): Binaural fusion of low- and high-frequency sounds. J. Acoust. Soc. Amer. 30, 322.

Leakey, D. M. (1959): Some measurement of the effects of interchannel intensity and time differences in two channel sound systems. J. Acoust. Soc. Amer. 31, 977–986.

Lee, Y. L. (1960): Statistical theory of communication. John Wiley, New York.

Lehmann, P. (1976): Über die Ermittlung raumakustischer Kriterien und deren Zu-sammenhang mit subjektiven Beurteilungen der Hörsamkeit [On the development of spatial acoustic criteria and their connection with subjective judgments of listenability]. Dissertation, Technische Universität, Berlin.

Lehmann, P., and H. Wilkens (1980): Zusammenhang subjektiver Beurteilungen von Konzertsälen mit raumakustischen Kriterien [The relationship of subjective judgments of concert halls to spatial acoustic criteria]. Acustica 45, 256–268.

Lehnert, H., and J. Blauert (1989): A concept for binaural room simulation. In: Proc. IEEE ASSP Worksh. Application of Signal Processing to Audio and Acoustics, New Paltz NY.

Lehnert, H. (1990): Erzeugung von virtuellen akustischen Umgebungen [Generation of virtual auditory environments]. In: Fortschr. Akust. DAGA '90, DFG-GmbH, Bad Honnef, pp. 895–898.

Lehnert, H., and J. Blauert (1991a): Berechnung von langen Impulsantworten durch ein schnelles Strahlverfolgungsverfahren [Calculation of long impulse responses with a fast ray tracing algorithm]. In: Fortschr. Akust. DAGA '91, DPG-GmbH, Bad Honnef, pp. 637–640.

Lehnert, H., and J. Blauert (1991b): Virtual auditory environment. In: Proc. 5th Int. Conf. Advanced Robotics IEEE/ICAR, Pisa, pp. 211–216.

Lehnert, H. (1992a): Binaurale Raumsimulation: Ein Computermodell zur Erzeugung virtueller auditiver Umgebungen. [Binaural room simulation: A computer model for the creation of virtual auditory environment]. Verlag Shaker, Aachen.

Lehnert, H. (1992b): Systematic errors of the ray-tracing algorithm. J. Appl. Acoust. **38**, 207–221.

Lehnert, H., and J. Blauert. (1992): Principles of binaural room simulation. J. Appl. Acoust. **36**, 259–291.

Lehnert, H. (1993a): Auditory spatial impression. In: Proc. 12th Int. AES Conf., Audio Engr. Soc., New York, pp. 40–46.

Lehnert, H. (1993b): Real-time generation of interactive virtual auditory environments. In: IEEE Worksh. Appl. Signal Processing, Audio, and Acoustics, New Paltz NY, paper 5.4.

Lehnert, H. (1993c): Virtuelle auditive Umgebung mittels binauraler Raumsimulation [Virtual auditory environments using binaural room simulation]. In: H. J. Warnecke and H.-J. Bullinger (Eds.), Virtual Reality '93: Anwendungen und Trends, Springer, New York, pp. 143–151.

Lehnert, H. (1994a): Analyse zur Realisierbarkeit von interaktiven virtuellen auditive Umgebungen in nicht-trivialen Geometrien [Analysis of the realizability of interactive virtual auditory environments in nontrivial geometries]. In: Fortschr. Akust. DAGA '94, DPG-GmbH, Bad Honnef, pp. 233–236.

Lehnert, H. (1994b): Fundamentals of auditory virtual environment. In: N. Magnenat, and D. Thalmann (Eds.), Virtual reality and artificial life, John Wiley and Sons, Chichester, pp. 161–172.

Lehnert, H. (1995): Vereinfachung von binauralen Impulsantworten zur Auralisierung von Rückwürfen [Simplification of binaural impulse responses to be used for the auralization of reflected sounds]. In: Fortschr. Akust. DAGA '95, Deutsch. Ges. Akust., Oldenburg, pp. 303–306.

Lehnert, H., and F. Giron (1995): Vocal communication in virtual environments. Virtual Reality World '95, Mecklermedia, London, pp. 279–273.

Lehnert, H., and M. Richter (1995): Auditory virtual environment: Simplified binaural treatment of reflections. In: Proc. Int. Congr. Acoust. ICA '95, TAPIR, Trondheim, pp. 265–268.

Lehnhardt, E. (1960): Über das Richtungshören des Menschen. Elektroakustische Versuche mit kleinsten Zeitdifferenzen [On human directional hearing. Electroacoustical experiments with very small time differences]. HNO **8**, 353–357.

Lehnhardt, E. (1961): Die akustische Korrelation [Acoustical correlation]. Arch. Ohren-Nasen-Kehlkopfheilk. **178**, 493–497.

Lerche, E., and P. Plath (1961): Zur Lokalisation von Schallquellen bei Kopfhörerempfang [On the localization of sound sources with headphones]. Pflügers Arch. **274**, 91.

Levitt, H., and L. R. Rabiner (1967a): Binaural release from masking for speech and gain in intelligibility. J. Acoust. Soc. Amer. **42**, 601–608.

Levitt, H., and L. R. Rabiner (1967b): Predicting binaural gain in intelligibility and release from masking for speech. J. Acoust. Soc. Amer. **42**, 820–829.

Licklider, J. C. R. (1948): The influence of interaural phase relations upon the masking of speech by white noise. J. Acoust. Soc. Amer. **20**, 150–159.

Licklider, J. C. R., and J. C. Webster (1950): The discriminability of interaural phase relations in two-component tones. J. Acoust. Soc. Amer. **22**, 191–195.

Licklider, J. C. R. (1951): A duplex theory of pitch perception. Experientia **7**, 128–134.

Licklider, J. C. R. (1956): Audio frequency analysis. In: C. Cherry (Ed.), Information theory, 3d London symp., Butterworth, London, pp. 253–268.

Licklider, J. C. R. (1959): Three auditory theories. In: S. Koch (Ed.), Psychology: A study of a science, vol. 1, McGraw-Hill, New York, pp. 41–144.

Licklider, J. C. R. (1962): Periodicity pitch and related auditory process models. Int. Audiol. 1, 11–36.

Lim, J. S. (1983): Speech enhancement, Prentice Hall, New Jersey.

Lindemann, W. (1982): Evaluation of interaural signal differences. In: O. S. Pedersen and T. Paulsen (Eds.), Binaural effects in normal and impaired hearing, Scandinavian Audiol. Suppl. 15.

Lindemann, W., and J. Blauert (1982): Die Anwendung eines Modells binauraler Signalverarbeitung auf Schallfelder in Räumen [Application of a model of binaural signal processing to the sound field in rooms]. In: Fortschr. Akust. FASE/DAGA '82, Göttingen, pp. 1182–1185.

Lindemann, W. (1985): Die Erweiterung eines Kreuzkorrelationsmodells der binauralen Signalverarbeitung durch kontralaterale Inhibitionsmechanismen [Extension of a cross-correlation model of binaural signal processing by means of contralateral inhibition mechanisms]. Dissertation, Bochum.

Lindemann, W., J. Blauert, K. Gruber, and U. Breuer (1985): Die räumliche Verteilung der Hörereignisse als Funktion des interauralen Korrelationsgrades [Spatial distribution of auditory events as a function of the interaural degree of correlation]. In: Fortschr. Akust. DAGA '85, DPG-GmbH, Bad Honnef, pp. 499–502.

Lindemann, W. (1986a): Extension of a binaural cross-correlation model by means of contralateral inhibition, I: Simulation of lateralization of stationary signals. J. Acoust. Soc. Am. 80, 1608–1622.

Lindemann, W. (1986b): Extension of a binaural cross-correlation model by means of contralateral iinhibition, II: The law of the first wave front. J. Acoust. Soc. Am. 80, 1623–1630.

Lochner, J. P. A., and J. F. Burger (1958): The subjective masking of short time delayed echoes, their primary sounds, and their contribution to the intelligibility of speech. Acustica 8, 1–10.

Lochner, J. P. A., and W. deV. Keet (1960): Stereophonic and quasistereophonic reproduction. J. Acoust. Soc. Amer. 32, 393–401.

Lungwitz, H. (1923): Die Entdeckung der Seele-Allg. Psychobiol. [The discovery of the soul — General psychobiology]. Brücke Verlag Kurt Schmersow, Kirchhain N. L.

Lungwitz, H. (1933a): Lehrbuch der Psychobiologie [Textbook of psychobiology], vol. 1. Walter de Gruyter, Berlin.

Lungwitz, H. (1933b): Lokalisation der akustischen Gegenstände [The localization of acoustical objects]. In: Lehrbuch der Psychobiologie, vol. 2, Walter de Gruyter, Berlin.

Mach, R. (1865): Bemerkungen über den Raumsinn des Ohres [Remarks on the spatial sense of the ear]. Poggendorfs Ann. 128, 5th series, vol. 6, 331–333.

Makita, Y. (1962): On the directional localization of sound in the stereophonic sound field. Europ. Broadcasting Union Rev. Part A, 73, 102–108.

Mallock, A. (1908): Note on the sensitivity of the ear to the direction of explosive sounds. Proc. Roy. Soc. Med. 80, 110ff.

Marshall, A. H. (1967): A note on the importance of room cross-section in concert halls. J. Sound and Vibration 5, 100–112.

Marshall, A. H. (1979): Aspects of acoustical design and properties of Christchurch town hall, New Zealand. J. Sound and Vibration 62, 181–194.

Marshall, A. H., and J. R. Hyde (1979): Some preliminary acoustical considerations in the design for the proposed Wellington (New Zealand) town hall. J. Sound and Vibration 63, 201–211.

Matsudaira, T. K., and T. Fukami (1973): Phase difference and sound image localization. J. Audio Eng. Soc. 21, 792–797.

Matsumoto, M. (1897): Research on acoustic space. Yale Psychol. Lab. Studies 5, 1–75.

Matzker, J. (1958): Versuch einer Erklärung des Richtungshörens auf Grund feinster Zeitunterschiedsregistrierungen [An attempt to explain directional hearing on the basis of very fine time difference discrimination]. Acta Oto-laryngol. 49, 483–494.

Matzker, J. (1964): Das Leitsymptom aller zentralen Hörstörungen: Die Beeinträchtigung der exakten akustischen Rechts-Links-Balance [The characteristic symptom of all central hearing disturbances: The disturbance of exact acoustical right–left balance]. Arch. Ohr.-Nas.-Kehlk.-Heilk. 183, 261–270.

*Matzker, J. (1965): Die zerebralen Hörstörungen und ihre Diagnostik [Cerebral hearing disturbances and relevant diagnostic techniques]. Stud. Gen. 18, 682–700.

Maxfield, J. P. (1933): Some physical factors affecting the illusion in sound motion pictures. J. Acoust. Soc. Amer. 4, 69–80.

McFadden, D. (1968): Masking level differences determined with and without interaural disparities. J. Acoust. Soc. Amer. 44, 212–213.

McFadden, D. (1969): Lateralization and detection of a tonal signal in noise. J. Acoust. Soc. Amer. 45, 1505–1509.

McFadden, D., L. A. Jeffress, and H. L. Ermey (1971): Differences of interaural phase and level in detection and lateralization: 250 Hz. J. Acoust. Soc. Amer. 50, 1484–1493.

McFadden, D., and E. G. Pasanen (1976): Lateralization at high frequencies based on interaural time differences. J. Acoust. Soc. Amer. 59, 634–639.

McFadden, D., and C. M. Moffitt (1977): Acoustic integration for lateralization at high frequencies. J. Acoust. Soc. Amer. 61, 1604–1608.

McFadden, D., and E. G. Pasanen (1978): Binaural detection at high frequencies with time-delayed waveforms. J. Acoust. Soc. Amer. 63, 1120–1131.

McGamble, E. A. (1909): Intensity as a criterion in estimating the distance of sounds. Psychol. Rev. 16, 416–426.

McKinley, R. L., M. A. Erickson, and W. R. D'Angelo (1994): 3-dimensional auditory displays: Development, applications and performance. Aviation, Space, Environm. Med., A31–A38

Mehrgardt, S., and V. Mellert (1973): Zur Ermittlung der Übertragungscharakteristik des Gehörs — Vergleich von Hörschwellen- und Sondenmikrophonmessung [On the representation of the transfer characteristic of the human auditory apparatus — Comparisons of auditory thresholds and probe microphone measurements]. In: Fortschritte der Akustik, DAGA '73, VDI-Verlag, Düsseldorf, pp. 459–462.

Mehrgardt, S. (1976): Messungen der interauralen Übertragungsfunktion und der Trommelfellimpedanz mit dem Impulsmessverfahren [Measurement of the interaural transfer function and the eardrum impedance using an impulse procedure]. In: Fortschritte der Akustik, DAGA '76, VDI-Verlag, Düsseldorf, pp. 613–616.

Mehrgardt, S., and V. Mellert (1977): Transformation characteristics of the external human ear. J. Acoust. Soc. Amer. **61**, 1567–1576.

Mellert, V. (1971): Richtungshören in der Medianebene und Schallbeugung am Kopf [Directional hearing in the median plane and diffraction of sound around the head]. Dissertation, Universität Göttingen.

Mellert, V. (1972): Construction of a dummy head after new measurements of the threshold of hearing. J. Acoust. Soc. Amer. **51**, 1359–1361.

Mellert, V., K. F. Siebrasse, and S. Mehrgardt (1974): Determination of the transfer function of the external ear by an impulse response measurement. J. Acoust. Soc. Amer. **56**, 1913–1915.

Mellert, V. (1975): Verbesserte Schallfeldabbildung mit einem neuen Kunstkopf [Improved representation of the sound field with a new dummy head]. In: Fortschritte der Akustik, DAGA '75, Physik-Verlag, Weinheim, pp. 433–436.

Mellert, V. (1976): Die Normung kopfbezogener Stereo-Aufnahmen und ihre Wiedergabe über Lautsprecher [The normalization of head-related stereo signals and their reproduction over loudspeakers]. Fernseh-Kinotech. **30**, 86–88.

Mellert, V. (1978): Die Mikrophonanordnung beim Kunstkopfbau [Incorporating microphones into the dummy head]. Rundfunktech. Mitt. **22**, 196–198.

Mertens, H. (1960): An energy theory of directional hearing and its application in stereophony. Europ. Broadcasting Union Rev. Part A, **59**, 22–33.

Mertens, H. (1965): Directional hearing in stereophony: Theory and experimental verification. Europ. Broadcasting Union Rev. Part A, **92**, 1–14.

Metz, O. (1946): The acoustic impedance measured in normal and pathological ears. Acta Oto-laryngol. Suppl. **63**.

Metz, O. (1951): Studies on the contraction of the tympanic muscles as indicated by changes in the impedance of the ear. Acta Oto-laryngol. **27**, 399–405.

Meurmann, Y., and O. H. Meurmann (1954): Do the semicircular canals play a part in directional hearing? Acta Oto-laryngol. **44**, 542–555.

Meyer, E. (1925): Über das stereoakustische Hören [On 3-dimensional hearing]. Elektrotech. Z. **46**, 805–807.

Meyer, E., and G. R. Schodder (1952): Über den Einfluss von Schallrückwürfen auf Richtungslokalisation und Lautstärke bei Sprache [On the influence of reflected sound on directional localization and loudness of speech]. Nachr. Akad. Wiss. Göttingen, Math. Phys. Klasse IIa, **6**, 31–42.

Meyer, E., and R. Thiele (1956): Raumakustische Untersuchungen in zahlreichen Konzertsälen und Rundfunkstudios unter Anwendung neuerer Messverfahren [Investigations of the room acoustics of numerous concert halls and broadcast studios, using new measurement procedures]. Acustica **6**, 425–444.

Meyer, E., and H. Kuttruff (1964): Zur Raumakustik einer grossen Festhalle [On the room acoustics of a large concert hall] Acustica **14**, 138–147.

Meyer, E., W. Burgtorf, and P. Damaske (1965): Eine Apparatur zur elektroakustischen Nachbildung von Schallfeldern. Subjektive Hörwirkungen beim Übergang Kohärenz–Inkohärenz [An apparatus for the electroacoustical simulation of sound fields. Subjective auditory effects at the transition between coherence and incoherence]. Acustica **15**, 339–344.

Meyer, E., and E. G. Neumann (1967): Physikalische und technische Akustik [Physical and Technical Acoustics]. F. Vieweg & Sohn, Braunschweig.

Meyer, J. (1980): Akustik und musikalische Aufführungspraxis [Acoustics and the practice of musical performance]. Verlag Das Musikinstrument, Frankfurt.

Meyer, K., H. L. Applewhite, and F. A. Biocca (1992): A survey of position trackers, Presence 1, 173–200.

Meyer zum Gottesberge, A. (1940): Physiologisch-anatomische Elemente der Schall-richtungsbestimmung [Physiological and anatomical elements of the determination of the direction of sound]. Arch. Ohren-Nasen-Kehlkopfheilk. 147, 219–249.

Meyer zum Gottesberge, A. (1968): Eine funktionelle Studie über die Pneumatisation des Schläfenbeins [A functional study of the air-filled porosity of the temporal bone]. Acta Oto-laryngol. 65, 216–223.

Middlebrooks, J. C. and D. M. Green (1990): Directional dependence of interaural envelope delays. J. Acoust Soc. Amer. 87, 2149–2162

Mills, A. W. (1958): On the minimum audible angle. J. Acoust. Soc. Amer. 30, 237–246.

Mills, A. W. (1960): Lateralization of high-frequency tones. J. Acoust. Soc. Amer. 32, 132–134.

*Mills, A. W. (1972): Auditory localization. In: J. Tobias (Ed.), Foundations of modern auditory theory, vol. 2, Academic Press, New York, pp. 301–345.

Mitchell, M., C. Ross, and G. Yates (1971): Signal processing for a cocktail-party effect. J. Acoust. Soc. Am. 50, 656–660.

Mizuno, I. (1960): Experimentelle Studien zur Schallokalisation [Experimental studies of sound localization]. Oto-Rhino-Laryngol. Clin. (Kyoto), cited in. Zbl. Hals-Nasen-Ohrenheilk. 69, 234.

Mohrmann, K. (1939): Lautheitskonstanz im Entfernungswechsel [Constancy of loudness with changes in distance]. Z. Psychol. 145, 145–199.

Molino, J. A. (1974): Psychophysical verification of predicted interaural differences in localizing distant sound sources. J. Acoust. Soc. Amer. 55, 139–147.

Møller, A. R. (1959): An apparatus for measuring the acoustic impedance of the ear. Proceedings, 3d Int. Congr. on Acoustics, Stuttgart, vol. 1, pp. 29–33.

Møller, A. R. (1960): Improved technique for detailed measurements of the middle ear impedance. J. Acoust. Soc. Amer. 32, 250.

Møller, A. R. (1962): Acoustic reflex in man. J. Acoust. Soc. Amer. 34, 1524–1534.

Møller, H. (1992): Binaural technology — fundamentals. J. Appl. Acoust. 36, 171–218.

*Moore, B. C. J. (1977): Introduction to the psychology of hearing. Macmillan, London.

Möricke, K. B., and W. Mergenthaler (1959): Biologie des Menschen [Human biology]. Quelle und Meyer, Heidelberg.

Morimoto, M., Y. Ando, and Z. Maekawa (1975): A note on head-related transfer functions. Oral presentation, meeting of the Acoustical Society of Japan.

Morimoto, M., and Y. Ando (1977): Localization in the median plane of sound sources simulated by a digital computer. Proceedings, 8th Int. Congr. on Acoustics, Madrid, vol. 1, p. 371.

Morimoto, M., and Y. Ando (1982): Simulation of sound localization. In: R. W. Gatehouse (Ed.), Localization of sound: Theory and application, The Amphora Press, Groton, CT, pp. 85–89.

Morse, P. M. (1948): Vibration and sound. McGraw-Hill, New York.

Morton, J. Y., and R. A. Jones (1956): The acoustical impedance presented by some human ears to hearing aid earphones of the insert type. Acustica **6**, 339–345.

Moushegian, G., and L. A. Jeffress (1959): Role of interaural time and intensity differences in the lateralization of low-frequency tones. J. Acoust. Soc. Amer. **31**, 1441–1445.

Muir, D. (1982): The development of human auditory localization in infancy. In: R. W. Gatehouse (Ed.), Localization of sound: Theory and Application, Amphora Press, Groton CT, pp. 220–243.

Müller, S. (1970): Die Wirkung des akustischen Reflexes bei Impulsbelastung [The effect of the acoustical reflex in connection with impulse loading]. Acustica **23**, 223–229.

Muncey, R. W., A. F. B. Nickson, and P. Dubout (1953): The acceptability of speech and music with a single artificial echo. Acustica **3**, 168–173.

Münsterberg, H. (1889): Raumsinn des Ohres [The spatial sense of hearing]. Cited in Beitr. exp. Psychol. **2**, 182.

Münsterberg, H., and A. H. Pierce (1894): The localization of sound. Psychol. Rev. **1**, 461–476.

Myers, C. S. (1914): The influence of timbre and loudness on the localization of sounds. Proc. Roy. Soc. London **B88**, 267–284.

Nasse, H., U. Sieben, and R. E. Gerlach (1980): Die Maskierungswirkung eines kontralateralen Maskierers bei diotischen Rauschen [The masking effect of a contralateral masker with diotic noise]. In: Fortschritte der Akustik, DAGA '80, VDE-Verlag, Berlin, pp. 599–601.

Niese, H. (1956/57): Untersuchungen für die Richtcharakteristik des Aufnahmemikrophons bei raumakustischen Impulsmessungen [Investigations to determine an appropriate directional characteristic for a microphone used in spatial acoustic impulse measurements]. Hochfrequenztech. u. Elektroakustik **65**, 192–200.

*Nordlund, B. (1962): Physical factors in angular localization. Acta Oto-laryngol. **54**, 75–93.

Nordlund, B., and G. Liden (1963): An artificial head. Acta Oto-laryngol. **56**, 493–499.

Nordmark, J. O. (1968): Some analogies between pitch and lateralization phenomena. J. Acoust. Soc. Amer. **35**, 1544–1547.

Nordmark, J. O. (1970): Time and frequency analysis. In: J. V. Tobias (Ed.), Foundations of modern auditory theory, vol. 1, Academic Press, New York, pp. 55–84.

Nordmark, J. O. (1976): Binaural time discrimination. J. Acoust. Soc. Amer. **60**, 870–880.

Norman, D. A., R. Phelps, and F. Whightman (1972): Some observations on underwater hearing. J. Acoust. Soc. Amer. **50**, 544–548.

Nuetzel, J. M., and E. R. Hafter (1976): Lateralization of complex waveforms: Effects of fine structure, amplitude and duration. J. Acoust. Soc. Amer. **60**, 1339–1346.

Nuetzel, J. M., and E. R. Hafter (1981): Discrimination of interaural delays in complex waveforms: Spectral effects. J. Acoust. Soc. Amer. **69**, 1112–1118.

Nyquist, H., and S. Brand (1930): Measurement of phase distortion. Bell Syst. Tech. J. **7**, 522–549.

Olson, H. F. (1959): Stereophonic sound reproduction. Proceedings, 3d Int. Congr. on Acoustics, Stuttgart, vol. 1, pp. 791–795.

Onchi, Y. (1949): A study of the mechanism of the middle ear. J. Acoust. Soc. Amer. 21, 404–410.

Onchi, Y. (1961): Mechanism of the middle ear. J. Acoust. Soc. Amer. 33, 794–805.

Ortmeyer W. (1966a): Über die Lokalisierung von Schallquellen bei Zweikanalstereophonie [On the localization of sound sources in connection with two-channel stereophony]. Hochfrequenztech. u. Elektroakustik 75, 77–87.

Ortmeyer, W. (1966b): Schallfelduntersuchungen bei Zweikanalstereophonie [Investigations of sound fields in two-channel stereophony]. Hochfrequenztech. u. Elektroakustik 75, 137–145.

Osman, E. (1971): A correlation model of binaural masking level differences. J. Acoust. Soc. Amer. 50, 1494–1511.

Parker, D. E., H. E. von Gierke, and M. F. Reschke (1968): Studies of acoustical stimulation of the vestibular system. Aerospace Med. 39, 1321–1325.

Parker, D. E., and H. E. von Gierke (1970): Vestibular nerve response to pressure changes in the external auditory meatus of the guinea pig. Acta Oto-laryngol. 71, 456–461.

Patterson, J. H., and D. M. Green (1970): Discrimination of transient signals having identical energy spectra. J. Acoust. Soc. Amer. 48, 894–905.

Patterson, J. H. (1971): Masking of tones by transient signals having identical energy spectra. J. Acoust. Soc. Amer. 50, 1126–1130.

Paulsen, J., and H. W. Ewertsen (1966): Audio-visual-reflex. Acta Oto-laryngol. Suppl. 224, 217–221.

Peissig, J., and B. Kollmeier (1990): Echtzeitsimulation digitaler Hörgerätealgorithmen [Real-time simulation of digital algorithms for hearing aids]. In: Fortschr. Akust. DAGA '90, DPG-GmbH, Bad Honnef, pp. 1007–1010.

Peissig, J. (1993): Binaurale Hörstrategien in komplexen Störschallsituationen [Binaural hearing strategies in complex noise situations], vol. 88, series 17: Biotechnik, VDI-Verlag, Düsseldorf.

Perekalin, W. E. (1930): Über akustische Orientierung [On acoustical orientation]. Z. Hals-Nasen-Ohren-Heilk. 25, 443–461.

Perrott, D. R., and L. F. Elfner (1968): Monaural localization. J. Auditory Res. 8, 185–193.

Perrott, D. R. (1969): Role of signal onset in sound localization. J. Acoust. Soc. Amer. 45, 436–445.

Perrott, D. R., and M. A. Nelson (1969/70): Limits for the detection of binaural beats. J. Acoust. Soc. Amer. 46, 1477–1481; 47, 663–664.

Perrott, D. R., R. Briggs, and S. Perrott (1970): Binaural fusion: Its limits as defined by signal duration and signal onset. J. Acoust. Soc. Amer. 47, 565–568.

Perrott, D. R., and B. J. Baars (1974): Detection of interaural onset and offset disparities. J. Acoust. Soc. Amer. 55, 1290–1292.

Perrott, D. R., and A. D. Musicant (1977a): Rotating tones and binaural beats. J. Acoust. Soc. Amer. 61, 1288–1292.

Perrott, D. R., and A. D. Musicant (1977b): Minimum auditory movement angle: Binaural localization of moving sources. J. Acoust. Soc. Amer. 62, 1463–1466.

Perrott, D. R. (1979): Studies in the perception of auditory motion. In: R. W. Gatehouse (Ed.), Localization of Sound: theory and application, The Amphora Press, Groton, CT, pp. 169–193.

Perrott, D. R. (1984): Binaural resolution of the size of an acoustic array: Some experiments with stereophonic arrays. J. Acoust. Soc. Am. **76**, 1704–1712.

Perrott, D. R., T. Z. Strybel, and C. L. Manligas (1987): Conditions under which the Haas precedence effect may or may not occur. J. Audit. Res. **27**, 59–72.

Perrott, D. R., K. Marlborough, and P. Merrill (1988): Minimum-audible-angle thresholds obtained under conditions in which the precedence effect is assumed to operate. J. Acoust. Soc. Am. **85**, 282–288.

Peterson, J. (1916): The nature and probable origin of binaural beats. Psychol. Rev. **23**, 333–351.

Petri, J. (1932): Über Aufbau und Leistung der Ohrmuschel [On the structure and function of the pinna]. Z. Hals-Nasen-Ohren-Heilk. **30**, 605–608.

Petzold, F. (1927): Elementare Raumakustik [Elementary room acoustics]. Bauwelt-Verlag, Berlin.

Pickett, J. M. (1959): Backward masking. J. Acoust. Soc. Amer. **31**, 1613–1615.

Pickles, J. O. (1982): An introduction to the physiology of hearing. Academic Press, London.

*Pierce, A. H. (1901): Studies in auditory and visual space perception, vol. 1: The localization of sound. Longmans, Green, New York.

Pinheiro, M. L., and H. Tobin (1969): Interaural intensity difference for intercranial lateralization. J. Acoust. Soc. Amer. **46**, 1482–1487.

Plath, P. (1969): Das Hörorgan und seine Funktion: Einführung in die Audiometrie [The organ of hearing and its functioning: An introduction to audiometry]. C. Marhold Verlag, Berlin.

Plath, P., J. Blauert, and G. Klepper (1970): Untersuchungen über die Trägheit des Richtungshörens bei Gesunden und Patienten [Investigations of the persistence of directional hearing in health and disease]. Arch. klin. u. exp. Ohren-Nasen-Kehlkopfheilk. **196**, 212–215.

Platte, H.-J., J. Blauert, and P. Laws (1973): Anordnung zur Messung von Aussenohr-Übertragungsfunktionen nach der Impulsmethode [Apparatus for the measurement of external-ear transfer functions using the impulse method]. In: Fortschritte der Akustik, DAGA '73, VDI-Verlag, Düsseldorf, pp. 463–466.

Platte, H.-J., P. Laws, and H. vom Hövel (1975): Anordnung zur genauen Reproduktion von Ohrsignalen [Apparatus for the exact reproduction of ear input signals]. In: Fortschritte der Akustik, DAGA '75, Physik-Verlag, Weinheim, pp. 361–364.

Platte, H.-J., and P. Laws (1976a): Ein Beitrag zum Problem der Messung der menschlichen Trommelfellimpedanz [A contribution on the problem of measuring the human eardrum impedance]. In: Fortschritte der Akustik, DAGA '76, VDI-Verlag, Düsseldorf, pp. 621–624.

Platte, H.-J., and P. Laws (1976b): Die Vorne-Ortung bei der kopfbezogenen Stereophonie [Forward positioning in head-related stereophony]. Radio Mentor Electronic **42**, 97–100.

Platte, H.-J., and P. Laws (1978): Technische Probleme beim Einsatz kopfbezogener sterephoner Übertragungsverfahren [Technical problems in the application of head-related stereophonic reproduction processes]. Rundfunktech. Mitt. **22**, 22–27.

Platte, H.-J. (1979): Zur Bedeutung der Aussenohrübertragungseigenschaften für den Nachrichtenempfänger "menschliches Gehör" [On the meaning of external-ear transfer properties for the receiver of information known as the "human auditory system"]. Dissertation, Technische Hochschule, Aachen.

Platte, H.-J., and K. Genuit (1980): Ein Beitrag zum Verständnis der Summenlokalisation [A contribution to the understanding of summing localization]. In: Fortschritte der Akustik, DAGA '80, VDE-Verlag, Berlin, pp. 595–598.

Platte, H.-J., and H. vom Hövel (1980): Zur Deutung der Ergebnisse von Sprachverständlichkeitsmessungen mit Störschall im Freifeld [On the interpretation of the results of the intelligibility of speech with interfering signals in a free field]. Acustica 45, 139–150.

Plenge, G. (1971a): Über die Hörbarkeit kleiner Änderungen der Impulsantwort eines Raumes [On the audibility of small changes in the impulse response of a room]. Acustica 25, 315–325.

Plenge, G. (1971b): Ein Beitrag zur Erklärung der Im-Kopf-Lokalisation [A contribution to the explanation of inside-the-head locatedness]. In: Gemeinschaftstagung für Akustik und Schwingungstechnik, Berlin 1970, VDI-Verlag, Düsseldorf, pp. 411–416.

Plenge, G., and G. Brunschen (1971): Signalkenntnis und Richtungsbestimmung in der Medianebene bei Sprache [A priori knowledge of the signal when determining the direction of speech in the median plane]. Proceedings, 7th Int. Congr. on Acoustics, Budapest, 19 H 10.

*Plenge, G. (1972): Über das Problem der Im-Kopf-Lokalisation [On the problem of inside-the-head locatedness]. Acustica 26, 241–252.

Plenge, G., and G. Romahn (1972): Electroacoustic reproduction of "perceived reverberation" for comparison in architectural acoustic investigations. J. Acoust. Soc. Amer. 51, 421–424.

Plenge, G. (1973): Über das Problem der intracranialen Ortung von Schallquellen bei der akustischen Wahrnehmung des Menschen [On the problem of intracranial localization of sound sources in human acoustical perception]. Dissertation, Technische Universität, Berlin.

Plenge, G. (1974): On the difference between localization and lateralization. J. Acoust. Soc. Amer. 56, 944–951.

Plenge, G., P. Lehmann, R. Wettschurek, and H. Wilkens (1975): New methods in architectural investigations to evaluate the acoustic qualities of concert halls. J. Acoust. Soc. Amer. 57, 1292–1299.

Plenge, G. (1978): Probleme bei der Einführung der Kunstkopfstereophonie beim Hörrundfunk [Problems in introducing dummy-head stereophony in broadcasting]. Rundfunktech. Mitt. 22, 216–218.

Plomp, R. (1976): Binaural and monaural speech intelligibility of connected discourse in reverberation as a function of azimuth of a single competing sound source (speech or noise). Acustica 34, 200–211.

Plomp, R., and A. M. Mimpen (1981): Effect of the orientation of the speaker's head and the azimuth of a noise source or the speech-reception threshold for sentences. Acustica 48, 325–328.

Politzer, A. (1876): Studien über die Paracusis loci [Studies of the paracusis loci]. Arch. Ohren-Nasen-Kehlkopfheilk. 11, 231–236.

Pollack, I. (1948): Monaural and binaural threshold sensitivity for tones and white noise. J. Acoust. Soc. Amer. 20, 52–57.

Pollack, I., and J. M. Pickett (1958): Stereophonic listening and speech intelligibility against voice babble. J. Acoust. Soc. Amer. **30**, 131–133.

Pollack, I., and W. Trittipoe (1959): Interaural noise correlations: Examination of variables. J. Acoust. Soc. Amer. **31**, 1616–1618.

Pollack, I. (1971): Interaural correlation detection of auditory pulse trains. J. Acoust. Soc. Amer. **49**, 1213–1216.

Pollack, I. (1977): Limiting interaural switching periods. In: E. F. Evans and J. P. Wilson (Eds.), Psychophysics and physiology of hearing, Academic Press, London, pp. 165–170.

Pollack, I. (1978): Temporal switching between binaural information sources. J. Acoust. Soc. Amer. **63**, 500–558.

Pompetzki, W., and J. Blauert (1990): Binaural recording and reproduction for documentation and evaluation. In: The Sound of Audio, In: Proc. 8th Int. AES Conf., Audio Engr. Soc., New York, pp. 225–229.

Pompetzki, W. (1993): Psychoakustische Verifikation von Computermodellen zur binauralen Raumsimulation [Psychoacoustical verification of computer models for binaural room simulation]. Dissertation, Bochum.

Pompetzki. W., and J. Blauert (1994): A study on the perceptual authenticity of binaural room simulation. In: Proc. Wallace-Clement-Sabine-Centennial Symp., Acoust. Soc. Am., Woodbury NY, 81–84.

Popper, A. N. and R. R. Fay (Eds), (1992): The mammalian auditory pathway. Springer, New York.

Pösselt, Ch. (1987): Binaurale Raumsimulation für Kopfhörerwiedergabe [Binaural simulation for reproduction via headphones]. In: Fortschr. Akust. DAGA '87, DPG-GmbH, Bad Honnef, pp. 725–728.

Pösselt, Ch., Ch. Jaffe, K. Genuit, and J. Blauert (1988a): Application of physical- and computer-modeling tools in the process of planning room acoustics. In: Proc. Spring Conf. Inst. Acoust., Edinburgh.

Pösselt, Ch., M. Morimoto, and Y. Yamasaki (1988b): Raumakustische Messungen in verschiedenen europäischen Konzertsälen [Room-acoustical measurements in different European concert halls]. In: Fortschr. Akust. DAGA '88, DPG-GmbH, Bad Honnef, pp. 739–732.

Pralong, D., and S. Carlile (1994): Measuring the human head-related transfer functions: A novel method for the construction and calibration of a miniature "in-ear" recording system, J. Acoust. Soc. Amer. **94**, 111–123.

Pratt, C. C. (1930): The spatial character of high and low tones. J. Exp. Psychol. **13**, 278–285.

*Preibisch-Effenberger, R. (1966a): Die Schallokalisationsfähigkeit des Menschen und ihre audiometrische Verwendung zur klinischen Diagnostik [The human faculty of sound localization and its audiometric application to clinical diagnostics]. Dissertation, Technische Universität, Dresden.

Preibisch-Effenberger, R. (1966b): Zur Methodik der Richtungsaudiometrie: Prüfung der Schallokalisationsfähigkeit durch elektroakustische Verzögerungskette oder Messungen im freien Schallfeld? [On the techniques of directional audiometry: Tests of the faculty of sound localization by using an electronic delay line or by measurements in a free sound field?]. Arch. klin. u. exp. Ohren-Nasen-Kehlkopfheilk. **187**, 588–592.

Preyer, W. (1887): Die Wahrnehmung der Schallrichtung mittels der Bogengänge [The perception of the direction of sound by means of the semicircular canals]. Pflügers Arch. **40**, 586–619.

Purkyne (1859): Cited by Eiselt in the Vierteljahresschrift für praktische Heilkunde Med. Fak., Prag **17** (1860).

Quante, F. (1973): Die Verständlichkeit von Sprachübertragungen aus einem lärmer-füllten Raum [The intelligibility of reproduced speech in a noisy room]. In: Fortschritte der Akustik, DAGA '73, VDI-Verlag, Düsseldorf, pp. 493–496.

Raab, D. H. (1961): Forward and backward masking between acoustic clicks. J. Acoust. Soc. Amer. **33**, 137–139.

Raatgever, J. (1974): On the frequency regions for lateralization. Proceedings, 8th Int. Congr. on Acoustics, London, vol. 1, p. 166.

Raatgever, J. (1976): Lateralization of broad-band signals with conflicting spectral regions. Proceedings, XIII Int. Congr. of Audiology, Firenze, p. 154.

Raatgever, J., and F. A. Bilsen (1977): Lateralization and dichotic pitch as a result of spectral pattern recognition. In: E. F. Evans and J. P. Wilson (Eds.), Psychophysics and physiology of hearing, Academic Press, London, pp. 441–453.

Raatgever, J. (1980a): On the binaural processing of stimuli with different interaural phase relationships. Dissertation, Technical Institute, Delft.

Raatgever, J. (1980b): Binaural time processing and time-intensity trading. In: G. van den Brink and F. A. Bilsen (Eds.), Psychophysical, physiological and behavioural studies in hearing, Delft University Press, Delft, pp. 425–428.

Rabiner, L. R., C. L. Laurence, and N. I. Durlach (1966): Further results on binaural unmasking and the EC-Model. J. Acoust. Soc. Amer. **40**, 62–70.

Rabinowitz, W. M. (1977): Acoustic reflex effects on the input admittance and transfer characteristics of the human middle ear. Dissertation, MIT, Cambridge, MA.

Rakert, B., and W. M. Hartman (1985): Localization of sound in rooms, II: The effect of a simple reflecting surface. J. Acoust. Soc. Am. **78**, 524–533.

Rakert, B., and W. M. Hartman (1986): Localization of sound in rooms, III: Onset and duration effects. J. Acoust. Soc. Am. **80**, 1695–1706.

Rakert, B., and Hartman, W. M. (1992): Precedence effect with and without binaural differences: Sound localization in three planes. J. Acoust. Soc. Am. **92**, 2296.

Rauch, M. (1922): Über die Lokalisation von Tönen und ihre Beeinflussung durch Reizung der Vestibularis [On the localization of sinusoidal tones and the influence of stimulation of the vestibular apparatus on it]. Monatsschr. Ohrenheilk. **56**, 176–182.

Lord Rayleigh (1877): Acoustical observations. Phil. Mag. **3**, 6th series, 456–464.

Lord Rayleigh (1904): On the acoustic shadow of a sphere. Phil. Transact. Roy. Soc. London **203A**, 87–99. Also in: The theory of sound, McMillan, London, 1929.

Lord Rayleigh (1907): On our perception of sound direction. Phil. Mag. **13**, 6th series, 214–232.

Reichardt, W., and W. Schmidt (1966): Die hörbaren Stufen des Raumeindrucks bei Musik [The audible steps of spatial impression in music]. Acustica **17**, 175–179.

Reichardt, W. (1968): Grundlagen der technischen Akustik [Fundamentals of technical acoustics]. Akademische Verlagsgesellschaft, Leipzig.

Reichardt, W., and B.-G. Haustein (1968): Zur Ursache des Effektes der "Im-Kopf-Lokalisation" [On the cause of the inside-the-head locatedness effect]. Hochfrequenztech. u. Elektroakustik **77**, 183–189.

Reichardt, W., and U. Lehmann (1976): Sind Raumeindruck und Durchsichtigkeit des Hörerlebnisses im Konzertsaal Gegensätze? [Are the spatial impression and clarity of the auditory experience opposite to one another in concert halls?]. Appl. Acoustics **9**, 139–150.

Reichardt, W., and U. Lehmann (1978a): Raumeindruck als Oberbegriff von Räumlichkeit und Halligkeit. Erläuterung der Raumeindrucksmasses R [The spatial impression as a broad concept including spaciousness and reverberance. Defining the index of spatial impression R]. Acustica **40**, 277–289.

Reichardt, W., and U. Lehmann (1978b): Definition eines Raumeindruckmasses R zur Bestimmung des Raumeindrucks bei Musikdarbietungen auf der Grundlage subjektiver Untersuchungen [Definition of an index R to define the spatial impression in music presentations on the basis of subjective investigations]. Appl. Acoustics **11**, 99–127.

Reichardt, W., and U. Lehmann (1981): Optimierung von Raumeindruck und Durchsichtigkeit von Musikdarbietungen durch Auswertung von Impulsschalltests [Optimization of the spatial impression and clarity of music presentations by evaluating impulse tests]. Acustica **48**, 174–185.

Reschke, M. F., D. E. Parker, and M. E. von Gierke (1970): Stimulation of the vestibular apparatus in the guinea pig by static pressure changes: Head and eye movements. J. Acoust. Soc. Amer. **48**, 913–923.

Retjö, H. (1938): Reizen die Schallwellen auch den statischen Apparat? [Do sound waves also stimulate the static apparatus?]. Monatsschr. Ohrenheilk. **72**, 34–39.

Rimski-Korsakov, A. V. (1962): Correlation of binaural noise signals and sound image localization. Proceedings, 4th Int. Congr. on Acoustics, Copenhagen, H 57.

Robinson, D. E., and L. S. Whittle (1960): The loudness of directional sound fields. Acustica **10**, 74–80.

Robinson, D. E., and L. A. Jeffress (1963): Effect of varying the interaural noise correlation on the detectability of tone signals. J. Acoust. Soc. Amer. **35**, 1947–1952.

Robinson, D. E. (1971): The effect of interaural signal–frequency disparity on signal detectability. J. Acoust. Soc. Amer. **50**, 568–571.

Robinson, D. E., and I. Pollack (1971): Forward and backward masking testing a discrete perceptual-moment hypothesis in audition. J. Acoust. Soc. Amer. **50**, 1512–1519.

Robinson, D. E., and C. S. Jackson (1972): Psychophysical methods. In: J. V. Tobias (Ed.), Foundations of modern auditory theory, vol. 2, Academic Press, New York, pp. 99–128.

Robinson, D. E., and J. P. Egan (1974): Lateralization of an auditory signal in correlated noise and in uncorrelated noise as a function of signal frequency. Percept. Psychophys. **15**, 281–284.

Rodgers, C. A. P. (1981): Pinna transformations and sound reproduction. J. Audio Eng. Soc. **29**, 226–234.

Roffler, S. K., and R. A. Butler (1968a): Localization of tonal stimuli in the vertical plane. J. Acoust. Soc. Amer. **43**, 1260–1266.

Roffler, S. K., and R. A. Butler (1968b): Factors that influence the localization of sound in the vertical plane. J. Acoust. Soc. Amer. **43**, 1255–1259.

Rosenzweig, M. R., and W. A. Rosenblith (1950): Some electrophysiological correlates of the perception of successive clicks. J. Acoust. Soc. Amer. **22**, 878–880.

*Rosenzweig, M. R. (1961): Development of research on the physiological mechanism of auditory localization. Psychol. Bull. **58**, 376–389.

Röser, D. (1960): Die zentralen Vorgänge beim Richtungshören [Central processes in directional hearing]. Arch. Ohren-Nasen-Kehlkopfheilk. **177**, 57–72.

Röser, D. (1965): Schallrichtungsbestimmung bei krankhaft verändertem Gehör [The determination of the direction of sound with defective hearing]. Dissertation, Technische Hochschule, Aachen.

Röser, D. (1966a): Das Richtungsgehör des Schwerhörigen [Directional hearing of the hard-of-hearing person]. Z. Laryngol. Rhinol. Otol. **45**, 423–440.

Röser, D. (1966b): Die Lokalisationsempfindung des Schwerhörigen bei Stereophonie [The sensation of localization of the hard-of-hearing person for stereophony]. Arch. klin. u. exp. Ohren-Nasen-Kehlkopfheilk. **187**, 599–605.

Röser, D. (1966c): Der Einfluss der Entfernung auf das Richtungshören [The influence of distance on directional hearing]. Arch. klin. u. exp. Ohren-Nasen-Kehlkopfheilk. **186**, 356–364.

Röser, D. (1969): Die Richtungsempfindlichkeit für Schall innerhalb der Medianebene [The sensitivity to the direction of sound in the median plane]. Arch. klin. u. exp. Ohren-Nasen-Kehlkopfheilk. **194**, 473–477.

Ross, S. (1968): Impedance at the eardrum, middle-ear transmission, and equal loudness. J. Acoust. Soc. Amer. **43**, 491–505.

Rowland, R. C. J., and J. V. Tobias (1967): Interaural intensity difference limen. J. Speech and Hearing Res. **10**, 745–756.

Ruotolo, B. R., R. M. Stern, and H. S. Colburn (1979): Discrimination of symmetric time–intensity traded binaural stimuli. J. Acoust. Soc. Amer. **66**, 1733–1737.

Russell, I. J., and P. M. Sellick (1978): Intracellular studies of hair cells in the mammalian cochlea. J. Physiol. **284**, 261–290.

Ryan, T. A., and F. Schehr (1941): Influence of eye movement and position on auditory localization. Amer. J. Psychol. **54**, 243–252.

Saberi, K., and D. R. Perrott (1990): Lateralization threshold obtained under conditions in which the precedence effect is assumed to operate. J. Acoust. Soc. Am. **87**, 1732–1737.

Sakai, H., and T. Inoue (1968): Lateralization of high-frequency complex stimuli. Proceedings, 6th Int. Congr. on Acoustics, Tokyo, A-3-9.

Sakamoto, N., T. Gotoh, and Y. Kimura (1976): On "out-of-head localization" in head-phone listening. J. Audio Eng. Soc. **24**, 710–715.

Sakamoto, N., T. Gotoh, Y. Kimura, and A. Kurahashi (1977): A consideration of distance perception in binaural hearing. Proceedings, 9th Int. Congr. on Acoustics, Madrid, vol. 1, p. 370.

Sakamoto, N., T. Gotoh, T. Kogure, M. Shimbo, and A. Clegg (1978): On the advanced stereophonic reproducing system "ambience stereo." 60th Convention, Audio Eng. Soc., Los Angeles, preprint 1361 (G-3).

Sandel, T. T., D. C. Teas, W. E. Feddersen, and L. A. Jeffress (1955): Localization of sound from single and paired sources. J. Acoust. Soc. Amer. **27**, 842–852.

Searle, C. L., L. D. Braida, D. R. Cuddy, and M. F. Davis (1975): Binaural pinna disparity: Another auditory localization cue. J. Acoust. Soc. Amer. **57**, 448–455.

Searle, C. L., L. D. Braida, M. F. Davis, and H. S. Colburn (1976): Model for auditory localization. J. Acoust. Soc. Amer. **60**, 1164–1175.

Seashore, C. E. (1899): Localization of sound in the median plane. Univ. of Iowa Stud. Psychol. **2**, 46–54.

Seraphim, H. P. (1961): Über die Wahrnehmbarkeit mehrerer Rückwürfe von Sprachschall [On the perceptibility of multiple reflections of speech sounds]. Acustica **11**, 80–91.

Seraphim, H. P. (1963): Raumakustische Nachbildungen mit elektroakustischen Hilfsmitteln [Simulation of room acoustics using electronic aids]. Acustica **13**, 75–85.

Sever, J. C., and A. M. Small (1979): Binaural critical masking bands. J. Acoust. Soc. Amer. **66**, 1343–1350.

Shannon, C. (1949): Communication in the presence of noise. Proc. IRE **37**, 10–21.

Shao, L. (1992): Untersuchung der computergestützten Simulation von Raumimpulsantworten mit der Monte-Carlo-Methode [Investigation into computer-aided simulation of room impulse responses using the Monte-Carlo method]. In: Fortschr. Akust. DAGA '92, DPG-GmbH, Bad Honnef, pp. 209–212.

Shaw, E. A. G., and J. E. Piercy (1962): Physiological noise in relation to audiometry. J. Acoust. Soc. Amer. **34**, 745.

Shaw, E. A. G. (1966): Ear canal pressure generated by a free sound field. J. Acoust. Soc. Amer. **39**, 465–470.

Shaw, E. A. G., and R. Teranishi (1968): Sound pressure generated in an external-ear replica and real human ears by a nearby sound source. J. Acoust. Soc. Amer. **44**, 240–249.

*Shaw, E. A. G. (1974a): The external ear. In: W. D. Keidel and W. D. Neff (Eds.), Handbook of sensory psychology, vol. 5, Springer-Verlag, Berlin–New York, pp. 455–490.

Shaw, E. A. G. (1974b): Transformation of sound pressure level from the free field to the eardrum in the horizontal plane. J. Acoust. Soc. Amer. **56**, 1848–1861.

Shaw, E. A. G. (1974c): Wave properties of the human ear and various physical models of the ear. J. Acoust. Soc. Amer. **56**, S3(A).

*Shaw, E. A. G. (1975): The external ear: New knowledge. In: S. Daalsgaard (Ed.), Earmolds and associated problems, Scand. Audiol. Suppl. 5, 24–48.

Shaw, E. A. G. (1977): Eardrum representation in middle-ear acoustical networks. J. Acoust. Soc. Amer. **62**, S12.

*Shaw, E. A. G. (1980): The acoustics of the external ear. In: G. Studebaker and I. Hochberg (Eds.), Acoustical factors affecting hearing aid performance, University Park Press, Baltimore, MD.

Shelton, B. R., and C. L. Searle (1978): Two determinants of localization acuity in the horizontal plane. J. Acoust. Soc. Amer. **64**, 689–691.

Shinn-Cunningham, B. G., P. M. Zurek, and N. I. Durlach (1993): Adjustment and discrimation measurements of the precedence effect. J. Acoust. Soc. Am. **93**, 2923–2932.

Shinn-Cunningham, B. G., H. Lehnert, G. Kramer, G., E. M. Wenzel, and N. I. Durlach (1996): Auditory displays. In: R. Gilkey, and T. Anderson (Eds.), Binaural and spatial hearing, Lawrence Erlbaum, Hilldale NJ, (in press).

Santon, F. (1989): Nouveaux resultats sur la coloration [New results on coloration]. In: Proc. 13th Int. Congr. Acoust. ICA '89, pp. 439–442.

Sayers, B. McA., and E. C. Cherry (1957): Mechanism of binaural fusion in the hearing of speech. J. Acoust. Soc. Amer. **29**, 973–987.

Sayers, B. McA. (1964): Acoustic-image lateralization judgement with binaural tones, J. Acoust. Soc. Amer. **36**, 923–926.

Sayers, B. McA., and F. E. Toole (1964): Acoustic-image lateralization judgements with binaural transients. J. Acoust. Soc. Amer. **36**, 1199–1205.

Sayers, B. McA., and P. A. Lynn (1968): Interaural amplitude effects in binaural hearing. J. Acoust. Soc. Amer. **44**, 973–978.

Schaefer, K. L. (1890): Zur interauralen Lokalisation diotischer Wahrnehmungen [On the interaural localization of diotic perceptions]. Z. Psychol. u. Physiol. Sinnesorg. **1**, 300–309.

Scharf, B. (1970): Critical bands. In: J. V. Tobias (Ed.), Foundations of modern auditory theory, vol. 1, Academic Press, New York, pp. 157–202.

Scharf, B. (1974a): Critical bandwidths in lateralization. Proceedings, 8th Int. Congr. on Acoustics, London, vol. 1, p. 159.

Scharf, B. (1974b): Localization of unlike tones from two loudspeakers. In: H. R. Moskowitz et al. (Eds.), Sensation and measurement, Reidel, Dordrecht, pp. 309–314.

Scharf, B., and M. Florentine (1975): Critical bandwidth in lateralization. J. Acoust. Soc. Amer. 57, S25(A).

Scharf, B., M. Florentine, and C. H. Meiselman (1976): Critical band in auditory lateralization. Sensory Processes **1**, 109–126.

Scharf, B., S. Quigley, C. Aoki, N. Peachey, and A. Reeves (1987): Focused auditory attention and frequency selectivity, Percept. Psychophys. **42**, 215–223.

Scharf, B., (1995): Adaptation and attention in psychophysics. In: G. A. Manley, G. M. Klump, C. Köppl, H. Fastl, and H. Oeckinghaus (Eds.), Advances in hearing research, World Science Publ., Singapore, pp. 365–386.

Schelhammer, G. C. (1684): De auditu liber unus. Lugduni Batavorum. Cited in von Békésy (1960).

Schenkel, K. D. (1964): Über die Abhängigkeit der Mithörschwellen von der interauralen Phasenlage des Testschalls [On the dependence of absolute thresholds of perception on the interaural phase angle of the test sound]. Acustica **14**, 337–346.

Schenkel, K. D. (1966): Die Abhängigkeit der beidohrigen Mithörschwellen von der Frequenz des Testschalls und vom Pegel des verdeckenden Schalles [The dependence of binaural masked thresholds on the frequency of the maskee and the level of the masker]. Acustica **17**, 345–356.

Schenkel, K. D. (1967a): Die beidohrigen Mithörschwellen von Impulsen [The binaural masked threshold of impulses]. Acustica **16**, 38–46.

*Schenkel, K. D. (1967b): Accumulation theory of binaural masked thresholds. J. Acoust. Soc. Amer. **41**, 20–30.

Scherer, P. (1959): Über die Ortungsmöglichkeit verschiedener stereophonischer Aufnahmeverfahren [On the ability of various stereophonic sound-collection processes to define position]. Nachrichtentech. Fachber. **15**, 36–42.

Scherer, P. (1966): Über den Einfluss gleich- und gegenphasiger Rauminformation in beiden Stereokanälen [On the influence of in- and out-of-phase information about the room in the two stereophonic channels]. Proceedings, 7th Conference of Audio Sound Engineers, Cologne, WDR Köln.

Schirmer, W. (1963): Die Richtcharakteristik des Ohres [The directional characteristics of the ear]. Hochfrequenztech. u. Elektroakustik 72, 39–48.

Schirmer, W. (1966a): Die Veränderung der Wahrnehmbarkeitsschwelle eines künstlichen Rückwurfes bei kopfbezüglicher stereophoner Übertragung [Change in the threshold of perceptibility of an artificial reflection in head-related stereophonic reproduction]. Hochfrequenztech. u. Elektroakustik 75, 115–123.

Schirmer, W. (1966b): Die Unterscheidbarkeit von Hörerplätzen mittels kopfbezüglicher stereophoner und monophoner Übertragung [The ability to distinguish the position of the listener in head-related stereophonic and monophonic reproduction]. Hochfrequenztech. u. Elektroakustik 75, 181–184.

Schirmer, W. (1966c): Zur Deutung der Übertragungsfehler bei kopfbezüglicher Stereophonie [On the explanation of errors in head-related stereophonic reproduction]. Acustica 17, 228–233.

Schlichthärle, D. (1978): Anwendung von Methoden der Digitalfiltertheorie auf das Cochlea-Leitungsmodell [Applications of digital filtering theory to a circuit model of the cochlea]. In: Fortschritte der Akustik, DAGA '78, VDE-Verlag, Berlin, pp. 523–526.

Schlichthärle, D. (1981): Modelle des Hörens – mit Anwendungen auf die Hörbarkeit von Laufzeitverzerrungen [Models of hearing – With applications to the audibility of delay distortions]. Dissertation, Ruhr-Universität Bochum.

Schmidt, P. H., A. H. M. van Gemert, R. J. de Fries, and J. W. Duyff (1953): Binaural threshold for azimuth difference. Acta Physiol. Pharmacol. Nederl. 3, 2–18.

Schmidt, W. (1978): Vergleich der objektiven Kriterien zur Messung des akustischen Raumeindruckes [Comparison of objective criteria for measurement of the acoustical spatial impression]. Paper presented at the 1978 meeting of the Federation of European Acoustical Societes, Warsaw.

Schodder, G. R. (1956a): Über die Verteilung der energiereichen Rückwürfe in Sälen [On the distribution of strong reflections in concert halls]. Acustica 6, 445–465.

Schodder, G. R. (1956b): Vortäuschen eines akustischen Raumeindrucks [Simulation of an acoustical impression of space]. Acustica 6, 482–488.

Schöne, P. (1980a): Der Signalstörabstand bei Kunstköpfen [Signal-to-noise ratio of dummy heads]. In: Fortschritte der Akustik, DAGA '80, VDE-Verlag, Berlin, pp. 835–838.

Schöne, P. (1980b): Zur Nutzung des Realisierungsspielraumes in der kopfbezogenen Stereofonie [On the use of the playback space in head-related stereophony]. Rundfunktech. Mitt. 28, 1–11.

Schöne, P. (1981): Ein Beitrag zur Kompatabilität raumbezogener und kopfbezogener Stereophonie [A contribution to the compatibility of room-related and head-related stereophony]. Acustica 47, 170–175.

Schroeder, M. R. (1958): An artifical stereophonic effect obtained from a single audio signal. J. Audio Eng. Soc. 6, 74–79.

Schroeder, M. R. (1961): Improved quasi-stereophony and "colorless" artificial reverberation. J. Acoust. Soc. Amer. 33, 1061–1064.

Schroeder, M. R., B. S. Atal, G. M. Sessler, and J. E. West (1966): Acoustical measurements in Philharmonic Hall (New York). J. Acoust. Soc. Amer. 40, 434–440.

Schroeder, M. R., D. Gottlob, and K. F. Siebrasse (1974): Comparative study of European concert halls: Correlation of subjective preference with geometric and acoustic parameters. J. Acoust. Soc. Amer. 56, 1195–1201.

Schroeder, M. R. (1980a): Advances in architectural acoustics. J. Acoust. Soc. Japan (E) 1, 71–77.

Schroeder, M. R. (1980b): Toward better acoustics for concert halls. Physics Today (Oct.) 24–30.

Schröter, J. (1976): Die Störung der Schallausbreitung einer ebenen Welle im Rohr durch eine schräg eingespannte Membran [The disturbance of sound propagation in a tube by a diagonally placed tensioned membrane. In: Fortschritte der Akustik, DAGA '76, VDI-Verlag, Düsseldorf, pp. 633–636.

Schröter, J. (1980): Catalog of transfer functions of the external ear. Unpublished paper, Ruhr-Universität Bochum.

Schröter, J., and H. Els (1980a): Die akustischen Eigenschaften des menschlichen Kopfes [The acoustical properties of the human head]. Progress report 239, German Federal Institute for Occupational Safety and Accident Research, Dortmund.

Schröter, J., and H. Els (1980b): New artificial head for measurement of hearing protectors. Proceedings, 10th Int. Congr. on Acoustics, Sydney, B-14.2.

Schröter, J., Ch. Pösselt, H. Opitz, P. Divenyi, and J. Blauert, (1986): Generation of binaural signals for research and home entertainment. In: Proc. 12th Int. Congr. Acoust., vol. 1, Toronto, B1–6.

Schubert, E. D., and M. C. Schultz (1962): Some aspects of binaural signal selection. J. Acoust. Soc. Amer. 34, 844–849.

Schubert, E. D., and J. Wernick (1969): Envelope versus microstructure in the fusion of dichotic signals. J. Acoust. Soc. Amer. 45, 1525–1531.

Schubert, P. (1966): Wahrnehmbarkeit von Einzelrückwürfen bei Musik [The perceptibility of individual reflections in music]. Electro-Acoustique 10, 39–44.

Schuster, K. (1936): Messung von akustischen Impedanzen durch Vergleich [Measurement of acoustical impedances using a comparison technique]. Elektr. Nachrichtentech. 13, 164–176.

Schwartzkopff, J. (1962a): Vergleichende Physiologie des Gehörs und der Lautäusserungen [Comparative physiology of hearing and sound production]. Fortschr. Zoolog. 15, 213–336.

Schwartzkopff, J. (1962b): Die akustische Lokalisation bei Tieren [Acoustical localization in animals]. Ergeb. Biol. 15, 136–176.

Schwartzkopff, J. (1968): Die Verarbeitung von akustischen Nachrichten im Gehirn von Tieren verschiedener Organisationshöhen [The processing of acoustical information in the brain in animals of different degrees of organization]. Arbeitsgem. Forsch. Nordrhein Westfalen 196, Westdeutscher Verlag, Cologne.

Schwarze, D. (1963): Die Lautstärke von Gausstönen [The loudness of Gaussian tone bursts]. Dissertation, Technische Universität, Berlin.

Schwarz, L. (1943): Zur Theorie der Beugung einer ebenen Schallwelle an einer Kugel [On the theory of the diffraction of a plane sound wave around a sphere]. Akust. Z. 8, 91–117.

Shutt, C. E. (1898): Experiments in judging the distance of sound. Kansas Univ. Quart. 7, 9–16.

Sieben, U., and R. E. Gerlach (1980): Interaction between two-tone complexes and masking noise. In: Psychophysical, Physiological and Behavioural Studies in Hearing (G. A. van den Brink and F. A. Bilsen, eds.), 433–437, Delft Univ. Press

Siebert, W. M. (1968): Stimulus transformation in the peripheral auditory system. In: P. Kolers and M. Eden (Eds.), Recognizing patterns, MIT Press, Cambridge, MA.

Siebrasse, K. F. (1973): Vergleichende subjektive Untersuchungen zur Akustik von Konzertsälen [Comparative subjective investigations of the acoustics of concert halls]. Dissertation, Universität Göttingen.

Siegel, S. (1956): Nonparametric statistics for the behavioral sciences. McGraw-Hill, New York.

Simpson, M. (1920): Experiments in binaural phase difference effects with pure tones. Phys. Rev., series II, 15, 421–424.

Sivian, L. J., and S. D. White (1933): On minimum audible sound fields. J. Acoust. Soc. Amer. 5, 288–321.

Sixtl, F. (1967): Messmethoden in der Psychologie [Psychological measuring techniques]. J. Beltz, Weinheim.

Skudrzyk, E. (1954): Die Grundlagen der Akustik [Fundamentals of acoustics]. Springer-Verlag, Vienna.

Slatky, H. (1994): Algorithmen zur richtungsselektiven Verarbeitung von Schallsignalen eines binauralen Cocktail-Party-Prozessors [Algorithms for direction-selective processing of sound signals by means of a binaural cocktail-party processor], vol. 286, series 10: Kommunikationstechnik, VDI-Verlag, Düsseldorf.

*Snow, W. (1953): Basic principles of stereophonic sound. J. Soc. Motion Picture and Television Eng. 61, 567–589.

Snow, W. B. (1954): Effects of arrival time on stereophonic localization. J. Acoust. Soc. Amer. 26, 1071–1074.

Sobotta, J., and H. Becker (1963): Atlas der Anatomie des Menschen [Atlas of human anatomy], 16th ed., part 3. Urban & Schwarzenberg, München.

Søhoel, T., G. Arnesen, and K. Y. Gjavenes (1964): Sound localization in free field and interaural threshold effects. Acta Oto-laryngol. Suppl. 188.

Somerville, T., C. L. S. Gilford, N. F. Spring, and R. D. M. Negus (1966): Recent work on the effects of reflectors in concert halls and music studios. J. Sound and Vibration 3, 127–134.

Sondhi, M. M., and N. Guttman (1966): Width of spectrum effective in the binaural release of masking. J. Acoust. Soc. Amer. 40, 600–606.

Sondhi, M. M., and B. Gopinath (1971): Determination of vocal-tract shape from impulse response at the lips. J. Acoust. Soc. Amer. 49, 1867–1873.

Sone, T., M. Ebata, and N. Tadamoto (1968): On the difference between localization and lateralization. Proceedings, 6th Int. Congr. on Acoustics, Tokyo, A-3-6.

Starch, D., and A. L. Crawford (1909): The perception of the distance of sound. Psychol. Rev. 16, 427–430.

Stefanini, A. (1922): Da che dipende il giudizio sulla direzione del suono [The dependence of orientation on the direction of sound incidence]. Arch. ital. oto-rino-laringol. 33, 155ff.; cited in Röser (1965).

Steinberg, J. C., and W. B. Snow (1934): Physical factors. Bell Syst. Tech. J. **13**, 245–258.

Steinberg, K. D. (1967): Richtungshören bei cerebralen Prozessen [Directional hearing in connection with cerebral processes]. Arch. klin. u. exp. Ohren-Nasen-Kehlkopfheilk. **188**, 438–442.

Steinhauser, A. (1877): Die Theorien des binauralen Hörens [Theories of binaural hearing]. Arch. Ohren-Nasen-Kehlkopfheilk. **12**, 62–66.

Steinhauser, A. (1879): The theory of binaural audition. Phil. Mag. **7**, 181–197, 261–274.

Stenzel, H. (1938): Über die von einer starren Kugel hervorgerufene Störung des Schallfeldes [On the disturbance of the sound field by rigid sphere]. Elektr. Nachrichtentech. **15**, 72–78.

Stern, R. M., Jr. (1976): Lateralization, discrimination and detection of binaural pure tones. Dissertation, MIT, Cambridge, MA.

Stern, R. M., Jr., and H. S. Colburn (1978): The theory of binaural interaction based on auditory-nerve data, IV. A model for subjective lateral position. J. Acoust. Soc. Amer. **64**, 127–140.

Stern, R. M., and C. Trahiotis (1996): Models of binaural perception. In: R. Gilkey, and T. Anderson,(Eds.), Binaural and spatial hearing, Lawrence Erlbaum, Hilldale NJ, (in press).

Stevens, S. S., and E. B. Newman (1936): The localization of actual sources of sound. Amer. J. Psychol. **48**, 297–306.

*Stevens, S. S., and H. Davis (1938): Hearing, its psychology and physiology. John Wiley, New York.

Stevens, S. S. (1951): Handbook of experimental psychology. John Wiley, New York.

Stevens, S. S. (1958): Problems and methods of psychophysics. Psychol. Bull. **55**, 177–196.

Stevens, S. S., and M. Guirao (1962): Loudness, reciprocality and partition scales. J. Acoust. Soc. Amer. **34**, 1466–1471.

Stewart, G. W. (1911): The acoustic shadow of a rigid sphere with certain applications in architectural acoustics and audition. Phys. Rev. **33**, 467–479.

Stewart, G. W. (1914): Phase relations in the acoustic shadow of a rigid sphere. Phys. Rev., series II, **2**, 252–258.

Stewart, G. W. (1916): Certain cases of the variation of sound intensity with distance. Phys. Rev., series II, **7**, 442–446.

Stewart, G. W. (1917): The theory of binaural beats. Phys. Rev., series II, **9**, 514–528.

Stewart, G. W. (1920): The function of intensity and phase in the binaural location of pure tones. Phys Rev., series II, **15**, 248, 425–431, 432–445.

Stiller, D. (1960): Lokalisationsvermögen [The faculty of localization]. Hochfrequenztech. u. Elektroakustik **71**, 76.

Stirnemann, A. (1978): Impedanzmessung am menschlichen Ohr mit Hilfe eines akustischen Bezugswiderstandes [Impedance measurement of the human ear with the aid of a reference acoustical impedance]. In: Fortschritte der Akustik, DAGA '78, VDE-Verlag, Berlin, pp. 601–604.

Stratton (1887): Psychol. Rev. **4**, cited in Güttich (1937).

Stumpf, C. (1905): Differenztöne und Konsonanz [Difference tones and consonance]. Z. Psychol. **39**, 269–283.

Stumpp, H. (1936): Experimentalbeitrag zur Raumakustik [An experimental contribution to spatial acoustics]. Beihefte Gesundheitsing., series II, no. 17.

Suchowerskyi, W. (1969): Personal correspondence.

Sujaku, Y., S. Kuwada, and T. C. T. Yin (1981): Binaural interaction in the cat inferior colliculus: Comparison of physiological data with a computer-simulated model. In: J. Syca and L. A. Aitkin (Eds.), Neuronal mechanisms of hearing, Plenum Press, New York, London, pp. 233–238.

Tachibana, H., Y. Yamasaki, M. Morimoto, Y. Hirasawa, Z. Maekawa, and Ch. Pösselt (1989): Acoustic survey of auditoriums in Europe and Japan. J. Acoust. Soc. Jpn. (E) **10**, 73–85.

Tarnóczy, T. (1958): Über den Vorwärts-Rückwärts-Eindruck [On the front-back impression]. Acustica **8**, 343.

Taylor, M. M., and D. P. J. Clarke (1971): Monaural detection with contralateral cue (MDCC), II. Interaural delay of cue and signal. J. Acoust. Soc. Amer. **49**, 1243–1253.

Teas, D. C. (1962): Lateralization of acoustic transients. J. Acoust. Soc. Amer. **34**, 1460–1465.

Theile, G., and G. Plenge (1977): Localization of lateral phantom sources. J. Audio Eng. Soc. **25**, 196–200.

Theile, G. (1978): Weshalb ist der Kammfiltereffekt bei Summenlokalisation nicht hörbar? [Why is the comb filter effect in summing localization inaudible?]. Paper presented to the 11th conference of audio engineers, Berlin.

Theile, G. (1980): Über die Lokalisation im überlagerten Schallfeld [On localization in a superimposed sound field]. Dissertation, Technische Universität, Berlin.

Theile, G. (1981a): Zur Kompatibilität von Kunstkopfsignalen mit intensitätssstereophonen Signalen bei Lautsprecherwiedergabe: Die Richtungsabbildung [On the compatibility of dummy-head signals with intensity stereophony signals in loudspeaker reproduction: Directional imaging]. Rundfunktech. Mitt. **25**, 67–73.

Theile, G. (1981b): Zur Kompatibilität von Kunstkopfsignalen mit intensitätssstereophonen Signalen bei Lautsprecherwiedergabe: Die Klangfarbe [On the compatibility of dummy-head signals with intensity stereophony signals in loudspeaker reproduction: Timbre]. Rundfunktech. Mitt. **25**, 146–154.

Theile, G. (1981c): Zur Theorie der optimalen Wiedergabe von stereophonen Signalen über Lautsprecher und Kopfhörer [On the theory of the optimal reproduction of stereophonic signals over loudspeakers and headphones]. Rundfunktech. Mitt. **25**, 155–169.

Thompson, P. O., and J. C. Webster (1963): The effect of talker–listener angle on word intelligibility. Acustica **13**, 319–323.

Thompson, S. P. (1877/78/81): On binaural audition, Parts I, II, III. Phil. Mag., 5th series, **4**, 274–277; **6**, 383–391; **12**, 351–355.

Thompson, S. P. (1879): The "pseudophone." Phil. Mag., 5th series, **8**, 385–390.

Thompson, S. P. (1882): On the function of the two ears in the perception of space. Phil. Mag., 5th series, **13**, 406–416.

Thurlow, W. R., and L. F. Elfner (1959): Pure-tone cross-ear localization effects. J. Acoust. Soc. Amer. **31**, 1606–1608.

Thurlow, W. R., and T. E. Parks (1961): Precedence suppression effects for two-click sources. Percept. Motor Skills 13, 7–12.

Thurlow, W. R., and A. E. Marten (1962): Perception of steady and intermittent sound with alternating noise-burst stimuli. J. Acoust. Soc. Amer. 34, 1853–1858.

Thurlow, W. R., and J. W. Mangels, and P. S. Runge (1967): Head movements during sound localization. J. Acoust. Soc. Amer. 42, 489–493, 1347.

Thurlow, W. R., and P. S. Runge (1967): Effects of induced head movements on localization of direct sound. J. Acoust. Soc. Amer. 42, 480–487, 1347.

Thurlow, W. R., and J. R. Mergener (1971): Effect of stimulus duration on localization of direction of noise stimuli. J. Speech and Hearing Res. 13, 826–838.

Thurlow, W. R., and Ch. E. Jack, (1973): Certain determinants of the "ventriloquism" effect. Percept. Motor Skills 36, 1171–1184.

Thurlow, W. R., and T. M. Rosenthal (1976): Further study of existence regions for the "ventriloquism" effect. J. Am. Audiol. Soc. 1, 280–286.

Tobias, J. V., and S. Zerlin (1959): Lateralization thresholds as a function of stimulus duration. J. Acoust. Soc. Amer. 31, 1591–1594.

Tobias, J. V. (1972): Curious binaural phenomena. In: J. V. Tobias (Ed.), Foundations of modern auditory theory, vol. 2, Academic Press, New York, pp. 463–486.

Tonndorf, J., et al. (1966): Bone conduction [A collection of seven papers]. Acta Otolaryngol. Suppl. 213.

Tonndorf, J., and S. M. Khanna (1970): The role of tympanic membrane in middle ear transmission. Ann. Otolog., Rhinolog., Laryngol. 79, 743–745.

Tonndorf, J. (1972): Bone conduction. In: J. V. Tobias (Ed.), Foundations of modern auditory theory, vol. 2, Academic Press, New York, pp. 195–238.

Tonning, F. M. (1970): Directional audiometry, I. Directional white noise audiometry. Acta Oto-laryngol. 69, 388–394.

Tonning, F. M. (1971): Directional audiometry, II. The influence of azimuth on the perception of speech. Acta Oto-laryngol. 72, 352–357.

Toole, F. E., and B. McA. Sayers (1965a): Lateralization judgements and the nature of binaural acoustic images. J. Acoust. Soc. Amer. 37, 319–324.

Toole, F. E., and B. McA. Sayers (1965b): Inferences of neural activity associated with binaural acoustic images. J. Acoust. Soc. Amer. 37, 769–779.

Toole, F. E. (1967): In-head localization of acoustic images. J. Acoust. Soc. Amer. 41, 1592.

Toole, F. E. (1969): Front–back discriminantion in free-field sound localization. J. Acoust. Soc. Amer. 46, 125.

Toole, F. E. (1970): In-head localization of acoustic images. J. Acoust. Soc. Amer. 48, 943–949.

Torick, E. L., A. di Mattia, A. J. Rosenheck, L. A. Abbagnaro, and B. B. Bauer (1968): An electric dummy for acoustical testing. J. Audio Eng. Soc. 16, 397–403.

*Trimble, O. C. (1928): The theory of sound localization: A restatement. Psychol. Rev. 35, 515–523.

Trimble, O. C. (1934): Localization of sound in the anterior–posterior and vertical dimensions of "auditory" space. Brit. J. Psychol. 24, 320–334.

Trincker, D., and C. J. Partsch (1957): Reizfolgeströme am Bogengang des Meerschweinchens [Electrical currents resulting from stimulation of the semicircular canal of the guinea pig]. Pflügers Arch. **266**, 77–78.

Tröger, J. (1930): Die Schallaufnahme durch das äussere Ohr [Collection of sound by the external ear]. Phys. Z. **31**, 26–47.

Tsujimoto, K. (1980): Equalization in artificial-head recording for loudspeaker reproduction. Proceedings, 10th Int. Congr. on Acoustics, Sydney, L-12.2.

Tullio, P. (1929): Das Ohr und die Entstehung von Sprache und Schrift [The ear and the origin of speech and writing]. Urban & Schwarzenberg, Berlin.

Unbehauen, R. (1969): Systemtheorie [Systems theory]. R. Oldenbourg-Verlag, München.

Upton, M. (1936): Differential sensitivity in sound localization. Proc. Nat. Acad. Sci. USA **22**, 409–412.

Urbantschitsch, V. (1889): Zur Lehre von den Schallempfindungen [On the science of sound sensations]. Pflügers Arch. **24**, 574–595.

van Bergeijk, W. A. (1962): Variation on a theme of Békésy: A model of binaural interaction. J. Acoust. Soc. Amer. **34**, 1432–1437.

van den Brink, G., K. Sintnicolaas, and W. S. van Stam (1976): Diotic pitch fusion. J. Acoust. Soc. Amer. **59**, 1471–1476.

van de Veer, R. A. (1957): Enige onderzockingen over het richtingshoeren [Some experiments on directional hearing]. Dissertation, University of Amsterdam.

van Gilse, P. H. G. (1928): Untersuchungen über die Lokalisation des Schalles [Investigations of the localization of sound]. Dutch Society of ENT Doctors, Amsterdam. Cited in Zentralblatt Hals-Nasen-Ohren-Heilk. **12**, 543.

van Gilse, P. H. G., and O. Roelofs (1937): Untersuchungen über die Schallokalisation [Investigations of sound localization]. Acta Oto-laryngol. **15**, 1.

van Soest, J. L. (1929): Richtungshooren bij sinusvormige geluidstrillingen [Directional hearing of sinusoidal sound waves]. Physica **9**, 271–282.

Veit, I. (1971): Das binaurale Hören mit Knochenleitungshören und seine praktive Verwendbarkeit für Knochenleitgeräte [Binaural hearing by bone conduction, and its practical applicability to bone-conduction devices]. Dissertation, Technische Hochschule, Aachen.

Veits, C. (1936): Hörraummessung bei einem Einohrigen [Measurement of auditory space by a one-eared person]. Z. Hals-Nasen-Kehlkopfheilk. **39**, 94–100.

Vermeulen, R. (1956): Stereo reverberation. Philips Tech. Rev. **17**, 258–266.

Vermeulen, R. (1958): Stereo reverberation. J. Audio Eng. Soc. **6**, 124–130.

Villchur, E. (1969): Free field calibration of earphones. J. Acoust. Soc. Amer. **46**, 1526–1534.

Voelcker, H. (1966): Towards a unified theory of modulation. Proc. IEEE **54**, 340–353, 735–755.

Vogel, A. (1975): Ein gemeinsames Funktionsschema zur Beschreibung von Lautheit und Rauhigkeit [A unified functional categorization of loudness and auditory roughness]. Biol. Cyber. **18**, 31–40.

vom Hövel, H., and H.-J. Platte (1980): Sprachverständlichkeit bei einer und mehreren unkorrelierten Störschallquellen im Freifeld [Intelligibility of speech for single and multiple uncorrelated interfering noise sources in a free sound field]. In: Fortschritte der Akustik, DAGA '80, VDE-Verlag, Berlin, pp. 615–619.

vom Hövel, H. (1981): Vorhersage der Sprachverständlichkeit unter Berücksichtigung der Eigenschaften des äusseren Gehörs und des binauralen Hörens [Prediction of the intelligibility of speech with respect to the properties of the external ear and of binaural hearing]. In: Fortschritte der Akustik, DAGA '81, VDE-Verlag, Berlin, pp. 713–716.

von Békésy, G. (1930a): Zur Theorie des Hörens: Über das Richtungshören bei einer Zeitdifferenz oder Lautstärkeungleichheit der beidseitigen Schalleinwirkungen [On the theory of hearing: On directional hearing in connection with a time difference or inequality of loudness of the effective sound between the two sides]. Phys. Z. **31**, 824–838, 857–868.

von Békésy, G. (1930b): Über das Fechnersche Gesetz und seine Bedeutung für die Theorie der akustischen Beobachtungsfehler und der Theorie des Hörens [On Fechner's law and its meaning in connection with the theory of acoustical errors of observation and the theory of hearing]. Ann. Phys. Lpz. **7**, 329–359.

von Békésy, G. (1931): Bemerkungen zur Theorie der günstigsten Nachhalldauer von Räumen [Notes on the theory of the ideal reverberation time of rooms]. Ann. Phys. **8**, 851–873.

von Békésy, G. (1932): Über den Einfluss der durch den Kopf und den Gehörgang bewirkten Schallfeldverzerrungen auf die Hörschwelle [On the influence of the distortions of the sound field by the head and the auditory canal on the threshold of hearing]. Ann. Phys. Lpz. **14**, 51–56.

von Békésy, G. (1933): Über den knall und die Theorie des Hörens [Clicks and the theory of hearing]. Phys. Zeits. **34**, 577–582.

von Békésy, G. (1935): Über akustische Reizung des Vestibularapparates [On acoustical stimulation of the vestibular apparatus]. Pflügers Arch. **236**, 59–76.

von Békésy, G. (1936a): Zur Physik des Mittelohres und über das Hören bei fehlerhaftem Trommelfell [On the physics of the middle ear and on hearing when the eardrum is defective]. Akust. Z. **1**, 13–23.

von Békésy, G. (1936b): Über die Herstellung und Messung langsamer sinusförmiger Druckschwankungen [On the generation and measurement of slow sinusoidal pressure variations]. Ann. Phys. Lpz. **26**, 554–566.

von Békésy, G. (1938): Über die Entstehung der Entfernungsempfindung beim Hören [On the origin of the sensation of distance in hearing]. Akust. Z. **3**, 21–31.

von Békésy, G. (1941): Über die Messung der Schwingungsamplitude der Gehörknöchelchen mittels der kapazitiven Sonde [On the measurement of the amplitude of oscillation of the ossicles by means of the capacitive probe]. Akust. Z. **6**, 1–16.

von Békésy, G. (1947): A new audiometer. Acta Oto-laryngol. **35**, 411–422.

von Békésy, G. (1949): The moon illusion and similar auditory phenomena. Amer. J. Psychol. **62**, 540–552.

*von Békésy, G. (1960): Experiments in hearing. McGraw-Hill, New York (contains all of the author's previous works).

von Békésy, G. (1971): Auditory backward inhibition in concert halls. Science **171**, 529–536.

von Betzold, W. (1890): Urteilstäuschungen nach Beseitungen einseitiger Harthörigkeit [Confusions of judgment after elimination of unilateral deafness]. Z. Psychol. u. Physiol. Sinnesorg. **1**, 486–487.

von Hornbostel, E. M., and M. Wertheimer (1920): Über die Wahrnehmung der Schallrichtung [On the perception of the direction of sound]. Sitzungsber. Akad. Wiss. Berlin, 388–396.

von Hornbostel, E. M. (1923): Beobachtungen über ein- und zweiohriges Hören [Observations on one- and two-eared hearing]. Psychol. Forsch. **4**, 64–114.

*von Hornbostel, E. M. (1926): Das räumliche Hören [Spatial hearing]. In: A. Bethe et al. (Eds.), Handbuch der normalen und pathologischen Physiologie, vol. 2, Springer-Verlag, Berlin, pp. 601–618.

von Kries, J. (1890): Über das Erkennen der Schallrichtung [On the recognition of the direction of sound]. Z. Psychol. u. Physiol. Sinnesorg. **1**, 235–251, 488.

von Wedel, H. (1979): Untersuchungen zum zeitlichen Auflösungsvermögen beim dichotischen Hören [Time resolution ability in dichotic hearing experiments]. Arch. Otorhinolaryngol. **222**, 133–144.

von Wedel, H. (1981): A psychoacoustical study on time resolution of brief intensity changes in dichotic hearing. Arch. Otorhinolarygol. **232**, 123–130.

von Wilmowsky, H. J. (1960): Dynamische Vorgänge beim Richtungshören [Dynamic processes in directional hearing]. Z. Naturforsch. (A), 132–135.

Vorländer, M. (1988a): Ein Strahlverfolgungs-Verfahren zur Berechnung von Schallfeldern in Räumen [A ray-tracing method for the calculation of sound fields in enclosed spaces]. Acustica **65**, 138–148.

Vorländer, M. (1988b): Die Genauigkeit von Berechnungen mit dem raumakustischen Schallteilchenmodell und ihre Abhängigkeit von der Rechenzeit [The accuracy of computations with the room-acoustical sound-particle model and its dependence on the computing time]. Acustica **66**, 90–96.

Waetzmann, E., and L. Keibs (1936a): Theoretischer und experimenteller Vergleich von Hörschwellenmessungen [Theoretical and experimental comparisons of measurements of auditory thresholds]. Akust. Z. **1**, 3–12.

Waetzmann, E., and L. Keibs (1936b): Hörschwellenbestimmungen mit dem Thermophon und Messungen am Trommelfell [Determining auditory thresholds with the thermophone and with measurements at the eardrum]. Ann. Phys. Lpz., 5th series, **26**, 141–144.

Wagenaars, W. M. (1990): Localization of sound in a room with reflecting walls. J. Audio Eng. Soc. **38**, 99–110.

Wagener, B. (1971): Räumliche Verteilungen der Hörrichtungen in synthetischen Schallfeldern [Spatial distribution of auditory directions in synthetic sound fields]. Acustica **25**, 203–219.

Wagner, H., T. Takahashi, and M. Konishi (1981): Representation of interaural time differences in the central nucleus of the barn owl's inferior colliculus. J. Neurosc. **7**, 3105–3116.

Wallach, H. (1938): Über die Wahrnehmung der Schallrichtung [On the perception of the direction of sound]. Psychol. Forsch. **22**, 238–266.

Wallach, H. (1940): The role of head movements and vestibular and visual cues in sound localization. J. Exp. Psychol. **27**, 339–368.

Wallach, H. (1949): On sound localization. J. Acoust. Soc. Amer. **10**, 270–274.

Wallach, H., E. B. Newman, and M. R. Rosenzweig (1949): The precedence effect in sound localization. Amer. J. Psychol. **57**, 315–336.

Wallerus, H. (1976): Richtungsauflösungvermögen des Gehörs für Sinustöne mit interauralen Pegelunterschieden [Directional resolution capability of the human auditory apparatus for sinusoidal signals with interaural level differences]. In: Fortschritte der Akustik, DAGA '76, VDI-Verlag, Düsseldorf, pp. 589–592.

Warncke H. (1941): Die Grundlagen der raumbezüglichen stereophonischen Übertragung im Tonfilm [The fundamentals of room-related stereophonic reproduction in sound films]. Akust. Z. 6, 174–188.

Warren, R. M. (1963): Are loudness judgements based on distance estimates? J. Acoust. Soc. Amer. 35, 613–614.

Watkins, A. J. (1978): Psychoacoustic aspects of synthesized vertical locale cues. J. Acoust. Soc. Amer. 63, 1152–1165.

Watkins, A. J. (1979): The monaural perception of azimuth: A synthesis approach. In: R. W. Gatehouse (Ed.), Localization of Sound: Theory and application, The Amphora Press, Groton, CT, pp. 194–206.

Weber, R., and V. Mellert (1978): Ein Kunstkopf mit ebenem Frequenzgang [A dummy head with a flat frequency response]. In: Fortschritte der Akustik, DAGA '78, VDE-Verlag, Berlin, pp. 645–648.

Webster, F. A. (1951): The influence of interaural phase on masked thresholds. J. Acoust. Soc. Amer. 23, 452–462.

Wendt, K. (1959): Die Wortverständlichkeit bei zweiohrigem Hören [Word intelligibility in two-eared hearing]. Nachrichtentech. Fachber. 15, 21–24.

Wendt, K. (1960a): Versuche zur Ortung von Intensitätsstereophonie [Experiments in the determination of position in intensity-difference stereophony]. Frequenz 14, 11–14.

Wendt, K (1960b): Die Übertragung der Rauminformation [The reproduction of information about a room]. Rundfunktech. Mitt. 4, 209–212.

*Wendt, K. (1963): Das Richtungshören bei der Überlagerung zweier Schallfelder bei Intensitäts- und Laufzeitstereophonie [Directional hearing with two superimposed sound fields in intensity- and delay-difference stereophony]. Dissertation, Technische Hochschule, Aachen.

Wendt, K (1964): Das Richtungshören bei Zweikanal-Stereophonie [Directional hearing in connection with two-channel stereophony]. Rundfunktech. Mitt. 8, 171–179.

*Wenzel, E. M. (1992): Localization in virtual acoustic displays. Presence 1, 80–107.

Werner, H. (1922): Erscheinungsformen gebundener Intensität [Forms in which intensity linkage occurs]. Z. Psychol. u. Physiol. Sinnesorg., Suppl. 10, 68–94.

West, J. E. (1966): Possible subjective significance of the ratio of height to width of concert halls. J. Acoust. Soc. Amer. 40, 1245.

West, J. E., J. Blauert, and D. J. McLean (1976): Teleconferencing, head-related acoustical system. Unpublished paper.

Wettschurek, R. (1971): Über Unterschiedsschwellen beim Richtungshören in der Medianebene [On difference thresholds in connection with directional hearing in the median plane]. In: Gemeinschaftstagung für Akustik und Schwingungstechnik, Berlin 1970, VDI-Verlag, Düsseldorf, pp. 385–388.

Wettschurek, R. (1973): Die absoluten Unterschiedswellen der Richtungswahrnehmung in der Medianebene beim natürlichen Hören, sowie beim Hören über ein Kunstkopf-Übertragungssystem [The absolute difference threshold of directional perception in the median plane in natural hearing and in hearing over a dummy-head reproducing system]. Acustica 28, 197–208.

Wettschurek, R. (1976): Über die Abhängigkeit raumakustischer Wahrnehmungen von der Lautstärke [On the dependence of spatial acoustic perceptions on loudness]. Dissertation, Technische Hochschule, Berlin.

Whitfield, I. C. (1970): Central nervous processing in relation to spatio-temporal discrimination of auditory patterns. In: R. Plomp and G. F. Smoorenburg (Eds.), Frequency analysis and periodicity detection in hearing, A. W. Sijthoff, Leiden, pp. 136–152.

Whitworth, R. H., and L. A. Jeffress (1961): Time versus intensity in the localization of tones. J. Acoust. Soc. Amer. **33**, 925–929.

Wiener, F. M., and D. A. Ross (1946): The pressure distribution in the auditory canal in a progressive sound field. J. Acoust. Soc. Amer. **18**, 401–408.

Wiener, F. M. (1947): On the diffraction of a progressive sound wave by the human head. J. Acoust. Soc. Amer. **19**, 143–146.

Wighman, E. R., and F. A. Firestone (1930): Binaural localization of pure tones. J. Acoust. Soc. Amer. **2**, 271–280.

Wightman, F. L. (1969a): Binaural masking with sine-wave maskers. J. Acoust. Soc. Amer. **45**, 72–78.

Wightman, F. L. (1969b): Masking level differences with narrow-band noise maskers. J. Acoust. Soc. Amer. **45**, 335.

Wightman, F. L. (1989): Headphone simulation of free-field listening I: Stimulus synthesis. J. Acoust. Soc. Amer. **85**, 858–867.

*Wightman, F. L., and D. J. Kistler (1993): Sound localization. In: W. A. Yost, N. Popper, and R. R. Fay (Eds.), Human psychophysics, Springer, New York, pp. 155–192.

Wilbanks, W. A., and J. K. Whitmore (1968): Detection of monaural signals as a function of interaural noise correlation and signal frequency. J. Acoust. Soc. Amer. **43**, 785–797.

Wilkens, H. (1971a): Subjektive Ermittlung der Richtcharakteristik des Kopfes und einer kopfbezogenen Aufnahme und Wiedergabeanordnung [Evaluation of the directional characteristics of the head and of a head-related sound-collection and reproduction apparatus by means of auditory experiments]. In: Gemeinschaftstagung für Akustik und Schwingungstechnik, Berlin 1970, VDI-Verlag, Düsseldorf, pp. 407–410.

Wilkens, H. (1971b): Beurteilung von Raumeindrücken verschiedener Hörerplätze mittels kopfbezogener Stereophonie [The judgment of spatial impression for various positions of the listener by means of head-related stereophony]. Proceedings, 7th Int. Congr. on Acoustics, Budapest, 24 S 5.

Wilkens, H., G. Plenge, and R. Kürer (1971): Wiedergabe von kopfbezogenen stereophonen Signalen durch Lautsprecher [The reproduction of head-related stereophonic signals over loudspeakers]. Convention '71, Audio Eng. Soc., Cologne.

Wilkens, H. (1972): Kopfbezügliche Stereophone, ein Hilfsmittel für Vergleich und Beurteilung verschiedener Raumeindrücke [Head-related stereophony, an aid in comparing and judging various spatial impressions]. Acustica **26**, 213–221.

Wilkens, H. (1975): Mehrdimensionale Beschreibung subjektiver Beurteilungen der Akustik von Konzertsälen [Multidimensional description of subjective judgments of the acoustics of concert halls]. Dissertation, Technische Universität, Berlin.

Wilson, H. A., and C. S. Myers (1908): The influence of binaural phase differences in the localization of sound. Brit. J. Psychol. **2**, 362–386.

Wittmann, J. (1925): Beiträge zur Analyse des Hörens bei dichotischer Reizaufnahme [Contributions to the analysis of hearing when stimuli are collected dichotically]. Arch. ges. Psychol. **51**, 21–122.

Wolf, S. (1987): Ein probabilistisches Modell zur Simulation binauraler Phänomene [A probabilistic model to simulate binaural phenomena]. In: Fortschr. Akust. DAGA '87, DPG-GmbH, Bad Honnef, pp. 533–536.

Wolf, S. (1988): Untersuchungen zum Gesetz der ersten Wellenfront [Investigations into the law of the first wavefront]. In: Fortschr. Akust. DAGA '88, 605–609, DPG-GmbH, Bad Honnef.

Wolf, S. (1990): Lokalisation in geschlossenen Räumen [Localization in enclosed spaces]. In: Fortschr. Akust. DAGA '90, DPG-GmbH, Bad Honnef, pp. 747–750.

Wolf, S. (1991): Lokalisation von Schallquellen in geschlossenen Räumen [Localization of sound sources in enclosed spaces]. Dissertation, Bochum.

Wolf, S., J. Blauert, and A. Persterer (1993): Human sound localization and the direction of gravity. Acta Acustica **1**, 57–59.

Wollherr, H. (1981): Mikrophonankopplung an das Aussenohr eines neuen Kunstkopfes [Microphone coupling to the external ear of a new dummy head]. Rundfunktech. Mitt. **4**, 141–145.

*Woodworth, R. S., and H. Schlosberg (1954): Experimental psychology. Holt, New York.

Wright, D., J. H. Hebrank, and B. Wilson (1974): Pinna reflections as cues for localization. J. Acoust. Soc. Amer. **56**, 957–962.

Wright, H. N. (1960): Measurement of perstimulatory auditory adaptation. J. Acoust. Soc. Amer. **32**, 1558–1567.

Xiang, N. (1988): Messung von Impulsantworten mit Maximalfolgen [Measurement of impulse responses with maximum-length sequences]. In: Fortschr. Akust. DAGA '88, DPG-GmbH, Bad Honnef, pp. 963–969.

Xiang, N. (1989): An ultrasonic electroacoustic transducer in cylindrical form using piezoelectric polyvinylidenefluoride films. In: Proc. Ultrasonics Int. '89, Cambridge Univ. Press, Cambridge, pp. 501–506.

Xiang, N., and D. Kopatz (1989): Leistungsfähige Lautsprecherboxen für den Ultraschallbereich [Efficent loudspeakers for the ultrasound range]. In: Fortschr. Akust. DAGA '89, DPG-GmbH, Bad Honnef, pp. 299–302.

Xiang, N. (1990): Ein Miniaturkunstkopf für binaurale Raumsimulation mittels eines verkleinerten raumakustischen Modells [A miniature dummy head for binaural room simulation with a scaled-down model]. In: Fortschr. Akust. DAGA '90, DPG-GmbH, Bad Honnef, pp. 831–834.

Xiang, N. (1991): A mobile universal measuring system for the binaural room-acoustic model technique, Schriftenr. Bundesanst. Arbeitsschutz, vol. Fb 611, Wirtschaftsverlag NW, Bremerhaven.

Xiang, N., and J. Blauert (1991a): A miniature dummy head for binaural evaluation of tenth-scale acoustic models. J. Appl. Acoust. **33**, 123–140.

Xiang, N., and J. Blauert (1991b): Computer-aided tenth-scale modelling for binaural auralization in room-acoustics design. 91th AES Conv., Audio Engr. Soc., New York, preprint 3120.

Xiang, N., and J. Blauert (1992): Auditorium-acoustics prediction using binaural tenth-scale modelling. In: Proc. Inst. Acoust. 14, part 2, Birmingham, pp. 57–64.

Xiang, N., and J. Blauert (1993): Binaural scale modelling for auralization and prediction of acoustics in auditoria. J. Appl. Acoust. **38**, 267–290.

Yamaguchi, Z., and N. Sushi (1956): Real ear response of receivers. J. Acoust. Soc. Japan **12**, 8–13; cited by Shaw and Teranishi (1967).

Yin, T. C. T. (1994): Psychological correlates of the precedence effect and summing localization in the inferior colliculus of the cat. J. Neurosc. 14, 5170–5186.

Yin, T. C. T., J. C. K. Chan, and L. H. Carney (1987): Effects of interaural time delays of noise stimuli on low-frequency cells in the cat's inferior colliculus,. III: Evidence for cross correlation. J. Neurophysiol. **58**, 562–583.

Yost, W. A., F. L. Wightman, and D. M. Green (1971): Lateralization of filtered clicks. J. Acoust. Soc. Amer. **50**, 1526–1531.

Yost, W. A. (1974): Discrimination of interaural phase differences. J. Acoust. Soc. Amer. **55**, 1299–1303.

Yost, W. A. (1975): Comments on the paper "Lateralization and the monaural masking level difference." J. Acoust. Soc. Amer. **57**, 1214–1215.

Yost, W. A. (1976): Lateralization of repeated filtered transients. J. Acoust. Soc. Amer. **60**, 178–181.

Yost, W. A., and J. Walton (1977): Hierarchy of masking-level differences obtained for temporal masking. J. Acoust. Soc. Amer. **61**, 1376–1379.

Yost, W. A. (1981): Lateral position of sinusoids presented with interaural intensive and temporal differences. J. Acoust. Soc. Amer. **70**, 397–409.

Yost, W. A., and D. R. Sonderquist (1984): The precedence effect: revisited. J. Acoust. Soc. Am. **76**, 1377–1383.

*Yost, W. A., and G. Gourevitch (Eds.) (1987): Directional hearing. Springer, New York.

Young, L. L., and R. Carhart (1974): Time-intensity trading functions for pure tones and a high-frequency AM signal. J. Acoust. Soc. Amer. **56**, 605–609.

Young, P. T. (1931): The role of head movements in auditory localization. J. Exp. Psychol. **14**, 95–124.

Zelinsky, R. (1988): A microphone array with adaptive post-filtering for noise reduction in reverberant rooms. In: Proc. ICASP '88, New York, pp. 2578–2581.

Zerlin, S. (1959): The interaural time disparity threshold as a function of interaural correlation. J. Acoust. Soc. Amer. **31**, 127.

Zurek, P. M. (1976): The binaural perception of echoed sound. Dissertation, Arizona State University, Tempe.

Zurek, P. M. (1979): Measurement of binaural echo suppression. J. Acoust. Soc. Amer. **66**, 1750–1757.

Zurek, P. M. (1980): The precedence effect and its possible role in the avoidance of interaural ambiguities. J. Acoust. Soc. Amer. **67**, 952–964.

Zurek, P. M. (1987): The precedence effect. In: W. A. Yost and G. Gourevitch (Eds.), Directional Hearing, Springer, New York, pp. 85–105.

Zwicker, E., and R. Feldtkeller (1967): Das Ohr als Nachrichtenempfänger [The ear as a receiver of information]. S. Hirzel Verlag, Stuttgart.

Zwicker, E. (1968): A model describing temporal effects in loudness and threshold. Proceedings, 6th Int. Congr. on Acoustics, Tokyo, vol. 1, A-3-4.

Zwicker, E. (1977): Procedure for calculating loudness of temporally variable sounds. J. Acoust. Soc. Amer. **62**, 675–682.

Zwislocki, J., and R. S. Feldman (1956): Just noticeable differences in dichotic phase. J. Acoust. Soc. Amer. **28**, 860–864.

Zwislocki, J. (1957a): Some impedance measurements on normal and pathological ears. J. Acoust. Soc. Amer. **29**, 1312–1317.

Zwislocki, J. (1957b): Some measurements of the impedance at the eardrum. J. Acoust. Soc. Amer. **29**, 349–356.

*Zwislocki, J. (1962): Analysis of the middle-ear function, I: Input impedance. J. Acoust. Soc. Amer. **34**, 1514–1532.

Author Index

Subject Index